AVOIDING COMMON OBSTETRICS AND GYNECOLOGY ERRORS

AVOIDING COMMON OBSTETRICS AND GYNECOLOGY ERRORS

EDITORS

CARLA P. ROBERTS, MD, PhD
Assistant Professor
Division of Reproductive Endocrinology and Infertility
Residency Program Director and Associate Chief of Service
Grady Memorial Hospital
Department of Gynecology and Obstetrics
Emory University School of Medicine
Atlanta, Georgia

DIANA BROOMFIELD, MD, MBA, FACOG, FACS
Vice Chair, Assistant Professor
Director, Residency Program
Chief, Division of Reproductive Endocrinology and Infertility
Department of Obstetrics & Gynecology
Howard University Hospital
Howard University, College of Medicine
Washington, District of Columbia

SERIES EDITOR

LISA MARCUCCI, MD
Associate Professor of Surgery
University of Kentucky
Lexington, Kentucky

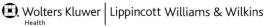

Wolters Kluwer | Lippincott Williams & Wilkins
Health
Philadelphia · Baltimore · New York · London
Buenos Aires · Hong Kong · Sydney · Tokyo

Acquisitions Editor: Sonya Seigafuse
Product Manager: Nicole Walz
Vendor Manager: Alicia Jackson
Senior Manufacturing Manager: Benjamin Rivera
Marketing Manager: Kimberly Schonberger
Design Coordinator: Holly Reid McLaughlin
Production Service: SPi Technologies

Printed in China

Library of Congress Cataloging-in-Publication Data
  Avoiding common obstetrics and gynecology errors / [edited by] Carla P. Roberts, Diana P. Broomfield.
     p. ; cm.
  Includes bibliographical references.
  ISBN 978-0-7817-9143-4 (pbk.)
  1. Obstetrical errors—Prevention—Handbooks, manuals, etc. 2. Gynecologic errors—Prevention—Handbooks, manuals, etc. I. Roberts, Carla P. II. Broomfield, Diana P.
  [DNLM: 1. Medical Errors—prevention & control—Handbooks. 2. Obstetrics—methods—Handbooks. 3. Gynecology—methods—Handbooks. WQ 39]
  RG103.8.A96 2010
  618.10028'9—dc22
                                                                                    2010034584

Care has been taken to confirm the accuracy of the information presented and to describe generally accepted practices. However, the authors, editors, and publisher are not responsible for errors or omissions or for any consequences from application of the information in this book and make no warranty, expressed or implied, with respect to the currency, completeness, or accuracy of the contents of the publication. Application of the information in a particular situation remains the professional responsibility of the practitioner.

 The authors, editors, and publisher have exerted every effort to ensure that drug selection and dosage set forth in this text are in accordance with current recommendations and practice at the time of publication. However, in view of ongoing research, changes in government regulations, and the constant flow of information relating to drug therapy and drug reactions, the reader is urged to check the package insert for each drug for any change in indications and dosage and for added warnings and precautions. This is particularly important when the recommended agent is a new or infrequently employed drug.

 Some drugs and medical devices presented in the publication have Food and Drug Administration (FDA) clearance for limited use in restricted research settings. It is the responsibility of the health care provider to ascertain the FDA status of each drug or device planned for use in their clinical practice.

To purchase additional copies of this book, call our customer service department at (800) 638-3030 or fax orders to (301) 223-2320. International customers should call (301) 223-2300.

Visit Lippincott Williams & Wilkins on the Internet: at LWW.com. Lippincott Williams & Wilkins customer service representatives are available from 8:30 am to 6 pm, EST.

                                                                    10 9 8 7 6 5 4 3 2 1

RRS1010

DEDICATIONS

To Dr. John Rock, a wonderful mentor and an even greater role model. To my colleagues (residents and faculty members) at Emory University who helped make this book possible. To my daughter, Cally, and my husband, Al, who have never wavered in their support for me as I pursue my interests.

CARLA P. ROBERTS

I dedicate this book first in memoriam of my father, Pastor Joshua I. Broomfield's, who although is deceased, undying belief in excellence continues to inspire me to do my best in whatever my heart and mind conceives and strives for. To my husband and my three children, James, Jovan, and Joiliana, I thank you for your patience and tolerance, and for you love in allowing me the time, space, and opportunity to work on this book. To my mother, Mrs. Verna Broomfield, for providing me with the time to write and edit by taking care of my children and managing the daily activities of our household and for always believing in me and supporting my every effort. To my five siblings Franklyn, Anthony, Sherlita, Vernita, and especially to Ramon, who has worked endlessly to manage our Journal, *Fertility Today Magazine,* and my medical practice, Maryland IVF, so that I may have the time to write and edit, I thank you all. I also dedicate this book to all my family living and those who have gone on to await the second coming of our Lord; it is because of their sacrifices, love, support, guidance, and encouragement that I have developed into the woman, friend, daughter, sister, cousin, aunt, wife, mother, educator, colleague, professor, leader, and physician that I am today. Lastly, I dedicate this book to all our patients whose lives will ultimately be touched directly or indirectly through this educational tool for physicians around the world.

DIANA BROOMFIELD

The realities of today's practice in Obstetrics and Gynecology require careful attention to efficiencies and high quality care. Physicians must have cultural sensitivity and competency for diverse patient populations to effectively work in complex community settings. The creation of well coordinated patient care teams will provide a comprehensive care plan addressing the social determinants of health and significantly improve health outcomes. In *Common Errors in Obstetrics and Gynecology*, the authors use a case-based format review the management of acute and chronic conditions in women. The text carefully outlines common management errors in logical sequence and list important take home points illustrated in each chapter. This innovative text underscores the importance of a comprehensive view of illness in women and stresses the need for a carefully integrated health care plan.

This is a first edition of a textbook that is a valuable addition to the personal library of any physician who cares for women. This up to date, comprehensive, socially relevant text will undoubtedly undergo many revisions over the next decades as practitioners demand resources that address the importance of comprehensive, integrated patient care.

JOHN A. ROCK, MD
Founding Dean, and Senior Vice President for Medical Affairs
Herbert Wertheim College of Medicine
Florida International University
Miami, Florida

From the beginning of medical education, health care providers have learned to find mentors who divulge years of practical and learned experience. The years spent learning the basic sciences, such as anatomy, physiology, histology, embryology, and pathology to name a few, must come together in a way that seamlessly cares for women of all ages. This book provides the reader with countless clinical examples within the breadth and depth of gynecology and obstetrics. The contributing authors developed each section with thought toward common clinical experiences that any health care provider would face when caring for the female patient.

When the topics discussed on these pages were developed, we instructed the authors to think of an average day when residents and medical students were under their watchful guidance. We tasked the authors to select those topics that, at the end of the day, they told their student protégées, "if you learned nothing else from me today, never ever do the following if you want to prevent an error." The topics flowed freely and easily!

We are certain that we have developed an excellent educational source for those who are beginning in the field of gynecology and obstetrics as well as those who are looking for a quick review of any or all of the topics covered within these covers. We hope the readers enjoy reviewing the material presented here as much as we have enjoyed developing it!

CARLA P. ROBERTS

This book was intended to be a guide for residents and physicians who give a brief synopsis on how to avoid common error in the fields of obstetrics and gynecology. One of the difficulties encountered in writing many of the chapters in this book was how to keep it simple and succinct, while keeping it evidenced based.

DIANA BROOMFIELD

The editors are pleased to accept comments, corrections, and suggestions and request they be sent to: insidesurgery@gmail.com

ACKNOWLEDGMENTS

Many thanks to Lisa Consoli, Nicole Walz, Kerry Barrett, and Sonya Seigafuse for their support and guidance during the development of this book. Their patience is unparalleled.

CARLA P. ROBERTS

I want to thank my Howard University OB/GYN Residency Program Coordinator, Mrs. Deittra Hall, for her support and assistance in gathering the necessary ancillary information from my residents and faculty for this book and for never hesitating when asked for her assistance whether the request is delineated in her "Job Description" or whether it was just a request to facilitate me doing my job better or just because I asked. I thank her and appreciate ALL her efforts!

I also want to thank my colleague, friend, and coeditor, Dr. Carla Roberts, not only for believing in me and giving me, my residents, and faculty this opportunity to write so many chapters in this book but also for her selfless willingness and decision to share the editorial role of this book.

DIANA BROOMFIELD

CONTRIBUTORS

RONY A. ADAM, MD
Vice Chair, Quality and Performance
  Improvement
Department of Obstetrics and Gynecology
Geisinger Medical Center
Danville, Pennsylvania

SAMEENA AHMED, MD
Fellow/Associate
Department of Gynecology and Obstetrics
Emory University
Atlanta, Georgia

JOHN-CHARLES AKODA, MD
Resident
Department of Obstetrics & Gynecology
Howard University Hospital
Howard University, College of Medicine
Washington, District of Columbia

JESSICA C. ARLUCK, MD, MPH
Associate Program Director
Assistant Professor
Department of Gynecology and Obstetrics
Emory University
Emory University Hospital Midtown
Atlanta, Georgia

ALBERT ASSANTE, MD, MPH
Resident
Department of Gynecology and Obstetrics
Emory University
Atlanta, Georgia

MARTINA L. BADELL, MD
Associate
Department of Gynecology and Obstetrics
Emory University
Atlanta, Georgia

DAPHNE P. BAZILE, MD
Instructor
Department of Obstetrics & Gynecology
Howard University Hospital
Howard University, College of Medicine
Washington, District of Columbia

PAVNA K. BRAHMA, MD
Clinical Fellow
Division of Reproductive Endocrinology
  and Infertility
Department of Gynecology and
  Obstetrics
Emory University
Emory University Hospital Midtown
Atlanta, Georgia

AIMEE SCHICKEDANZ BROWNE, MD, MSc
Assistant Professor, Reproductive
  Endocrinology and Infertility
Department of Gynecology and Obstetrics
Emory University Hospital Midtown
Atlanta, Georgia

ALEXANDRA BUFORD, DO
Resident
Department of Obstetrics and
  Gynecology
Howard University Hospital
Howard University, College of Medicine
Washington, District of Columbia

PENNY CASTELLANO, MD
Associate Professor
Department of Gynecology and
  Obstetrics
Chief Medical Officer for Clinical
  Operations
Chief Quality Officer
The Emory Clinic
Atlanta, Georgia

TARA P. CLEARY, MD
Associate/Fellow
Department of Gynecology and Obstetrics
Emory University
Fellow
Department of Gynecology and Obstetrics
Grady Memorial Hospital
Atlanta, Georgia

ELIZABETH COLLINS, MD, MPH
Resident
Department of Gynecology and Obstetrics
Emory University
Atlanta, Georgia

SUSANNAH COPLAND, MD, MSc
Assistant Professor
Department of Obstetrics and Gynecology
Duke University
Durham, North Carolina

CARRIE CWIAK, MD, MPH
Assistant Professor and Family Planning
   Division Director
Department of Gynecology and Obstetrics
Emory University School of Medicine
Atlanta, Georgia

THINH DUONG, MD
Assistant Professor
Department of Gynecology and Obstetrics
Emory University
Atlanta, Georgia

JANE ELLIS, MD, PhD
Assistant Professor
Department of Gynecology and Obstetrics
Emory University
Atlanta, Georgia

CHARLENE EMMANUEL, MD
Resident
Department of Gynecology and Obstetrics
Emory University
Atlanta, Georgia

RICHARD ENCHILL, MD
Resident
Department of Obstetrics & Gynecology
Howard University Hospital
Howard University, College of Medicine
Washington, District of Columbia

ERIC I. FELNER, MD, MSCR
Associate Professor of Pediatrics
Department of Pediatrics
Emory University School of Medicine
Attending Physician
Children's Healthcare of Atlanta
   (CHOA)—Egleston
Atlanta, Georgia

VICTOR M. FELDBAUM, MD
Resident
Department of Gynecology and
   Obstetrics
Emory University
Atlanta, Georgia

AEVA GAYMON-DOOMES, MD
Private Practice (Psychiatry)
Silver Spring, Mary Land

ALFRED GENDY, MD
Assistant Professor/Director of
   Gynecology
Obstetrics and Gynecology Department
School of Community Medicine
University of Oklahoma-Tulsa
Assistant Professor
Department of Obstetrics and
   Gynecology
Hillcrest Medical Center
Tulsa, Oklahoma

FREZGHI GHEBREAB, MD
Resident
Department of Obstetrics & Gynecology
Howard University Hospital
Howard University, College of Medicine
Washington, District of Columbia

PIERRE GORDON, MD
Resident
Department of Obstetrics & Gynecology
Howard University Hospital
Howard University, College of Medicine
Washington, District of Columbia

VICTORIA GREEN, MD, MHSA, MBA, JD
Associate Professor
Department of Gynecology and Obstetrics
Emory University
Atlanta, Georgia

TIA M. GUSTER, MD
Resident
Department of Gynecology and Obstetrics
Emory University
Atlanta, Georgia

RUSSELL HILL, MD
Assistant Professor
Department of Obstetrics & Gynecology
Howard University Hospital
Howard University, College of Medicine
Washington, District of Columbia

SHUNA E.R. ISOM, MD
Research Fellow
Women's Health Institute
Howard University Hospital
Washington, District of Columbia

CALEB B. KALLEN, MD, PHD
Assistant Professor
Division of Reproductive Endocrinology
  and Infertility
Department of Gynecology and Obstetrics
Emory University School of Medicine
Atlanta, Georgia

JENNIFER FAY KAWWASS, MD
Chief Administrative Resident
Department of Gynecology and Obstetrics
Emory University
Atlanta, Georgia

VITALY A. KUSHNIR, MD
REI Fellow
Department of Gynecology and Obstetrics
Emory University
Emory Reproductive Center
Atlanta, Georgia

FRANCIS KWARTENG, MD
Department of Obstetrics and Gynecology
Clinic Director Mirian Worthy Women
  Health Center
Phoebe Putney Memorial Hospital/Albany
  Area Primary Health Care
Albany, Georgia

MARK P. LEONDIRES, MD
Medical Director
Reproductive Medicine Associates of
  Connecticut
Norwalk, Connecticut

KERRY M. LEWIS, MD
Professor
Department of Obstetrics and
  Gynecology
Howard University Hospital
Howard University, College of Medicine
Washington, District of Columbia

SANJAY LOGANI, MD
Incyte Pathology
Spokane Valley, Washington

BHAGIRATH MAJMUDAR, MD
Professor
Pathology and Laboratory Medicine
Emory University
Atlanta, Georgia

LYDIA MAYIDA, MD
Resident
Department of Obstetrics & Gynecology
Howard University Hospital
Howard University, College of Medicine
Washington, District of Columbia

MARK S. NANES, MD, PHD
Professor
Medical Endocrinology
Emory University
Atlanta, Georgia
Active Chief of Medicine
Chief of Endocrinology
Internal Medicine/Endocrinology
Atlanta VA Medical Center
Decatur, Georgia

LONG NGUYEN, MD
Resident
Department of Obstetrics & Gynecology
Howard University Hospital
Howard University, College of Medicine
Washington, District of Columbia

OSUEBI OKECHUKWU, MD
Resident
Department of Obstetrics & Gynecology
Howard University Hospital
Howard University, College of Medicine
Washington, District of Columbia

KENAN OMURTAG, MD
Resident
Department of Gynecology and
  Obstetrics
Emory University
Atlanta, Georgia

**GABRIELA M.
OPREA-ILIES, MD**
Assistant Professor
Pathology and Laboratory Medicine
Emory University
Atlanta, Georgia

EZEKIEL OSUNTOGUN, MD
Resident
Department of Obstetrics & Gynecology
Howard University Hospital
Howard University, College of Medicine
Washington, District of Columbia

MICHAEL OWOLABI, MD
Resident
Department of Obstetrics & Gynecology
Howard University Hospital
Howard University, College of Medicine
Washington, District of Columbia

JOHN K. PARK, MD, MSC
Carolina Conceptions
Raleigh, North Carolina

SAMUEL A. PAULI, MD
Clinical Fellow
Division of Reproductive Endocrinology
  and Infertility
Department of Gynecology and Obstetrics
Emory University School of Medicine
Clinical Fellow
Emory Reproductive Center
Emory University Hospital Midtown
Atlanta, Georgia

MONIQUE POWELL-DAVIS, MD
Department of Obstetrics and Gynecology
Howard University Hospital
Howard University, College of Medicine
Washington, District of Columbia

B. DENISE RAYNOR, MD, MPH
Fellow
Preventive and Family Medicine
Emory School of Medicine
Atlanta, Georgia

INEZ REEVES, MD
Assistant Professor
Department of Obstetrics & Gynecology
Howard University Hospital
Howard University, College of Medicine
Washington, District of Columbia

SPENCER S. RICHLIN, MD
Surgical Director
Reproductive Medicine Associates of
  Connecticut
Norwalk, Connecticut

NURU ROBI, MD
Resident
Department of Obstetrics & Gynecology
Howard University Hospital
Howard University, College of Medicine
Washington, District of Columbia

COURTNEY ROWLAND, MD
Resident
Department of Gynecology and Obstetrics
Emory University
Atlanta, Georgia

NAA SACKEY, MD
Resident
Department of Obstetrics & Gynecology
Howard University Hospital
Howard University, College of Medicine
Washington, District of Columbia

HEMANT SATPATHY, MD
Associate
OBGYN, Division of MFM
Emory University
Atlanta, Georgia

PATRICIA LEE SCOTT, MD
Fellow, Maternal Fetal Medicine
Department of Obstetrics and Gynecology
Wake Forest University
Winston-Salem, North Carolina

DONNA R. SESSION, MD
Associate Professor
Department of Gynecology and Obstetrics
Emory University School of Medicine
Chief
Division of Reproductive Endocrinology
  and Infertility
Emory University School of Medicine
Atlanta, Georgia

HOLLY SHEN, MD
Resident
Department of Gynecology and Obstetrics
Emory University
Atlanta, Georgia

KEVIN SCOTT SMITH, MD, FACOG
Assistant Professor
Department of Obstetrics & Gynecology
Howard University Hospital
Howard University, College of Medicine
Washington, District of Columbia

JESSICA B. SPENCER, MD, MSc
Assistant Professor
Division of Reproductive Endocrinology
  and Infertility
Department of Gynecology and
  Obstetrics
Emory University School of Medicine
Emory Reproductive Center
Emory University Hospital Midtown
Atlanta, Georgia

SUMATHI SRIVATSA, MD, FACE
Assistant Professor
Division of Endocrinology
Department of Medicine
Emory University
Physician
Division of Endocrinology
The Emory Healthcare/Emory Hospital
Atlanta, Georgia

ROBERT N. TAYLOR, MD, PHD
Leach-Hendee Professor and Vice Chair for
  Research
Director, Reproductive Endocrinology and
  Infertility Fellowship
Department of Gynecology and
  Obstetrics
Emory University School of Medicine
Atlanta, Georgia

A. JASON VAUGHT, MD
Resident
Department of Gynecology and
  Obstetrics
Emory university
Atlanta, Georgia

EKTA VISHWAKARMA, MD
Resident
Department of Obstetrics & Gynecology
Howard University Hospital
Howard University, College of Medicine
Washington, District of Columbia

STEPHEN H. WEISS, MD, MPH
Assistant Professor
Department of Gynecology and Obstetrics
Emory University Hospital Midtown
Atlanta, Georgia

NIKKIA HENDERSON WORRELL, MD
Resident
Department of Gynecology and Obstetrics
Emory university
Atlanta, Georgia

EDOM YARED, MD
Resident
Department of Obstetrics & Gynecology
Howard University Hospital
Howard University, College of Medicine
Washington, District of Columbia

MICHAL A. YOUNG, MD, FAAP
Associate Professor
Department of Obstetrics & Gynecology
Howard University Hospital
Howard University, College of Medicine
Washington, District of Columbia

CONTENTS

SECTION II: LABOR

SECTION III: POST-PARTUM

SECTION X: VULVAR LESIONS

SECTION XI: FAMILY PLANNING

SECTION XII: GYNECOLOGIC ONCOLOGY AND PATHOLOGY

SECTION XIII: UROGYNECOLOGY

SECTION XIV: PEDIATRIC AND ADOLESCENT GYNECOLOGY

SECTION XVII: MENOPAUSE

SECTION XVIII: SURGERY

```
                        1
```

FETAL KICK COUNTS: KICKING IS NOT JUST FOR FOOTBALL AND SOCCER

JANE ELLIS, MD, PhD

A 32-year-old, G3P0020 female who is 34 weeks pregnant comes to the office for a routine antenatal visit. She reports that she is nervous because she has had two previous miscarriages. Although her fundal height is appropriate, she reports that 3 days ago she noticed that the baby seemed much less active. She denies any vaginal bleeding or uterine cramping. She was told the baby is probably just sleeping and to not worry as her fundal height is measuring the appropriate age and fetal heart tones are present. She is sent home and told to return for her next routine visit in 2 weeks.

Many clinicians instruct their obstetric patients to perform fetal kick counts on a daily basis at home as an informal type of antenatal testing, which assesses the frequency of fetal movement. These fetal movement counts rely on the mother's perception of and ability to count the movements of her fetus. The mother is usually instructed to start these daily counts at 28 to 32 weeks and continue until delivery. A mother's perception that her fetus' movements are decreased may portend fetal demise, possibly within hours to days. In addition, patients should be asked at each prenatal visit for their assessment of fetal movement and reminded that a perceived decrease in fetal movement should be evaluated immediately.

There are several methods by which a patient can assess fetal movement, and there is no evidence that one method is superior to any other. A commonly used protocol involves having the patient lie on her side and count each perceived movement. If she detects ten movements in a 2-hour period, then she may stop counting and be reassured of fetal well-being. The mother may also count fetal movements for 1 hour three times per week. The test is reassuring if the number of movements equals or exceeds the number noted on earlier counts. Patients may be given "kick count cards" to record the daily fetal movement. The card can be reviewed at each visit to determine if the movements are normal and that the mother is performing the counts correctly.

TAKE HOME POINTS

- The goal of antenatal testing is to reduce morbidity and mortality in fetuses at risk for intrauterine distress or demise.
- Fetal movement counts, or "kick counts," are assessments of fetal movement performed by the mother on a daily basis.

SUGGESTED READINGS

Moore TR, Piacquadio K. A prospective evaluation of fetal movement screening to reduce the incidence of antepartum fetal death. *Am J Obstet Gynecol.* 1989;160:1075–1080.
Neldam S. Fetal movements as an indicator of fetal well-being. *Dan Med Bull.* 1983;30: 274–278.

ANTENATAL TESTING: YOU SEE MOM EVERY WEEK... DO NOT FORGET TO EXAMINE THE BABY

JANE ELLIS, MD, PHD

Antenatal tests frequently used in clinical practice include the nonstress test (NST); the biophysical profile (BPP); the modified BPP, which includes an NST and measurement of amniotic fluid index (AFI); the contraction stress test (CST) or oxytocin challenge test (OCT); and various Doppler studies, including the umbilical artery blood flow velocity or middle cerebral artery (MCA) velocity.

Basic to the interpretation of fetal assessment is an understanding of the physiology of fetal heart rate patterns and fetal behavioral state changes. Research involving human and animal fetuses revealed that hypoxemia and acidemia can markedly affect the fetal heart rate pattern, the activity level, and the muscle tone. Developing or increasing hypoxemia and/or acidemia may be reflected by changes in fetal heart rate, breathing, movement, tone, or velocity of blood flow.

THE NONSTRESS TEST

The main thrust behind the NST is that heart rate reactivity, which reflects the status of the fetus' autonomic nervous system, is a reliable indicator of fetal well-being. To obtain the fetal heart rate tracing, the patient is placed in a comfortable reclining position with a left lateral tilt. A transducer is placed on the maternal abdomen over the fetal heart to record its rate. The baseline fetal heart rate is noted, with normal being between 120 and 160 beats per minute. A second transducer is placed over the uterine fundus to detect contractions. If the fetal heart rate tracing is noted to contain accelerations that peak at least 15 beats per minute above the baseline, last 15 seconds from baseline to baseline, and occur at least twice in a 20-minute period, then it is considered to be reactive. Decelerations may be noted as a drop in the fetal heart rate below its previous baseline. Decelerations may take different forms and represent cord compression or uteroplacental insufficiency, among other things. The NST is considered nonreactive if it does not contain fetal heart rate accelerations over a 40-minute period.

Gestational age may affect reactivity; in general, normal fetuses between 24 and 28 weeks of gestation may have a nonreactive NST up to 50% of the time. As mentioned previously, a nonreactive NST or an NST that contains decelerations may require additional fetal assessment or delivery. The fetal heart rate tracing may also be nonreactive when the fetus is in a sleep cycle, but it could also be indicative of impending acidosis. The response to such a NST, whether it be additional testing or delivery, will depend on the overall clinical scenario, which includes the gestational age of the fetus, potential for complications relating to prematurity, the indication for fetal testing, and any maternal or fetal complications such as maternal hypertension or intrauterine growth restriction (IUGR). A nonreactive stress test requires additional evaluation of the fetus, usually by the BPP, if delivery is not anticipated.

THE CONTRACTION STRESS TEST

The CST is performed in a manner very similar to the NST. With the patient in a reclining position and comfortably in a left lateral tilt and transducers in place, the baseline fetal heart rate is obtained for 10 to 20 minutes. If the heart rate is reassuring, the test is started. If three contractions occur spontaneously in a 30-minute period, then the test is complete. If fewer than three or no contractions occur in that time period, then uterine stimulation to elicit contractions is needed. The uterus can be stimulated by having the patient gently rub one nipple through her clothing for 2 to 3 minutes or until a contraction begins. If no contractions occur, she can repeat the stimulation after a 5-minute rest and may repeat the cycle of stimulation-rest until an adequate contraction pattern is obtained. If this fails to produce the desired contraction pattern, then an intravenous line can be placed and low-dose oxytocin can be started at the rate of 0.5 to 1.0 mU per minute and increased every 20 minutes until the desired contraction pattern of three contractions in a 10-minute period is obtained.

The interpretation of the CST depends on the response of the fetal heart rate to uterine contractions. If no significant decelerations occur after the contractions, the CST is read as negative. If decelerations are noted following >50% of the contractions, then the CST is positive. The CST is equivocal if hyperstimulation of the uterus (more than three contractions in a 10-minute period or contractions lasting longer than 90 seconds) results in decelerations in the heart tracing due to inability of the fetus to recover following hyperstimulation or if decelerations are noted after fewer than 50% of the contractions. If the contraction pattern is not adequate, then the CST is unsatisfactory. At this point, an alternative method of testing should be considered.

The CST is not as widely used now as it has been previously. One reason for this is that it is time-consuming and labor intensive for staff members who administer the test. A labor and delivery suite or a perinatal center that performs a high volume of testing may find this method impractical.

A second reason the CST is used less often is that it cannot be used in patients in whom uterine contractions are undesirable. These include patients at risk for preterm delivery, history of a classical uterine incision, preterm premature rupture of membranes, and known or suspected placenta previa.

THE BIOPHYSICAL PROFILE

The biophysical profile, or BPP, incorporates the NST with four ultrasound measures. These measures include (a) fetal breathing movement, defined as one or more episodes of fetal breathing movements lasting 30 seconds or more; (b) fetal movement, defined as three or more discrete body or limb movements; (c) fetal tone, defined as one or more episodes of extension of a fetal extremity with return to flexion or opening or closing of a hand; and (d) assessment of the amniotic fluid volume, where the detection of a single vertical pocket of fluid exceeding 2 cm is considered adequate. The NST is the fifth component.

Each component is given a score of 0 or 2. Zero is given if the measure is abnormal or absent; a score of 2 is given if the component is normal. If the NST is reactive, then a score of 2 is given. A nonreactive NST receives a 0. The NST may be eliminated from the BPP if the other components are each normal without affecting the validity of the test. If the total score from all components is 8 or 10, the BPP is considered normal and is reassuring. A score of 6 is considered equivocal and generally indicates that follow-up testing is needed. A score of 4 or less is abnormal. Depending on the gestational age, delivery may be indicated with this abnormal score or repeat testing if fetal status is suspected to improve. In the very premature fetus, follow-up testing, administration of steroids to enhance fetal lung development, and close surveillance may be indicated in preparation for possible delivery.

The BPP must be conducted for a full 30 minutes if one or more of the ultrasound measures are abnormal. For many healthy fetuses, however, all four components may be obtained quickly within the first few minutes of the examination.

Documentation of amniotic fluid volume of ≤2 cm, indicative of oligohydramnios, requires further evaluation of the fetus. Decreased amniotic fluid may suggest rupture of membranes, fetal anomaly involving the gastrointestinal or genitourinary tract, a chromosomal or infectious etiology, or uteroplacental insufficiency.

THE MODIFIED BIOPHYSICAL PROFILE

This test combines the NST and the amniotic fluid volume in assessing fetal well-being. In the late second and third trimesters, amniotic fluid volume is maintained primarily by fetal urine production. Decreased fetal renal perfusion may reflect placental dysfunction and lead to decreased fluid volume via decreased fetal urination. The idea behind the modified BPP is that the NST is a short-term indicator of the fetal acid-base status while the amniotic fluid volume reflects long-term placental functioning. To estimate the amniotic fluid volume, the deepest umbilical cord–free pocket of fluid is measured by ultrasound in each of four abdominal quadrants. An AFI of >5 cm is considered adequate. Therefore, if the NST is reactive and the AFI is >5 cm, the test is considered reassuring.

UMBILICAL ARTERY DOPPLER VELOCIMETRY

This is a noninvasive ultrasound procedure in which blood flow through the umbilical arteries is assessed. It has become a popular test for assessing the status of a fetus in which IUGR has either been documented or is suspected. This technique is based on the finding that blood flow velocity is different in the growth-restricted fetus and the normally growing fetus. It has been observed that in a growth-restricted fetus the diastolic flow through the umbilical artery is diminished, whereas in a normally grown fetus blood flow is characterized by high-velocity diastolic flow. In some cases, the blood flow in fetuses with severe IUGR may be absent or reversed, a finding that suggests that the growth-restricted fetus may be at high risk for perinatal mortality. When umbilical artery Dopplers are performed, three commonly measured flow indices include the systolic-to-diastolic ratio (S/D), the resistance index, and the pulsatility index. The values are gestational-age dependent. When a study is performed, the values obtained are compared with those available in gestational age–based normative values that are widely available and are generally reported as multiples of the median (MoM). If the values are <1.50 MoM, then fetal status is reassuring. It is important for any Doppler studies that the measurements be accurate. The technique for correct measurement of blood flow by Doppler requires specific training and is beyond the scope of this chapter.

MIDDLE CEREBRAL ARTERY DOPPLERS

MCA Dopplers are another noninvasive ultrasound test becoming popular in assessing fetal status in Rh D-alloimmunized pregnancies. In these pregnancies, fetuses may experience mild to severe hemolytic anemia, hydrops fetalis, and fetal demise. The use of anti-D immunoglobulin such as RhoGAM has dramatically decreased the number of isoimmunized pregnancies. However, when these protocols are not followed or when patients present from outside of the United States where the immunoglobulin is not available, isoimmunization may occur. In the past, amniocentesis was performed to measure the level of bilirubin in amniotic fluid, which provides an indirect measure of fetal hemolysis.

Recent studies have suggested that the same information can be obtained by assessing Doppler velocity through the fetal middle cerebral arteries. Measurement of the peak systolic velocity (PSV) has proven to be the most accurate Doppler method to use in determining if a fetus is at risk for anemia. The PSV is gestational-age dependent. To determine if a fetus is at risk for anemia, PSV is compared with values in widely available tables based on gestational age. If the PSV derived by ultrasound exceeds 1.50 MoM, then moderate to severe anemia is suspected. Suspected anemia would require additional procedures such as periumbilical blood sampling to determine directly the fetal hematocrit. Chronic placental abruption would be another complication where fetal well-being in the face of suspected anemia could be assessed by MCA Dopplers. Many clinicians, however, still consider the role of MCA Dopplers to be investigational.

TAKE HOME POINTS

- The goal of antenatal testing is to reduce morbidity and mortality in fetuses at risk for intrauterine distress or demise.
- Various forms of antenatal testing are available. The form selected should be determined by the indication for testing, the maternal/fetal status, the gestational age of the fetus, and the potential for complications if preterm delivery is considered when testing is abnormal.
- Antenatal testing has been widely incorporated into clinical practice for a number of maternal and fetal conditions. A practitioner should keep in mind, however, that no randomized clinical trials clearly demonstrate improved perinatal outcomes from this assessment.
- The NST and CST rely on the interpretation of the fetal heart rate tracing, while the BPP, the modified BPP, and Doppler velocimetry incorporate ultrasound-derived measurements.
- The response to a test result, whether normal or abnormal, should depend in part on the gestational age of the fetus and the indication for testing. Consultation with a specialist such as a maternal-fetal medicine physician or a neonatologist should be obtained if a practitioner is not certain of appropriate follow-up.
- A number of controversies still exist in this area, including the appropriate gestational age to begin testing, the exact test to choose, the frequency of testing, and, in many cases, the best response to an abnormal test.
- Despite these unresolved issues, most clinicians and patients will continue to utilize these tests to help ensure the well-being of a fetus.

SUGGESTED READINGS

American College of Obstetricians and Gynecologists (ACOG), Committee on Practice Bulletins—Obstetrics. Antepartum fetal surveillance. ACOG Practice Bulletin No. 9. Washington, DC: ACOG; October 1999.

Boddy K, Dawes GS, Fisher R, et al. Foetal respiratory movements, electrocortical and cardiovascular responses to hypoxaemia and hypercapnia in sheep. *J Physiol*. 1974;243: 599–618.

Freeman RK. The use of the oxytocin challenge test for antepartum clinical evaluation of uteroplacental respiratory function. *Am J Obstet Gynecol*. 1975;121:481–489.

Freeman RK, Anderson G, Dorchester W. A prospective multi-institutional study of antepartum fetal heart rate monitoring. 1. Risk of perinatal mortality and morbidity according to antepartum fetal heart rate test results. *Am J Obstet Gynecol*. 1982;143: 771–777.

Huddleston JF, Sutliff G, Robinson D. Contraction stress test by intermittent nipple stimulation. *Obstet Gynecol*. 1984;63:669–673.

Karsdorp VH, van Vugt JM, van Geijn HP, et al. Clinical significance of absent or reversed end diastolic velocity waveforms in umbilical artery. *Lancet*. 1994;344:1664–1668.

Lavin JP Jr, Miodovnik M, Barden TP. Relationship of nonstress test reactivity and gestational age. *Obstet Gynecol*. 1984;63:338–344.

Manning FA, Morrison I, Lange IR, et al. Fetal biophysical profile scoring: selective use of the nonstress test. *Am J Obstet Gynecol*. 1987;156:709–712.

Manning FA, Platt LD. Maternal hypoxemia and fetal breathing movements. *Obstet Gynecol*. 1979;53:758–760.

Murata Y, Martin CB Jr, Ikenoue T, et al. Fetal heart rate accelerations and late decelerations during the course of intrauterine death in chronically catheterized rhesus monkeys. *Am J Obstet Gynecol*. 1982;144:218–223.

Natale R, Clewlow F, Dawes GS. Measurement of fetal forelimb movements in the lamb in utero. *Am J Obstet*. 1981;140:545–551.

Pearson JF, Weaver JB. Fetal activity and fetal wellbeing: an evaluation. *Br Med J*. 1976;1(6021): 1305–1307.

Roberts AB, Mitchell JM, Lake Y, et al. Ultrasonographic surveillance in red blood cell alloimmunization. *Am J Obstet Gynecol*. 2001;184:1251–1255.

Rutherford SE, Phelan JP, Smith CV, et al. The four-quadrant assessment of amniotic fluid volume: an adjunct to antepartum fetal heart rate testing. *Obstet Gynecol*. 1990;162: 703–709.

Vyas S, Nicolaides KH, Campbell S. Doppler examination of the middle cerebral artery in anemic fetuses. *Am J Obstet Gynecol*. 1990;162:1066–1068.

3

KNOW WHAT YOU ARE LOOKING AT: AMNIOTIC FLUID VOLUME

FREZGHI GHEBREAB, MD AND DIANA BROOMFIELD, MD, FACOG, FACS

A 19-year-old G3P0020 female at a gestational age of 34 weeks with no medical problems and uneventful pregnancy was found to have a fundal height that measured only 30 cm. She denied leakage of vaginal fluid and had normal fetal movement. Sonogram revealed that the amniotic fluid volume was 8.2 cm with normal fetal anatomic survey and fetal biometric assessment consistent with the date.

Normally, amniotic fluid volume increases to about a liter by 36 weeks of gestation and decreases thereafter to only 100 to 200 mL or less postterm. Diminished amniotic fluid volume is termed oligohydramnios, and amniotic fluid volume of >2 L is arbitrarily considered excessive and is termed hydramnios or polyhydramnios.

MEASUREMENT

The amniotic fluid volume can be assessed either quantitatively or qualitatively at the time of sonographic examination. The most accurate methods for determining total amniotic fluid volume are direct measurement at the time of hysterotomy and dye-dilution techniques. However, neither is clinically applicable, and in clinical practice, ultrasound is used to assess the volume of the amniotic fluid. Commonly used sonographic methods of assessing amniotic fluid volume include the following: (1) Subjective assessment of amniotic fluid volume: the sonographic visual evaluation of amniotic fluid volume without any objective measurements. The sonographer then reports the amniotic fluid volume as oligohydramnios, normal, or polyhydramnios based upon subjective interpretation. (2) Largest vertical pocket: oligohydramnios has a depth of 0 to 2 cm, normal has a depth of 2.1 to 8 cm, and polyhydramnios has a depth >8 cm. (3) Amniotic fluid index: it is the sum of the vertical depths of largest pocket in each of four equal uterine quadrants. Oligohydramnios has a sum of 0 to <5 cm, normal has a sum of 5 to 25 cm, and polyhydramnios has a sum of >25 cm.

KNOW HOW TO FIX IT: WHEN THE FLUID IS LOW

Oligohydramnios refers to amniotic fluid volume that is less than expected for gestational age. An adequate volume of amniotic fluid is essential for normal fetal movement and growth, as well as to provide a cushion for the fetus and the umbilical cord. General conditions associated with oligohydramnios are listed below:

- *Fetal*: chromosomal abnormalities, congenital abnormalities, growth restriction, fetal demise, postterm, and ruptured membranes.
- *Maternal*: uteroplacental insufficiency from chronic hypertension, preeclampsia, diabetes, and collagen-vascular diseases.
- *Placental*: placental abruption and twin-to-twin transfusion syndrome.
- *Drugs*: prostaglandin synthetase inhibitors and angiotensin-converting enzymes.
- *Idiopathic*: the majority of women with mild to moderate oligohydramnios have no known identifiable cause.

Oligohydramnios developing in early pregnancy is less common and frequently has a bad prognosis in part due to the association with congenital anomalies and preterm delivery. Even normal infants may suffer the consequences of early-onset severe oligohydramnios including amniotic band syndrome with serious deformities, musculoskeletal deformities such as clubfoot, and pulmonary hypoplasia. Oligohydramnios is also associated with increased frequency of labor induction, nonreassuring fetal heart tracing, cesarean delivery, still birth, neonatal intensive care admission, meconium aspiration, growth restriction, malformation, and cord compression in labor.

There is no proven effective long-term treatment for oligohydramnios. Short-term improvement in amniotic fluid volume may be achieved through the use of maternal hydration, amnioinfusion, and fetal membrane sealants. Oligohydramnios in the first trimester carries an ominous prognosis, and the mother should be counseled as such. Oligohydramnios in the second trimester depends on the degree of severity and the underlying etiology. Management includes a sonogram to look for fetal malformations and subsequent serial sonograms to evaluate amniotic fluid volume, fetal growth, and fetal well-being, and rupture of the membranes should be ruled out. While pregnancies with isolated mild to moderate idiopathic oligohydramnios do well, those with severe oligohydramnios often end in fetal or neonatal death. The management of oligohydramnios in late pregnancy depends on the clinical situation. The pregnancy should be evaluated for anomalies. In the presence of intrauterine growth restriction, nonreassuring fetal testing, or pregnancy reaching 37 to 38 weeks, delivery is recommended. Oligohydramnios detected before 36 weeks in the presence of normal anatomy and growth may be managed expectantly in conjunction with antepartum surveillance.

TAKE HOME POINTS

- Oligohydramnios occurring early in pregnancy carries a poor prognosis.
- Ruptured membranes should always be ruled out.
- Oligohydramnios detected before 36 weeks in the presence of normal anatomy and growth may be managed expectantly in conjunction with antepartum testing.

SUGGESTED READINGS

Barss VA. Assessment of amniotic fluid volume. UpToDate. September 26, 2008.

Chamberlain PF, Manning FA, Morrison I, et al. Ultrasound evaluation of amniotic fluid: volume I: the relationship of marginal and decreased amniotic fluid volumes to perinatal outcome. *Am J Obstet Gynecol.* 1984;150:245.

Clinical Management Guidelines for Obstetrician-Gynecologists. Management of postterm pregnancy. ACOG Practice Bulletin No.55. American College of Obstetricians and Gynecologists. *Obstet Gynecol* 2004;104:639–46.

Cunningham FG, Leveno KL, Bloom SL, et al. *Williams Obstetrics.* 22nd ed. New York, NY: McGraw-Hill; 2005.

Magann E, Perry KG Jr, Chauhan SP, et al. The accuracy of ultrasound evaluation of amniotic fluid volume in singleton pregnancies: the effect of operator experience and ultrasound interpretative technique. *J Clin Ultrasound.* 1997;25:249.

Rutherford SE, Phelan JP, Smith CV, et al. The four-quadrant assessment of amniotic fluid volume: an adjunct to antepartum fetal heart rate testing. *Obstet Gynecol.* 1987;70:353.

4

MANAGEMENT OF THE FETUS IN TRANSVERSE LIE

FREZGHI GHEBREAB, MD AND DIANA BROOMFIELD, MD, FACOG, FACS

A 32-year-old G5P4004 female presented with ruptured membranes at 36 weeks. On admission to labor and delivery, it was noted that the uterus appeared transversely ovoid and there was no ballottable fetal part in the fundus or in the lower pole of the uterus. The fetal heart tracing was reassuring and some irregular contractions were noted. Pelvic examination confirmed rupture of the membranes. The cervix was 2 cm dilated, and no fetal part was felt. Sonogram confirmed transverse lie. The patient was taken for cesarean section. At cesarean section, attempts to deliver the baby through a transverse lower segment incision failed and the baby was delivered through an inverted T-incision.

The fetus is in a transverse lie when its long axis is perpendicular to the long axis of the mother. When the long axis of the fetus forms an acute angle, it is termed an oblique lie, which usually is transitory and changes to a transverse or a longitudinal lie once labor starts.

A transverse lie can occur as back-up, or dorsosuperior, when the fetal back is facing upward and the small parts present at the cervix. A back-down, or dorsoinferior, position is seen when the fetal back is oriented downward so that the fetal shoulder presents at the cervix.

Transverse lie occurs with 1 in 300 deliveries and the frequency is much higher in early pregnancy. Most transverse lie pregnancies convert to a cephalic or breech presentation by term. Predisposing factors for transverse lie include prematurity, high parity, placenta previa–contracted pelvis, uterine anomalies or tumors, polyhydramnios, fetal anomaly, and multiple pregnancies.

Pregnancies with a transverse lie are at increased risk of maternal and perinatal morbidity related to placenta previa, umbilical cord prolapse, fetal trauma, and prematurity. The diagnosis may be suspected on inspection of a uterus that is transversely ovoid and is easily made by Leopold maneuvers. A sonogram confirms the diagnosis and determines the precise position of the fetus.

Management is dependent on the gestational age, viability of the fetus, position of the placenta, and whether labor has begun or the membranes have ruptured. Either cesarean delivery or external version to a longitudinal lie is the option of management since spontaneous delivery of the fetus is impossible. If the diagnosis is made prior to the onset of labor at or

>37 weeks of gestation, in the absence of contraindications to vaginal delivery, external cephalic version followed by artificial rupture of membranes, while the head is held in position, and induction of labor may be considered. In the presence of placenta previa or ruptured membranes, cesarean delivery is recommended. In the previable or dead fetus, vaginal delivery with an internal podalic version may be attempted once placenta previa is ruled out.

At the time of cesarean section for a transverse lie with back-up position, delivery may be accomplished through a low transverse incision if the lower segment is well formed. Most obstetricians believe that a transverse incision cannot safely accommodate delivery of the back-down fetus, and consequently, a vertical incision is frequently used in these presentations and in cases where the lower segment is not well formed.

TAKE HOME POINTS

- For a transverse lie with a back-down fetus, a vertical incision is frequently required.
- The term fetus in a mentum posterior position, transverse lie and a brow presentation cannot deliver vaginally.

SUGGESTED READINGS

Bowes Jr WA, Lockwood CJ, Barss VA. Management of the fetus in transverse lie. UpToDate. July 11, 2008.

Cunningham FG, Leveno KL, Bloom SL, et al. *Williams Obstetrics*. 22nd ed. New York, NY: McGraw-Hill; 2005.

5

GESTATIONAL DIABETES MELLITUS: INAPPROPRIATE MANAGEMENT

KERRY M. LEWIS, MD

A 32-year-old G2P0010 female presents at 24 weeks of gestation for her routine prenatal visit. Fetal heart tones are normal and her fundal height is appropriate. Her blood pressure is 120/54, and she describes good fetal movement. She is instructed to proceed to the laboratory for a 1-hour glucola screen and to return for her next prenatal visit in 4 weeks.

The patient has her 1-hour glucola test performed 2 days after her prenatal visit, and the results are forwarded to the obstetrician's office with a value of 155 mg/dL. Given an abnormally elevated result, the patient is contacted to come into the office to have a 3-hour glucose challenge test performed. She performs the test the following day and the results are as follows: fasting, 86 mg/dL; 1 hour, 215 mg/dL; 2 hour, 186 mg/dL; and 3 hour, 106 mg/dL. She is informed that she has two elevated values and that she has gestational diabetes mellitus. The patient is scheduled to have diabetic teaching for dietary recommendations and monitoring. She is informed that she will need to be started on insulin and will require induction of labor if the fetus gets "too big." She is concerned and wonders if she needs insulin and what impact is this diagnosis going to have on her unborn child.

EPIDEMIOLOGY AND RISKS ASSOCIATED WITH GESTATIONAL DIABETES MELLITUS

Gestational diabetes mellitus complicates 2% to 5% of pregnancies and is common among women with a strong family history of diabetes mellitus, morbid obesity, and advanced maternal age. Pregnancy complications include fetal macrosomia, increased risk for cesarean delivery, delay in fetal lung maturation, and fetal trauma during delivery. Thirty percent of women with gestational diabetes will develop type II diabetes within 15 years, and 33% to 50% of women with gestational diabetes will have gestational diabetes in a subsequent pregnancy.

Diagnostic Parameters. Pregnant women routinely undergo a 1-hour glucose screening test for gestational diabetes between 24 and 28 weeks of gestation. A 1-hour glucose screening test value of >140 mg/dL is considered abnormal; however, using this value fails to diagnose 80% of women with gestational diabetes. Therefore, many institutions are adopting a 1-hour glucose screening test value of >135 as abnormal. Lowering the threshold to 135 mg/dL increases the number of 3-hour glucose tolerance tests by 42% while increasing the detection frequency of gestational diabetes mellitus to 99%. Following an abnormal 1-hour screening test (>135 to 140 mg/dL), the patient is instructed to proceed to a confirmatory 3-hour glucose tolerance test. The diagnosis of gestational diabetes is made based on two abnormal values in the 3-hour glucose tolerance test.

Management Considerations: Diet, Exercise, Insulin, and Oral Hypoglycemics. Once the diagnosis is made, the patient is instructed to achieve adequate blood sugar values by attempting to control her diet by restricting her carbohydrate intake. Adequate control is achieved when the patient has stable fasting blood sugars of 65 to 95 mg/dL and 1-hour postprandial blood sugars of 65 to 140 mg/dL or 2-hour postprandial blood sugars of 65 to 120 mg/dL. Limited exercise in addition to dietary adjustments may be helpful in achieving these goals.

The patient with gestational diabetes mellitus monitors her blood sugars at home using a glucose meter and records the results of her blood sugar tests: fasting and 1 or 2 hours after breakfast, lunch, and dinner. The available evidence does not support a clear recommendation as to the number of times glucose levels should exceed targets before medical management with an oral hypoglycemic agent or insulin. The goal of medical therapy is to achieve normoglycemic levels when dietary changes have been unsuccessful.

Many patients would like to avoid injections associated with insulin administration; therefore, glyburide is an alternative to insulin therapy and may be considered a first-line therapy in select cases. Glyburide is a well-tolerated and safe medication that can provide excellent glucose control in the appropriately selected patient. Patients with higher mean fasting blood sugars, earlier gestational age at diagnosis, and gravidas of increasing maternal age are at greater risk of failing glyburide therapy. Gestational diabetics who fail glyburide therapy or who are considered not to be good candidates for glyburide therapy are managed with insulin.

The initial dosage of insulin is calculated based on the patient's weight and is divided into split dosing. NPH insulin is relatively long-acting insulin that is administered in the morning, primarily to control the lunchtime postprandial blood sugars, and at night (9 to 11 PM), to control the overnight blood sugars, thereby avoiding fasting hyperglycemia. Regular insulin is given within 30 minutes prior to meals, usually at breakfast and dinner. On occasion, a dose of regular insulin may be given prior to lunch if morning NPH insulin is not effective in controlling postprandial lunch hyperglycemia. If adequate control of blood sugars continues to be unachieved, other options of management include dosage adjustments, incorporating more rapid-acting insulin such as Novalog or Humalog, or an insulin pump.

The need for rapid-acting insulin or an insulin pump suggests more complicated glucose intolerance and the possibility of undiagnosed pregestational diabetes. This diagnosis may also be considered if the hemoglobin A_{1c} value is elevated. Suspicion of pregestational diabetes necessitates more aggressive glucose control along with consultation for ophthalmologic evaluation and urologic evaluation for diabetic nephropathy. Given the association between pregestational diabetes and preeclampsia, a 24-hour urine collection for protein would also be helpful as a baseline to compare in the event that preeclampsia was to occur.

Timing and Mode of Delivery. In the patient whose blood sugars are well-controlled by diet and exercise, the pregnancy is managed as a normal pregnancy with no need for additional antenatal testing or more frequent prenatal visits. In the patient who requires medication to control her diabetes, the risks of adverse fetal and neonatal outcomes require closer surveillance of the pregnancy to include regularly scheduled ultrasounds to evaluate fetal growth and antenatal testing to evaluate fetal well-being. If elective delivery prior to 39 weeks of gestation is considered, amniocentesis for fetal lung maturity should be performed on those women on oral hypoglycemic agents or insulin. Size of the fetus is never an indication for expedited delivery or induction of labor. If the fetal weight is estimated to be greater than 4,500 g, the patient is offered a cesarean delivery; otherwise, a vaginal delivery can be attempted.

Importance of Postpartum Screening. Because some patients with gestational diabetes are undiagnosed pregestational diabetics, an evaluation for glucose intolerance should occur at the 6-week postpartum visit. This consists of a fasting blood sugar with a normal glucose level of <125 mg/dL or a 75-g glucose challenge test with a normal 2-hour value <200 mg/dL.

TAKE HOME POINTS

- Medications to manage elevated blood sugars are only necessary if diet and exercise fail.
- Glyburide is a safe and effective alternative to insulin in the management of gestational diabetes.
- Close monitoring of the pregnancy is necessary for patients on medication to control their blood sugars.

- If a patient is suspected of having pregestational diabetes mellitus, ophthalmologic and renal evaluations are indicated.
- Induction of labor should not be performed for suspected macrosomia
- At the 6-week postpartum visit, the patient with gestational diabetes should be evaluated for type II diabetes mellitus.

SUGGESTED READINGS

ACOG Practice Bulletin. Clinical Management Guidelines for Obstetrician-Gynecologists. Gestational diabetes. Number 30, September 2001.

American Diabetes Association. Nutritional management during pregnancy in preexisting diabetes. In: American Diabetes Association. *Medical Management of Pregnancy Complicated by Diabetes.* 3rd ed. Alexandria, VA: American Diabetes Association; 2000:70–86.

Conway DL, Langer O. Effects of the new criteria for type 2 diabetes on the rate of postpartum glucose intolerance in women with gestational diabetes. *Am J Obstet Gynecol.* 1999;181: 610–614.

Coustan DR. Gestational diabetes. In: National Institutes of Diabetes and Digestive and Kidney Diseases. *Diabetes in America.* 2nd ed. Bethesda, MD: NIDDK, 1995; NIH Publication No. 95-1468:703–717.

Gaudier FL, Hauth JC, Poist M, et al. Recurrence of gestational diabetes mellitus. *Obstet Gynecol.* 1992;80:755–758.

Kahn BF, Davies JK, Lynch AM, et al. Predictors of glyburide failure in the treatment of gestational diabetes. *Obstet Gynecol.* 2006;107(6):1303–1309.

Langer O, Conway DL, et al. A comparison of glyburide and insulin in women with gestational diabetes mellitus. *N Engl J Med.* 2000;343:1134–1138.

Langer O, Rodriguez DA, Xenakis EM, et al. Intensified versus conventional management of gestational diabetes. *Am J Obstet Gynecol.* 1994;170:1036–1047.

Moses RG. The recurrence rate of gestational diabetes in subsequent pregnancies. *Diabetes Care.* 1996;19:1348–1350.

Nicholson W, Bolen S, et al. Benefits and risks of oral diabetes agents compared with insulin in women with gestational diabetes: a systematic review. *Obstet Gynecol.* 2009;113:193–205.

Philipson EH, Super DM. Gestational diabetes mellitus: does it recur in subsequent pregnancy? *Am J Obstet Gynecol.* 1989;160:1324–1331.

Rochon M, Rand L, et al. Glyburide for the management of gestational diabetes: risk factors predictive of failure and associated pregnancy outcomes. *Am J Obstet Gynecol.* 2006;195(4):1090.

Solomon CG, Willett WC, Carey VJ, et al. A prospective study of pregravid determinants of gestational diabetes mellitus. *JAMA.* 1997;278:1078–1083.

6

PROGNOSIS FOR ALL CASES OF NONIMMUNE HYDROPS IS NOT THE SAME

HEMANT SATPATHY, MD

Hydrops fetalis is a diagnosis often made following obstetrical (OB) ultrasound (US). Its characteristic findings include ascites, pleural effusion, skin edema, and pericardial effusion. Two of these four US findings have to be present to make the diagnosis. It has two subtypes, immune and nonimmune. The latter accounts for 90% of all hydrops cases. Aneuploidy, structural anomalies, anemia, and infections are the most common etiologies for the nonimmune hydrops fetalis. It has high perinatal mortality in the range of 50% to 95%. But, when nonimmune hydrops results from cardiac arrhythmias or parvovirus infection, the prognosis is usually excellent.

Several infections during pregnancy could result in nonimmune hydrops. Out of these infective agents, parvovirus and Toxoplasmosis, Other infections (Hepatitis B, Syphilis, Varicella–Zoster Virus, HIV, and Parvovirus B19), Rubella, Cytomegalovirus, Herpes simplex virus (TORCH) are most common. The parvovirus is acquired by exposure to sick children at home, school, or day care. By the time the child is sick, it is too late and has already exposed the pregnant mothers around the child through skin contact or respiratory droplets. Though most of the adult pregnant patients are immune to the virus from prior exposure, we screen all these patients for possible infection. The common blood test ordered to make a diagnosis is IgM and IgG antibodies to parvovirus.

About 30% to 50% of the time, there is vertical transmission of the virus from the mother to the fetus. But, only 2% to 3% of the time this results in nonimmune hydrops from anemia. The mechanism behind the anemia is the suppression of erythroid precursor cells in the bone marrow. This drop in hemoglobin, if significant, could end up in high–output heart failure, hypoxic endothelial damage, and portal hypertension from increased hepatic erythropoiesis. These three above mentioned mechanisms contribute to third spacing of fluid in these hydrops babies.

As the prognosis is usually grim in hydrops cases, often the obstetric providers offer termination of pregnancy or just supportive care irrespective of the cause. This is medical malpractice. We know that the survival is nearly 75% to 95% in patients with documented parvovirus infection. So, one has to be aggressive in these patients in monitoring the effect of the virus.

Standard recommendation is monitoring for signs of hydrops by frequent US in 1 to 2 weeks interval along with Doppler assessment of peak systolic blood flow in middle cerebral artery (MCA). The latter depicts the severity of anemia in the fetus. The lower the hemoglobin, the higher the blood flows because of the reduced blood viscosity.

Once significant anemia is documented, intrauterine blood transfusion is the standard of care. This is done by percutaneous umbilical blood sampling to confirm anemia followed by appropriately matched blood transfusion. A timely blood transfusion in these infected babies could prevent hydropic changes or even bring regression of existing hydropic changes. Most of the time, there is a need for one-time transfusion. Thus, one should be aggressive in managing nonimmune hydrops patients resulting from parvovirus infection.

TAKE HOME POINTS

- Do not treat every hydrops patient the same way.
- Do not offer termination or just supportive care to nonimmune hydrops babies resulting from parvovirus infection.
- An extensive workup is highly recommended to find a cause for hydrops.
- Every pregnant patient exposed to parvovirus should be offered the serology testing to document maternal infection.
- Noninvasive testing such as MCA Doppler to document fetal anemia is highly recommended in pregnant patients infected with parvovirus.
- When significant anemia is documented in these parvovirus–affected babies, intrauterine blood transfusion is recommended.

SUGGESTED READINGS

Creasy and Resnik's Maternal-Fetal Medicine Principle and Practice. 6th ed. Philadelphia, PA: W.B. Saunders; 2009.
Cunningham FG, Leveno KL, Bloom SL, et al. *Williams Obstetrics.* 22nd ed. New York, NY: McGraw-Hill; 2005.

7

RENAL DISEASES IN PREGNANCY

NURU ROBI, MD AND DIANA P. BROOMFIELD, MD, MBA, FACOG, FACS

A 32-year-old G3P1011 female at an estimated gestational age of 22w3d presents with complaints of fever, chills, and back pain. On physical examination, her vitals are B/P:120/67, T: 100.6°F, and pulse: 103 per minute. Her abdomen is soft, nontender, and gravid with a fundal height of 20 cm. The FHR is 170 BPM, with moderate variability. She also complained of mild bilateral tenderness over the costovertebral angle (CVA). Upon reviewing her prenatal records, you noted that the patient had a positive urine culture (Klebsiella >100,000 CFU/mL), which has gone untreated. She was admitted, and empirical IV antibiotics were started pending urine sensitivity results. On the 2nd day of her hospital admission, she developed shortness of breath and pulse oximetry consistent with desaturation.

Pregnancy causes numerous changes in the body of a woman. Both hormonal and mechanical changes increase the risk of urinary stasis and vesicoureteral reflux. These changes, along with an already short urethra (~3 to 4 cm in females as compared to males) and difficulty emptying the bladder, increase the frequency of urinary tract infections (UTIs) in pregnant women.

Bacteriuria occurs in 2% to 7% of pregnancies, particularly in multiparous women; a similar prevalence is seen in nonpregnant women. The organisms are also similar in species and virulence in pregnant and nonpregnant women. Thus, the basic mechanism of entry of bacteria into the urinary tract is likely to be the same. However, the smooth muscle relaxation and subsequent ureteral dilatation that accompany pregnancy are thought to facilitate the ascent of bacteria from the bladder to the kidney. As a result, bacteriuria in pregnant women has a greater propensity to progress to pyelonephritis (up to 40%) than in nonpregnant women. Acute pyelonephritis is one of the most common medical complications in pregnancy. It occurs in 1% to 2% of pregnant women and may result in significant maternal morbidity as well as fetal morbidity and mortality. The clinical course of pyelonephritis in pregnancy was well described over 20 to 30 years ago. Bacteriuria is also associated with an increased risk of preterm birth, low birth weight, and perinatal mortality.

Early screening for and treatment of asymptomatic bacteriuria in pregnancy have both maternal and fetal benefits as suggested by a Cochrane review of 14 randomized trials of asymptomatic bacteriuria in pregnant women that compared the outcome with antibiotic therapy to that with placebo or no treatment. A common error in treating pregnant patients is to not check their urine for the presence of bacteria.

Treatment of bacteriuria during pregnancy reduces the incidence of these complications and lowers the long-term risk of sequelae following asymptomatic bacteriuria.

The following regimens can be used for treatment of asymptomatic bacteriuria:

1. Nitrofurantoin (100 mg PO twice daily for 5 to 7 days)
2. Cefpodoxime (100 mg PO every 12 hours for 3 to 7 days)
3. Amoxicillin–clavulanate (500 mg PO twice a day for 3 to 7 days)
4. Fosfomycin (3 g PO as a single dose)

Acute uncomplicated pyelonephritis is suggested by flank pain, nausea/vomiting, fever (>38°C), and/or costovertebral angle tenderness and may occur in the presence or absence of symptoms of cystitis.

Although the prevalence of asymptomatic bacteriuria in pregnant women is similar to that seen in nonpregnant women, as many as 30% to 40% of pregnant women with untreated asymptomatic bacteriuria will develop symptomatic UTI, including pyelonephritis, during pregnancy. This risk is reduced by 70% to 80% if bacteriuria is eradicated. It has been estimated that as many as 20% of women with severe pyelonephritis develop complications that include septic shock syndrome or its variants, such as acute respiratory distress syndrome (ARDS). Acute renal failure associated with microabscesses and suppurative pyelonephritis has been described in isolated cases, independent of sepsis. The hypothetical patient described above falls into this category.

As with nonpregnant patients with complicated pyelonephritis, pregnant women should have definite improvement within 24 to 48 hours after appropriate antibiotics administration. Once afebrile for 48 hours, patients can be switched to oral therapy (guided by culture susceptibility results) and discharged to complete 10 to 14 days of treatment.

If symptoms and fever persist beyond the first 24 to 48 hours of treatment, a repeat urine culture and urinary tract imaging studies should be performed to rule out persistent infection and urinary tract pathology.

Our patient above was diagnosed with ADRS and was transferred to ICU where she required respiratory support with positive pressure ventilation and further IV antibiotics therapy. The condition of the patient improved 1 week after hospital admission. She was then discharged. What is the further management of the patient?

As noted by Cunningham in 1994, in patients with a history of acute pyelonephritis, subsequent recurrent bacteriuria occurred in 28% of women and pyelonephritis recurred in 10% during the same pregnancy. As a result, low-dose antimicrobial prophylaxis, such as nitrofurantoin (50 to 100 mg PO at bedtime) or cephalexin (250 to 500 mg PO at bedtime), and periodic urinary surveillance for infection are recommended for the remainder of the pregnancy.

Sulfa drugs should be avoided in mothers with glucose-6-phosphate deficiency.

Some facts about lab values related to renal system during pregnancy need to be remembered. It is important for the practicing clinician to be cognizant of the various physiologic and anatomic changes involving the urinary system that are induced by pregnancy. Probably the most significant of these is the increase in glomerular filtration rate and renal plasma flow, which starts very early in pregnancy and exceeds nonpregnant levels by 50%. This, in turn, results in a significantly higher endogenous creatinine clearance (110 to 150 mL per minute) and lower serum creatinine (0.5 to 0.8 mg/dL) and serum urea nitrogen (9 to 12 mg/dL) levels. Anatomically, there is a slight increase in kidney size and marked dilation of the renal pelvis, calyces, and ureters. To compensate for a 10-mm reduction in PCO_2 (averages 28 to 30 mm Hg), the kidneys excrete more bicarbonate in pregnancy, which results in a 4 to 5 mEq/L decrease in serum bicarbonate (averages 20 to 22 mEq/L). Serum osmolality also decreases by approximately 10 mOsm/L (serum sodium 5 mEq/L).

TAKE HOME POINTS

- *Urinalysis* is essentially unchanged during pregnancy, except for occasional glucosuria.
- Although *protein excretion* normally is increased, it seldom reaches levels that are detected by usual screening methods. Higby and colleagues (1994) reported 24-hour protein excretion to be 115 mg with a 95% confidence level at 260 mg per day. There were no significant differences by trimester.
- Albumin constitutes only a small part of total protein excretion and ranges from 5 to 30 mg per day.
- Most investigators agree that proteinuria must exceed 300 to 500 mg per day to be considered abnormal for pregnancy. Stehman-Breen and associates (2002) found that 3% of 4,589 nulliparous women had *idiopathic hematuria* when screened before 20 weeks. They also reported that these women had a twofold risk of preeclampsia.
- If the serum creatinine persistently exceeds 0.9 mg/dL (75 mol/L), then intrinsic renal disease should be suspected.
- A carefully collected, timed urine specimen can be used to estimate the glomerular filtration rate by creatinine clearance.

SUGGESTED READINGS

American College of Obstetricians and Gynecologists. Antimicrobial therapy for obstetric patients. ACOG educational bulletin 245. 1998; Washington, DC.

Cunningham FG, Leveno KL, Bloom SL, et al. *Williams Obstetrics*. 22nd ed. New York, NY: McGraw-Hill; 2005.

Cunningham FG, Morris GB, Mickal A. Acute pyelonephritis of pregnancy: a clinical review. *Obstet Gynecol*. 1973;42:112–114.

Guberman C, Greenspoon JS, Goodwin TM. Renal/Urinary Tract, Gastrointestinal and Dermatologic Disorders in Pregnancy. In DeCherney AH, Nathan L, Goodwin TM, Laufer N, eds. *Current Diagnosis & Treatment: Obstetrics & Gynecology*. 10th ed. New York, NY: McGraw-Hill Medical; 2007, pages 374–385.

Gilstrap LC III, Cunningham FG, Whalley PJ. Acute pyelonephritis in pregnancy: an anterospective study. *Obstet Gynecol*. 1981;57:409–413.

Higby K, Suiter CR, Phelps JY, et al. Normal values of urinary albumin and total protein excretion during pregnancy. *Am J Obstet Gynecol*. 1994;171(4):984–9.

Hooton TM, Stamm WE. Urinary tract infections and asymptomatic bacteriuria in pregnancy. UpToDate. 2009.

Leticia AJ. Urinary tract infection in pregnancy. E-medicine. October 9, 2008.

Stehman-Breen CO, Levine RJ, Qian C, et al. Increased risk of preeclampsia among nulliparous pregnant women with idiopathic hematuria. *Am J Obstet Gynecol*. 2002;187(3):703–8.

Thompson C, Verani R, Evanoff G, et al. Suppurative bacterial pyelonephritis as a cause of acute renal failure. *Am J Kidney Dis*. 1986;8:271.

8

OH THE PRESSURE! CARDIAC VALVES AND HYPERTENSION IN PREGNANCY

NAA SACKEY, MD AND DIANA BROOMFIELD, MD

A 32-year-old G2P0010 white woman presents for her first prenatal visit. She is 10 weeks pregnant, and her past medical history is significant for systemic lupus erythematosus and cardiac valve prosthesis as a result of endocarditis. She is concerned about her current medication and wants information about the risk her medical history will have on the baby.

During the second trimester, she comes in with complaints of orthopnea, fatigue, shortness of breath, and edema. An EKG done in the office shows supraventricular tachycardia. What is the next step in management?

Cardiac disease in pregnancy remains one of the leading causes of maternal mortality and morbidity. During pregnancy, there are several normal physiological changes that impact the cardiac system. The total blood volume and plasma volume increase by 50% while the plasma volume decreases by 30%. To compensate for the increase in blood volume, there is a decrease of systemic vascular resistance and increase in cardiac output. This increased intravascular volume also predisposes pregnant women to a hypercoagulable state. Due to these changes, it is crucial to appropriately manage congenital or acquired cardiac diseases in pregnant women.

The management of cardiac valve prosthesis in pregnancy can be challenging. In pregnancy, it is important to determine if the cardiac valve prosthesis is a mechanical versus porcine valve. In pregnancy, the use of warfarin and other anticoagulation therapies is controversial. The American Heart Association recommends that heparin be used through the first trimester, warfarin be used until 36 weeks, and subcutaneous heparin be used from 36 weeks until delivery. Although heparin has been shown to have a fourfold increase in thromboembolism events over warfarin, warfarin crosses the blood-brain barrier and can cause teratogenic effects such as intra-uterine growth retardation (IUGR), nasal hypoplasia, vertebral and ophthalmologic abnormalities, and developmental delays. Mechanical valves and antithrombotics are reported to have an increased risk of miscarriages and thromboembolic events. Porcine valves do not require anticoagulation in pregnancy, but pregnancy has been shown to decrease the life span of porcine valves.

Many patients with mechanical heart valves have coexisting cardiac disease such as primary pulmonary hypertension (PPH). Although it is a pulmonary disease, it has serious effects on the right heart. PPH is described as persistently elevated pulmonary artery pressure. Mean arterial pressure is usually >25 mm Hg in pulmonary hypertension. Symptoms of pulmonary hypertension include shortness of breath, fatigue, hoarseness, and lower extremity edema. Diagnosis is usually made by an echocardiogram. The management of PPH includes treatments that improve vasodilatation, such as oxygen, nifedipine, intravenous prostacyclin, and nitric oxide. Anticoagulation should be considered to prevent cerebrovascular accidents, and early delivery around 32 to 34 weeks is strongly encouraged.

Hypertension in pregnancy is a common disorder and can be categorized by chronic hypertension or gestational hypertension. Gestational hypertension should be properly managed to avoid developing preeclampsia, which is hypertension associated with proteinuria. Chronic hypertension is diagnosed as documented high blood pressure prior to pregnancy and two measurements of blood pressure >140/90 prior to the 20th week of gestation. Severe hypertension can cause maternal cardiac arrest, renal failure, or stroke. For safe antihypertensive therapies in pregnancy, see *Table 8.1*.

Certain hypertensive drugs should be avoided in pregnancy, such as angiotensin-converting enzyme inhibitors, angiotensin receptor blockers, and most diuretics except furosemide and thiazides. Angiotensin-converting enzyme inhibitors can cause renal failure, especially during the second and third trimesters, oligohydramnios, fetal growth retardation, fetal hypotension, and hypoplastic lung development.

Dysrhythmia is also a major concern in pregnancy especially in the presence of preexisting heart diseases. Dysrhythmia can be treated with pharmacological interventions; the safest drugs to use in pregnancy include digoxin, quinidine, and propranolol. Digoxin, a digitalis preparation, is relatively safe; a common error physicians make is not diligently monitoring the digoxin levels. Digoxin has a low therapeutic range and toxicity is common. Symptoms of toxicity include dysrhythmias, nausea, vomiting, abdominal pain, confusion, headaches, visual disturbance, electrolyte abnormalities, and renal insufficiency.

Many of these cardiac conditions can lead to cardiopulmonary arrest or other cardiac events that may require cardioversion. Cardioversion in pregnancy should be performed in a left lateral tilt position to prevent aortocaval compression due to the gravid uterus. All fetal monitoring should be turned off during cardioversion. In the event of cardiac arrest, the decision to perform a perimortem cesarean section is critical; delivery should be performed 4 to 5 minutes after the cardiac event. Perimortem delivery can increase maternal survival by increasing cardiac output, therefore improving maternal perfusion, and improve the chance of a successful resuscitation.

TABLE 8.1. COMMON ANTIHYPERTENSIVE DRUGS USED IN PREGNANCY

DRUGS	MECHANISM	SIDE EFFECTS	OTHER
Methyldopa	Central acting α-agonist	Dry mouth Lethargy Fever Drowsiness Abnormal liver function Hemolytic anemia	First-line treatment in pregnancy
Labetalol	β-Blocker with α-blocking activities	Flushing Headaches Decreased placental perfusion	Avoid in pregnant women with asthma and congestive heart failure
Nifedipine	Calcium channel blocker	Headache Low blood pressure Increased heart rate	Rapid onset May be used as monotherapy
Clonidine	α_2 Agonist	Dry mouth Sedation Orthostatic hypotension	Used in mild to moderate hypertension
Hydralazine	Vasodilator	Flushing Headache Tachycardia Lupus-like syndrome	Used for hypertensive emergency
Thiazide	Diuretic	Electrolyte imbalance Volume depletion	Contraindicated in late pregnancy

TAKE HOME POINTS

- Pregnant women with cardiac valve prosthesis should be on anticoagulation therapy.
- Warfarin causes warfarin embryopathy and should be avoided in the first trimester.
- A common error made in pregnancy is not properly managing hypertension and being informed of medications to avoid in pregnancy.
- Digoxin has a low therapeutic index and should be prudently monitored in pregnancy to avoid digitalis toxicity.
- Cardioversion can be performed in pregnancy. If necessary, it should be performed in the left lateral position.

SUGGESTED READINGS

Atkinson B, Slotnick RN. Teratogens and birth defect. In: Evans AT, ed. *Manual of Obstetrics*. 7th ed. Philadelphia, PA: Lippincott Williams & Wilkins; 2007.

Gabbe SG, Niebyl JR, Simpson JL. *Obstetrics: Normal and Problem Pregnancies*. 4th ed. Philadelphia, PA: Churchill Livingstone; 2002.

Queenan JT, Spong CY, Lockwood CJ. *Management of High-Risk Pregnancy: An evidence-based Approach*. 5th ed. Malden, MA: Blackwell Publishing; 2007.

Sovndal S, Tabas JA. Cardiovascular disorders in pregnancy. In: Pearlman MD, Tintinalli JE, Dyne PL, eds. *Obstetric & Gynecologic Emergencies: Diagnosis and Management*. New York, NY: McGraw-Hill Medical; 2004.

9

IS THE STETHOSCOPE NECESSARY IN THE OBSTETRICAL PATIENT?

SHUNA E.R. ISOM, MD AND DIANA BROOMFIELD, MD, MBA, FACOG, FACS

A 22-year-old college graduate presents to her primary care physician for a complete physical examination, as requested by her new employer. She has a history of irregular menses. Her last menstrual period was 4 months prior to evaluation. On cardiac evaluation, a fixed splitting of the second heart sound is detected. She was noted to be at 22 weeks of gestation and was in utter surprise. She mentioned that she has a congenital opening in her heart that was never repaired and never caused any problems.

A common error, if not in practice, certainly in thinking is that an obstetrician does not require, much less uses, a stethoscope. All patients, especially the obstetric patient because of the tremendous major hemodynamic alterations that occur during pregnancy, during labor and delivery, and during the postpartum period, require that you judiciously use your stethoscope. It has been reported that cardiac diseases complicate 1% to 4% of pregnancies in women without preexisting cardiac abnormalities. These hemodynamic changes begin as early as during the first 5 to 8 weeks of pregnancy and reach their peak late in the second trimester. In patients with preexisting cardiac disease (especially those with larger defects), the cardiac decompensation begins with the peak in the second trimester. Recall that both blood volume increases 40% to 50% and cardiac output rises 30% to 50% above baseline during normal pregnancy peaking by the end of the second trimester and reaching a plateau up until delivery. Since the blood volume is greater than the increase in red blood cell mass, a fall in hemoglobin concentration occurs leading to what is described as "anemia of pregnancy." The increase in cardiac output is precipitated by three factors: (1) an increase in preload because of greater blood volume, (2) a reduced afterload (secondary to a decrease in the systemic vascular resistance), and (3) an increase in the maternal heart rate by 10 to15 beats per minute. These hemodynamic changes lead to an increase in the stroke volume during the first and second trimesters, which declines in the third trimester secondary to compression of the inferior vena cava by the gravid uterus. These normal cardiac changes lead to profound hemodynamic fluctuations during labor and delivery. There are many hemodynamic stressors that occur during labor and delivery. With each uterine contraction, 300 to 500 mL of blood enters into the general circulation. The increase in stroke volume results in a 50% increase in cardiac output with each contraction. Thus, there may be up to a 75% increase in cardiac output baseline during labor and delivery. Hemodynamic changes during the postpartum state are also very significant. The hemodynamic changes return to their baseline state during the 2 to 4 weeks following vaginal delivery and usually within 4 to 6 weeks following a cesarean delivery. These hemodynamic changes put the obstetric patient at significant risk, especially when an underlying (known or undiagnosed) cardiac abnormality exists. Avoid making the common error of not utilizing your stethoscope judicially.

ATRIAL SEPTAL DEFECT

During fetal life, there is a normal opening between the atria, the foramen ovale. This allows blood to detour away from the lungs before birth. However, after birth, the foramen ovale is no longer necessary and usually closes or becomes very small within several weeks or months. Sometimes, the foramen ovale is larger than normal and does not completely close after birth; however, typically during early childhood, it eventually closes in most individuals. Nevertheless, one in five healthy adults may still have a small patent foramen ovale noted as an atrial septal defect (ASD). The presence of an ASD allows mixing of pulmonary venous and systemic venous circulations. Due to the increased pressure of pulmonary flow, a left-to-right shunt emerges through the defect. This leads to increased work for the heart and the lungs. Due to the chronicity of this increased circulation, some patients develop progressive vascular changes, such as the equalization of systemic and pulmonary pressures due to increased pulmonary vasculature resistance. The ability of the right ventricle to acquire normal or near normal functioning depends on the duration of the overloaded circulation. Two primary complications, namely, pulmonary hypertension and Eisenmenger syndrome, can result if the defect is large.

Eisenmenger syndrome consists of cyanosis, pulmonary hypertension, and erythrocytosis. In patients with Eisenmenger syndrome, the pulmonary hypertension is chronic and leads to permanent and irreversible pulmonary damage. This syndrome may result from ASD, ventricular septal defect (VSD), patent ductus arteriosus (PDA), or atrioventricular canal (AV canal) defect. Obstetrical patients with small ASD usually tolerate pregnancy well without complications. However, patients with a large ASD or with Eisenmenger syndrome have higher obstetrical risks. Obstetrical patients with a larger defect are at risk for pulmonary or cardiac complications such as congestive heart failure, arrhythmias, or pulmonary hypertension. Pregnancy is contraindicated in patients with Eisenmenger syndrome. Maternal mortality in the presence of Eisenmenger syndrome may be as high as 30% to 50% intrapartum or the immediate postpartum period and fetal loss as high as 75%.

ASDs are differentiated in three subtypes: sinus venous defects (5% to 10%), partial AV canal defects (ostium primum defects), and ostium secundum defects (80%).

PATENT DUCTUS ARTERIOSUS

Embryologically, the ductus arteriosus is derived from the sixth aortic arch. It spans from the left or main pulmonary artery to the upper descending portion of the thoracic aorta, distal to the left subclavian artery. At birth, when there is a failure in its closure, the ductus arteriosus is referred to as being *persistently patent*. Such occurrences may arise in isolated physiological situations or in conjunction with complex congenital heart defects. In cases such as the latter, the PDA may be essential to either pulmonary or systemic circulatory flow, resulting in decompensation of the infant if its patency is not maintained (utilizing exogenous prostaglandin E2). Clinically, small persistent PDA is typically asymptomatic; however, larger defects may lead to cardiac and pulmonary complications such as pulmonary hypertension, Eisenmenger syndrome, congestive heart failure, endocarditis, and arrhythmias. Thus, pregnancy in the midst of these complications increases both maternal and fetal morbidity and mortality.

VENTRICULAR SEPTAL DEFECT

VSD is an opening between the left and right ventricles that permits a flow of circulation from the higher pressured left ventricle (LV) to the lower pressured right ventricle. As a result, right ventricular pressures are elevated to the same levels as systemic pressures. With the size of the defect determining the severity of the infant's symptoms, large VSDs produce a large increase in pulmonary flow, thus presenting a clinical picture of congenital heart failure. If left untreated, pulmonary hypertension will ensue with increased pulmonary vascular resistance, thus leading to a reversal of the left-to-right shunt, known as Eisenmenger syndrome.

VSDs are differentiated into four subtypes based on septal location: perimembranous VSD, AV canal defects (inlet defects), supracristal VSD (outlet VSD), and muscular VSD (anterior, midventricular, posterior, and apical).

EISENMENGER SYNDROME

The sequela of uncorrected large VSD, ASD, or PDA is chronic pulmonary hypertension. As pulmonary resistance increases, the left-to-right shunt that was initially present reverses. This new right-to-left shunt causes late cyanosis, that is, clubbing and polycythemia.

AORTIC STENOSIS

Aortic stenosis (AS) may lead to hindrance of flow to the left ventricular outflow tract due to the decreased aperture in the subvalvular, valvular, or supravalvular region. In utero, left ventricular damage, that is, hypertrophy and ischemia, results in left atrial hypertension. This results in decreased right–to–left flow across the foramen ovale. Cardiac output is maintained, yet the LV incurs progressive structural damage as the intercavitary pressure obstructs coronary outflow, eventually resulting in left ventricular infarction and subendocardial fibroelastosis. At birth, the presentation of the neonate is dependent on both the degree of LV dysfunction as well as how complete the transition from parallel to in–series circulation (with the closure of the ductus arteriosus and foramen ovale) is. In severe cases of AS leading to LV dysfunction, the LV outflow is compromised, thus resulting in circulatory collapse. If the ductus has closed, neonatal presentation may include dyspnea, tachycardia, narrowed pulse pressure, oliguria, and profound metabolic acidosis. However, if the ductus is still patent, systemic profusion will be moderately maintained by the right ventricle. Hemodynamic monitoring is recommended during both labor and delivery. Pregnant patients with AS are considered at high risk for morbidity and mortality.

MARFAN SYNDROME

Marfan syndrome is a hereditary autosomal dominant disorder that is the result of a mutation in the gene fibrillin-1 (FBN1) on chromosome 15q21.1. Irreversible changes in the body's elastic tissue then occur, particularly in the connective tissue of the eyes, skin, and cardiovascular (i.e., aorta) and skeletal systems. Affected individuals are often tall and slender, possessing arachnodactyly and hyperextensible joints. Approximately half of affected individuals will also have some form of visual disturbance, that is, ectopia lentis, myopia, glaucoma, or cataracts. Pregnant patients with Marfan syndrome with a normal aortic root are considered to be at an intermediate risk for morbidity and mortality; however, those with an abnormal aortic root are at high risk.

TETRALOGY OF FALLOT

Tetralogy of Fallot (TOF) is a congenital defect of the neonatal heart. Classified as a cyanotic cardiovascular disorder, the classic form involves four primary defects: ventricular septal defect, pulmonary stenosis, overriding aorta, and right ventricular hypertrophy. At birth, neonates may not exhibit signs of cyanosis. However, "tet spells" may occur in which the child exhibits a frightening bluish hue to the skin following crying and/or feeding. TOF is rare, occurring in approximately 5 out of 10,000 infants.

COARCTATION OF THE AORTA

Coarctation of the aorta (COA) is a constricted aortic segment composed of medial thickening as well as some medial infolding with neointimal superimposition. The localized constriction may form a shelflike structure with an eccentric opening or may resemble a curtain-like, membranous structure with either a concentric or an eccentric appearance. Coarctations may comprise a discrete region of the vessel (most common) or a long segment of the aorta. Classically, aortic coarctations are located in the thoracic region of the aorta, distal to the origin of the left subclavian artery. As a result, dilatation immediately distal to the constriction is usually present, known as poststenotic dilatation.

Due to the significant afterload placed on the LV by aortic coarctation, increased wall stress and compensatory LV hypertrophy ensue. As the ductus arteriosus constricts, LV afterload increases. Subsequently, both LV systolic and diastolic pressures increase, resulting in heightened LA pressure, which may be the stimulus for the foramen ovale's reopening. A left-to-right shunt then presents resulting in increased RA and RV pressures. In the event that the foramen ovale does not reopen, pulmonary artery and venous pressures increase, which still results in right heart dilatation. Patients with this disorder are considered at intermediate risk.

PULMONARY STENOSIS

There are three specific sites where this pathology may occur: subvalvular, valvular, and supravalvular. In subvalvular pulmonary stenosis, fibromuscular narrowing restricted to the right ventricle's outflow tract is quite rare and may be a part of the illness associated with a double-chambered right ventricle. Varying degrees of tract narrowing are commonly seen in association with right ventricular hypertrophy. In valvular presentation, the basic trileaflet anatomy is present yet with varying degrees of fibrosis and commissural fusion. In this orientation, the leaflets possess a limited range of movement during systole, producing a "fish mouth" appearance at the orifice. As a result of its long-standing presence, pulmonic stenosis can lead to dilatation of the pulmonic artery, right ventricular hypertrophy, and eventual right ventricular dilatation. Calcified and bicuspid valves are also possible etiologies of valvular pulmonic stenosis, yet both are rare. Supravalvular pulmonary stenosis is a rare de novo occurrence. Right ventricular pressure overload is seen at catheterization (of adults). Pulmonary arterial stenosis often occurs in association with other congenital cardiac and noncardiac defects, that is, TOF, Noonan syndrome, Williams syndrome, etc.

TAKE HOME POINTS

- Individuals undergoing ASD closure younger than the age of ten have better right ventricular function prognosis.
- Pregnancy is contraindicated in patients with Eisenmenger syndrome.
- A large PDA in pregnancy (especially with cardiac and/or pulmonary hypertension) increases both maternal and fetal morbidity and mortality.
- Physical findings of VSD may include cyanosis, clubbing, and polycythemia.
- Pregnant patients with AS are considered at high risk for morbidity and mortality and should be monitored during labor and delivery.
- Marfan syndrome is an autosomal dominant disorder with a mutation of fibrillin-1 gene on chromosome 15q21.1 resulting in irreversible changes in the body's elastic tissue properties. Those with an abnormal aortic root are at high risk and should be monitored during labor and delivery.
- Long-standing pulmonic stenosis can lead to right ventricular hypertrophy and dilatation.

SUGGESTED READINGS

Balentine J, Eisenhart A. www.emedicine.medscape.com

Bhushan V, Le TT, Ozturk A, et al. *First Aid for the USMLE Step 1*. McGraw-Hill Medical Publishing; 2007:242.

Brunicardi FC, Andersen D, Billiar T, et al. *Schwartz's Manual of Surgery*. 8th ed. McGraw-Hill Companies, Inc.; 2006.

Daliento L, Somerville J, Presbitero P, et al. Eisenmenger syndrome. Factors relating to deterioration and death. *Eur Heart J*. 1998;19:1845–1855.

Gleicher N, Midwall J, Hochberger D, et al. Eisenmenger's syndrome and pregnancy. *Obstet Gynecol Surg*. 1979;34:721–741.

Keane MG, Sutton St. John MG. *Clinical Manifestations of Pulmonary Stenosis*. www.uptodateonline.com

Maroo A, Russell R. *Pregnancy and Heart Disease, Cleveland Clinic*. http://www.clevelandclinicmeded.com

Mullins D. *501 Human Diseases*. 1st ed. Clifton Park, NY: Thomson Delmar Learning Publishing; 2006.

Rao PS, Seib P. www.emedicine.medscape.com/article/895502; www.nlm.nih.gov/medlineplus/marfansyndrome.html; www.nlm.nih.gov/medlineplus/ency/encyclopedia_T-Tn.htm

10

HEMATOLOGIC DISORDERS OF PREGNANCY: IS THE CARDIAC EXAM NORMAL?

NURU ROBI, MD AND DIANA BROOMFIELD, MD, MBA, FACOG, FACS

A 25-year-old G1P0 female at 28 weeks of gestation presented to a clinic complaining of shortness of breath on exertion. On physical examination, her pulse rate was 101 beats per minute, a systolic ejection murmur was heard at the aortic region, a third heart sound was appreciated, and the lungs were clear.

Pregnancy induces physiological changes that often confuse the diagnosis of hematological disorders and assessment of their treatment. This is especially true for anemia. Plasma volume increases by 10% to 15% at 6 to 12 weeks of gestation and expands rapidly until 30 to 34 weeks, after which time there is only a modest rise. The total gain at term averages 1,100 to 1,600 mL and results in a total plasma volume of 4,700 to 5,200 mL, which is 30% to 50% above that found in nonpregnant women.

Red blood cell mass begins to increase at 8 to 10 weeks of gestation and steadily rises by 20% to 30% (250 to 450 mL) above nonpregnant levels by the end of pregnancy in women taking iron supplements. Among women not on iron supplements, the red cell mass may only increase by 15% to 20%. A greater expansion of plasma volume relative to the increase in hemoglobin mass and erythrocyte volume is responsible for the modest fall in hemoglobin levels (i.e., physiological or dilutional anemia of pregnancy) observed in healthy pregnant women. The greatest disproportion between the rates at which plasma and erythrocytes are added to the maternal circulation occurs during the late second trimester to early third trimester (lowest hematocrit is typically measured at 28 to 36 weeks [up-to-date]). Anemia is defined as hemoglobin levels of <11 g/dL (hematocrit <33%) in the first and third trimesters and <10.5 g/dL (hematocrit <32%) in the second trimester. Women with hemoglobin values below these levels can be considered anemic and should undergo a standard evaluation. Sixteen to twenty-nine percent of pregnant women become anemic in the third trimester.

In a typical singleton gestation, maternal iron requirements average close to 1,000 mg over the course of pregnancy: approximately 300 mg for the fetus and placenta and approximately 500 mg, if available, for the expansion of the maternal hemoglobin mass. Two hundred milligrams is shed through the gut, urine, and skin. Since most women do not have adequate iron stores to handle the demands of pregnancy, iron is commonly prescribed as part of a prenatal multivitamin or as a separate supplement.

The two most common causes of anemia in pregnancy and puerperium are iron deficiency and acute blood loss. The currently recommended daily elemental iron supplementation is 30 mg for prophylaxis. If anemia is present, this dose should be increased to 60 to 120 mg of daily supplemental iron.

The lower limit of normal platelet counts in pregnancy has been reported to be 106,000 to 120,000 platelets/μL. The most significant obstetrical consideration concerning platelet physiology in pregnancy is thrombocytopenia, which may be related to complications of pregnancy (e.g., severe preeclampsia, HELLP syndrome), medical disorders (e.g., idiopathic thrombocytopenic purpura, thrombotic thrombocytopenic purpura, hemolytic uremic syndrome), or gestational or incidental events. Thrombocytopenia is characterized by mild asymptomatic thrombocytopenia occurring in the third trimester in a patient without any history of thrombocytopenia (other than in a prior pregnancy). It is not associated with maternal, fetal, or neonatal sequelae and spontaneously resolves postpartum. Platelet counts are typically >70,000/μL.

Pregnancy is associated with leukocytosis, primarily related to increased circulation of neutrophils. The neutrophil count begins to increase in the 2nd month of pregnancy and plateaus in the second or third trimester, at which time the total white blood cell count ranges from 9,000 to 15,000 cells/μL. The white blood cell count falls to the normal nonpregnant range by the 6th day postpartum. Dohle bodies (blue–staining cytoplasmic inclusions in granulocytes) are a normal finding in pregnant women. In healthy women with normal pregnancies, there is no change in the absolute lymphocyte count and no significant changes in the relative numbers of T and B lymphocytes. The monocyte count is generally stable, the basophil count may slightly decrease, and the eosinophil count may slightly increase. Normal pregnant women can have a small number of myelocytes or metamyelocytes in the peripheral circulation.

Normal pregnancy is a prothrombotic state. The circulating levels of several coagulation factors change during pregnancy. Protein S activity and free protein S antigen decrease due to estrogen–induced increases in the complement 4b–binding protein and possibly due to other mechanisms related to the hormonal changes of pregnancy. Resistance to activated protein C increases in the second and third trimesters. Fibrinogen and factors II, VII, VIII, and X increase by 20% to 200%. There is also an increase in von Willebrand factor and the activity of the fibrinolytic inhibitors, thrombin-activatable fibrinolytic inhibitor (TAFI), plasminogen activator inhibitor-1 (PAI-1), and plasminogen activator inhibitor-2 (PAI-2). Factors V and IX remain unchanged, and factor XI levels decrease by 30%. The net effect of these changes is to increase the tendency toward thrombus formation, extension, and stability. Normalization of coagulation parameters varies depending on the factor, but all should return to baseline by 8 weeks postpartum.

TAKE HOME POINTS

- The total gain in plasma volume at term averages 1,100 to 1,600 mL, which results in a total plasma volume of 4,700 to 5,200 mL; this represents 30% to 50% above that found in nonpregnant women.
- A greater expansion of plasma volume relative to the increase in hemoglobin mass and erythrocyte volume is responsible for the modest fall in hemoglobin levels during pregnancy.
- Sixteen to twenty-nine percent of pregnant women become anemic by the third trimester.
- In a typical singleton gestation, maternal iron requirements average close to 1,000 mg over the course of pregnancy (300 mg for the fetus and placenta and 500 mg, if available, for the expansion of the maternal hemoglobin mass; 200 mg is shed through the gut, urine, and skin).
- The two most common causes of anemia in pregnancy and puerperium are iron deficiency and acute blood loss.
- Pregnancy results in physiologic changes that may mimic certain hematologic disorders; thus, before attributing the condition to physiological alterations, possible disorders should be excluded.

SUGGESTED READINGS

American College of Obstetricians and Gynecologists. ACOG Practice Bulletin No. 95: Anemia in pregnancy. *Obstet Gynecol.* 2008;112:201.

Bernstein IM, Ziegler W, Badger GJ. Plasma volume expansion in early pregnancy. *Obstet Gynecol.* 2001;97:669.

CDC criteria for anemia in children and childbearing-aged women. *Morb Mortal Wkly Rep.* 1989;38:400.

Cunningham FG, Leveno KL, Bloom SL, et al., eds. *Williams Obstetrics.* 22nd ed. New York, NY: McGraw-Hill; Chapter 51, Hematological disorders.

Institute of Medicine. *Iron Deficiency Anemia: Recommended Guidelines for the Prevention, Detection, and Management Among US Children and Women of Childbearing Age.* Washington, DC: Institute of Medicine; 1993.

Lund CJ, Donovan JC. Blood volume during pregnancy. Significance of plasma and red cell volumes. *Am J Obstet Gynecol.* 1967;98:394.

Thame M, Lewis J, Trotman H, et al. The mechanism of low birth weight in infants of mothers with homozygous sickle cell disease. *Pediatrics.* 2007;120:e686.

Vichinsky EP. *Pregnancy in Sickle Cell Disease.* UpToDate.

Villers MS, Jamison MG, De Castro LM, et al. Morbidity associated with sickle cell disease in pregnancy. *Am J Obstetr Gynecol.* 2008;199:125.

Whittaker PG, Lind T. The intravascular mass of albumin during human pregnancy: a serial study in normal and diabetic women. *Br J Obstet Gynecol.* 1993;100:587.

11

HEMATOLOGIC DISORDERS OF PREGNANCY: IS THE PAIN FROM SICKLE CELL DISEASE?

NURU ROBI, MD AND DIANA BROOMFIELD, MD, MBA, FACOG, FACS

A 26-year-old G2P1001 woman at 8 weeks of gestation presents with severe abdominal and back pain. She had similar complaints in her previous pregnancy, which necessitated repeated hospital admission and treatment including multiple transfusions. On physical exam, the patient appears dehydrated, her BP is 98/60 mm Hg, her pulse is 108 beats per minute, and her temperature is 98.7°F. On abdominal examination, she has mild bilateral lower abdominal tenderness without rebound tenderness. Extremities are tender on palpation.

In this situation, one must consider early complications, such as ectopic pregnancy and abortion, appendicitis, acute pyelonephritis, and sickle cell crisis. After a complete workup, the patient in this example was found to have a vasoocclusive crisis due to underlying sickle cell disease (SCD). An important consideration in patients with known SCD is that the symptomatic woman may categorically be considered to be suffering from a sickle cell crisis. As a result, serious obstetrical or medical problems that cause pain, anemia, or both may be overlooked. Some examples are ectopic pregnancy, placental abruption, pyelonephritis, or appendicitis. The term "sickle cell crisis" should be applied only after all other possible causes of pain or fever or worsening anemia have been excluded.

During pregnancy, patients with SCD have an increased risk for antenatal hospitalization, hypertensive disorders, intrauterine growth restriction (IUGR), and cesarean. Despite the improvement in survival of both the mother and the fetus in the face of newer SCD therapies, remember that patients with sickle hemoglobinopathies remain at risk for renal insufficiency, cerebrovascular accident, cardiac dysfunction, leg ulcers, and sepsis, particularly from encapsulated organisms. Fetal complications are related to compromised placental blood flow and include spontaneous abortion, IUGR, increased rate of fetal death in utero, low birth weight, and preterm delivery.

Iron and folate supplements are necessary to avoid pregnancy complications. Iron stores are often markedly increased in these women due to chronic hemolysis and/or repeated blood transfusions. Accordingly, iron supplementation should not be given routinely and should only be given when iron studies (e.g., serum iron, transferrin, and ferritin levels) indicate the presence of low iron stores. All women should receive folate supplementation at a dose higher than that present in prenatal vitamin preparations (i.e., 4 mg per day PO). Although the routine use of prophylactic blood transfusions to reduce complications of pregnancy in patients with SCD has been recommended, this approach is controversial. A randomized, controlled trial in 72 patients found no significant difference in perinatal outcome between the offspring of mothers with SCD treated with prophylactic transfusions and those who were not. However, prophylactic transfusion significantly reduced the incidence of painful crises. This advantage must be weighed against the associated increases in cost, number of hospitalizations, and risk of alloimmunization. For these reasons, some recommend that transfusion therapy be reserved for patients with previous perinatal mortality, preeclampsia, acute chest syndrome, new-onset neurologic event, or severe anemia or those in preparation for surgical intervention.

Maternal crises are usually treated as in nonpregnant women. During the first trimester, prevention of dehydration and control of nausea may help to decrease the incidence of painful crises. Late in pregnancy, waiting for the spontaneous onset of labor at term is appropriate; induction and cesarean section should be performed only for the usual obstetrical indications. During labor and delivery, the woman should be well oxygenated and hydrated to prevent sickling, and the fetus should be monitored continuously. Analgesics or regional anesthesia is useful to reduce maternal cardiac demands secondary to pain and anxiety.

TAKE HOME POINTS

- Examine the patient with abdominal pain for obstetric, gynecologic, and nongynecologic causes.
- The term "sickle cell crisis" should be applied only after all other possible causes of pain or fever or worsening anemia have been excluded.
- Maternal crises are usually treated as in nonpregnant women.
- All women should receive folate supplementation at a dose higher than that present in prenatal vitamin preparations (i.e., 4 mg per day PO).

SUGGESTED READINGS

American College of Obstetricians and Gynecologists. ACOG Practice Bulletin No. 95: anemia in pregnancy. *Obstet Gynecol*. 2008;112:201.

Bernstein IM, Ziegler W, Badger GJ. Plasma volume expansion in early pregnancy. *Obstet Gynecol*. 2001;97:669.

CDC criteria for anemia in children and childbearing-aged women. *Morb Mortal Wkly Rep*. 1989;38:400.

Chakravarty EF, Khanna D, Chung L. Pregnancy outcomes in systemic sclerosis, primary pulmonary hypertension, and sickle cell disease. *Obstet Gynecol.* 2008;111(4):927–934.

Cunningham FG, Leveno KL, Bloom S, et al., eds. Hematological disorders. In: *Williams Obstetrics.* 22nd ed. 2005:1307–1338.

Institute of Medicine. Iron deficiency anemia: recommended guidelines for the prevention, detection, and management among US children and women of childbearing age. Washington, DC: Institute of Medicine; 1993.

Lund CJ, Donovan JC. Blood volume during pregnancy. Significance of plasma and red cell volumes. *Am J Obstet Gynecol.* 1967;98:394.

Thame M, Lewis J, Trotman H, et al. the mechanism of low birth weighting infants of mothers with homozygous sickle cell disease. *Pediatrics.* 2007;120:e686.

Vichinsky EP. Pregnancy in sickle cell disease. UpToDate.

Villers MS, Jamison MG, De Castro LM, et al. Morbidity associated with sickle cell disease in pregnancy. *Am J Obstet Gynecol.* 2008;199:125.

Whittaker PG, Lind T. The intravascular mass of albumin during human pregnancy: a serial study in normal and diabetic women. *Br J Obstet Gynecol.* 1993;100:587.

12

ABDOMINAL PAIN CAN BE
A NECROTIC FIBROID

ALEXANDRA BUFORD, DO AND DIANA BROOMFIELD, MD

A 36-year-old, G2P001, African American woman complains of lower abdominal pain for 1 day. She has a gestational age of 14 weeks and 5 days. Her pain is eight out of ten, nonradiating, and without aggravating or alleviating factors and began suddenly while she was resting. There is no associated vaginal bleeding and she states that she still feels the baby moving. She has never felt this pain before and she did not take anything for relief.

On physical exam, the left inferior periumbilical area is tender to palpation. The fetal heart tones are within normal limits. The patient is advised that it may be discomfort from uterine growth and is prescribed Tylenol and bed rest. She returns the next day with slightly worse pain, fever, and vaginal spotting.

Myomas are the most common benign tumors of the pelvis and occur in 30% to 50% of women over the age of 30. They are derived from smooth muscle cells and contain extracellular collagen and elastin. On the outside is a pseudocapsule of connective tissue. They are located in the submucosa, subserous, or intramural compartments of the uterus.

Two out of three females with myomas are asymptomatic. Menorrhagia is the most common complaint from symptomatic women. This intense heavy bleeding can lead to anemia. Increased pain with the menstrual cycle or dyspareunia is noted as well. Depending on the location of the myoma, women can experience urinary symptoms and less commonly constipation. In pregnant women, myomas can be associated with premature labor and delivery, fetal malpresentation, and early pregnancy bleeding.

Myomas can grow over time with an adequate blood supply. If this blood supply is outgrown, subserosal myomas can attach to other organs in search of a new blood source. These benign tumors can also necrose after outgrowing their blood supply. The least problematic type of necrosis is hyaline necrosis, while red, or carneous, infarction is the most acute form of degeneration. Acute muscular infarction causes severe pain and localized peritoneal irritation. This spontaneous degeneration is seen in 5% to 10% of gravid women with fibroids.

Abdominal ultrasound is used to gain further information about uterine myomas. While examining the myometrium, a lack of homogeneity and a focal mass will be seen. Transvaginal ultrasound improves the imaging of the uterus unless the fibroids have markedly enlarged the uterus. After a solid myoma has started to necrose, one will see mixed echodense and echolucent areas during ultrasound examination. In most cases, magnetic resonance imaging (MRI) provides improved imaging information regarding the size, number, and exact location of the myomas.

There are many different treatment options for a woman with myomas. Surgical options include myomectomy and hysterectomy. Forty percent of the hysterectomies in the United States are due to fibroids. Myomectomy can be performed if the patient wishes to maintain fertility. Pregnant women are not surgical candidates, and it is preferable to prescribe bed rest or be admitted to the hospital for observation of pain, bleeding, or threatened abortion.

Necrotic myomas are more frequently seen since the development of uterine artery embolization. Pain is common for the first 24 hours after the procedure but can last up to 2 weeks. The necrotic tissue, more commonly observed with submucosal myomas, sheds into the uterine cavity. As the uterus attempts to expel the material, one can have infection, fever, and abdominal pain.

TAKE HOME POINTS

- Necrotic fibroids occur in 5% to 10% of pregnant women.
- Red infarction is the most severe form of degeneration.
- Fibroids can cause fetal malpresentation.
- On ultrasound, necrotic fibroids will have mixed echodense and echolucency.
- Pregnant women with necrotic fibroids may need to be admitted for threatened abortion or preterm labor.

SUGGESTED READINGS

Arici A, Seli E, eds. *Non-Invasive Management of Gynecological Disorders*. UK: Informa; 2008:114–119.

Katz V, Lentz G, Lobo R, et al., eds. *Comprehensive Gynecology*. 5th ed. St. Louis, MO, Mosby: 2007.

Sheikh, HH. Uterine leiomyoma as rare cause of acute abdomen. *Am J Obstet Gynecol.* 1998:3:830–831.

Sokol A, Sokol E, eds. *General Gynecology*. St. Louis, MO, Mosby: 2007.

13

IS IT THE APPENDIX? PREGNANT WOMEN STILL HAVE ONE!

ALEXANDRA BUFORD, DO AND DIANA BROOMFIELD, MD

A 20-year-old primigravid female at 26 weeks of gestation presents with a 1-day history of right lower abdominal pain. She states she has never had this pain before. The pain is sharp, radiates to her inner right thigh, and is aggravated by movement. The patient states that she has nausea but has not vomited. She also denies constipation, diarrhea, fever, or chills. Her appetite has diminished since the pain began. There is a history of Chlamydia a few months ago at which time she had two different sexual partners. Currently, she is monogamous and is only taking iron pills. On physical exam, there are bowel sounds in all four quadrants and fetal heart tones are within normal limits. On pelvic exam, the cervix is noted to be mildly tender and there is right lower quadrant (RLQ) pain on rectal exam. The patient is suspected to have pelvic inflammatory disease and is started on antibiotics and observed.

The next day you notice that the patient looks sicker than yesterday, but the patient states she feels better. Her vital signs reveal tachycardia, fever of 102°F, and increased respiratory rate. Also noted on labs is an increase in white blood cells. An ultrasound is ordered, and the patient is noted to have a perforated appendix.

Abdominal pain can be a symptom of many different inflammatory or disease processes. One must be sure to have the patient try to characterize the pain, determine the exact location, and state if the pain radiates to another location. Visceral pain is the result when a hollow organ gets obstructed. This obstruction then causes the smooth muscle to stretch and cause pain. This is commonly seen in early appendicitis, early pelvic inflammatory disease, and bowel obstruction. The somatic pain fibers found in the skin, parietal peritoneum, and abdominal wall can cause the patient to have well-localized, sharp, constant pain. Somatic pain is found in appendicitis and as pelvic inflammatory disease progresses.

RLQ pain in a female can be a sign of abdominal, pelvic, or genitourinary pathology. A practitioner must use the most important aspect of the patient encounter, the history and physical exam, to narrow down the differential diagnoses. In early ovarian torsion and pelvic inflammatory disease, it is unlikely to elicit rebound tenderness. However, on rectal exam, you can find RLQ pain to be reproduced if the patient is suffering from appendicitis, pelvic inflammatory disease, or ectopic pregnancy. Also, referred pain to the inner thigh (innervated by T11-12 and L1) can indicate pelvic inflammatory disease or appendicitis.

Appendicitis has a 7% lifetime occurrence and is common between ages 10 and 30 years. Fifty percent of patients have a history of pain that begins in the periumbilical area but later migrates to the RLQ. The patient may also give a history of not eating, fever or chills, and nausea and vomiting. The different physical exam findings that may be elicited are psoas sign, obturator sign, Rovsing sign, or Dunphy sign. A delay in the diagnosis can increase the risk of perforation and further complications.

Pelvic inflammatory disease can mimic appendicitis as can ovarian torsion or ectopic pregnancy. Female patients with the complaint of lower abdominal pain should get a β-hCG and a pelvic exam done as well. On pelvic exam, the presence of cervicitis and chandelier sign should be noted. This could help determine if the patient is suffering from appendicitis or a gynecologic disorder. If pelvic inflammatory disease is suspected, antibiotic treatment should be started to avoid future infertility.

Ordering studies may help guide you toward a final diagnosis. Laboratory studies are not always helpful. An elevated white blood cell count could indicate appendicitis, pelvic inflammatory disease, or a urinary tract infection. A urinary analysis can help rule in or out any urinary tract infections. Diagnostic studies can aid in confirming the diagnosis of appendicitis when the history and physical exam do not provide a definite answer. Ultrasound and CT are the two most common modalities used. Ultrasound is safer in pregnant patients, but CT provides more anatomical information.

TAKE HOME POINTS

- A good history and physical exam can shorten a list of differential diagnoses.
- All RLQ pain is not appendicitis.
- Prompt diagnosis of appendicitis decreases the risk of perforation.
- An elevated white blood cell count with RLQ pain is not always appendicitis.
- CT scan is preferred to ultrasound to confirm appendicitis.

SUGGESTED READINGS

Close R. In: Tintinalli J, ed. *Emergency Medicine: A Comprehensive Study Guide*. 6th ed. New York, NY, McGraw-Hill; 2004:653–655.

Curtin KR, Fitzgerald SW, Hoff FL, et al. CT diagnosis of acute appendicitis: imaging findings. *Am J Roentgenol*. 1995:164:905–909.

Hardin DM. Acute appendicitis: review and update. *Am Fam Physician*. 1999;60(7):2027–34.

14

WHEN VAGINAL DISCHARGE IS A SEXUALLY TRANSMITTED DISEASE

ALEXANDRA BUFORD, DO AND DIANA BROOMFIELD, MD

A 25-year-old, G1P0, white female presents with a 1-week history of vaginal discharge. The patient is currently at the beginning of her second trimester. She denies any sexual activity in the past 2 weeks. The discharge, as described by the patient, has a slight fishy odor. She denies any itching or burning on urination and states she is unsure of the color of the discharge. She has a history of Chlamydia as a teenager, which was treated and cleared. After wet mount and examination under a microscope, she is sent home with instructions to return if the discharge gets worse. Two weeks later, she returned with her fiancé for her prenatal visit and wanted to discuss the discharge again.

Normal vaginal pH ranges from 3.8 to 4.5. This acidic environment is maintained by the lactic acid that is produced by lactobacilli normally found in the vagina. This discharge is comprised of water, normal bacterial flora, electrolytes, and cervical and vaginal epithelial cells. Some women have occasional physiologic vaginal discharge, while others have daily physiologic vaginal discharge. During pregnancy, the amount of normal vaginal discharge increases due to the increase in estrogen.

When the normal vaginal flora gets disturbed, the pH of the vagina changes. This can occur after sexual intercourse, douching, or after menses. The changes seen in the discharge can include color, odor, texture, or quantity. There can also be associated symptoms of itching or burning as well as pain during sexual intercourse.

Bacterial vaginosis (BV) is found in 800,000 pregnant women a year in the United States. It occurs when the vaginal pH becomes more basic or >5.0. It can occur after sexual intercourse or after menses. Patients normally have a thin, white discharge that may have a fishy odor. On wet mount, clue cells will be present on >20% of the vaginal epithelial cells. When potassium hydroxide is added to the discharge, an amine odor is present. In the pregnant patient, BV can place the patient at risk for preterm labor.

Vaginal discharge with a pH of 5.0 or greater can also indicate a sexually transmitted disease (STD). *Trichomonas*, a parasitic flagellated protozoan, is a highly contagious STD that affects both men and women. There are between 5 and 8 million cases a year and 50% of females are asymptomatic.

A patient with symptoms may complain of foul-smelling discharge. Ten to twenty-five percent of patients will have a frothy discharge. Pruritus and dysuria may also be noted by the patient. Edema and erythema of the vulva are noted on physical exam. *Trichomonas* is best viewed under the high-power setting of a microscope. There will be an increase in white cells and motile trichomonads on the wet mount slide. As with BV, *Trichomonas* increases a patient's risk of preterm labor.

Gonorrhea most commonly affects the endocervix and is caused by the microorganism *Neisseria gonorrhoeae*. In a nonpregnant patient, there will be vaginal discharge, dysuria, intermenstrual bleeding, pelvic discomfort, or menorrhagia. Pregnant patients may complain of an increase in vaginal discharge and dysuria. Interestingly, *N. gonorrhoeae* is cultured on Thayer-Martin medium, which inhibits the growth of most other microorganisms.

Chlamydia is known as a "silent" disease because about three quarters of infected women have no symptoms. When symptoms occur, they may be an abnormal vaginal discharge or a burning sensation when urinating. When the infection spreads from the cervix to the fallopian tubes, some women still have no signs or symptoms; others have lower abdominal pain, low back pain, nausea, fever, pain during intercourse, or bleeding between menstrual periods. Nucleic acid amplification tests (NAATs), such as polymerase chain reaction (PCR), transcription-mediated amplification (TMA), and the DNA strand displacement amplification (SDA), now are the mainstays for the diagnosis. NAAT for *Chlamydia* may be performed on swab specimens collected from the cervix or urethra, on self-collected vaginal swabs, or in voided urine.

Untreated chlamydial infections can lead to premature delivery. Infants born to infected mothers can get early infant pneumonia and newborn conjunctivitis.

Differentiating between normal vaginal discharge and STD is not always clear. Obtaining a detailed history and physical exam including the number of sexual partners is important. A pregnant patient complaining of an increase in vaginal discharge can have normal leucorrhea, BV, *Trichomonas*, or another STD. Early diagnosis and treatment, even if the patient is asymptomatic, may decrease the risk of preterm labor.

TAKE HOME POINTS

- Normal vaginal pH is 3.8 to 4.5.
- Small amounts of vaginal discharge are normal in most women.
- Vaginal discharge increases during pregnancy.
- Vaginal infections can increase the risk of preterm labor.

- In asymptomatic patients, it may be difficult to decide to sample the discharge.
- Foul-smelling discharge can indicate *Trichomonas*.

SUGGESTED READINGS

Corey J, Klebanoff M, Hauth J, et al. Metronidazole to prevent preterm delivery in pregnant women with asymptomatic bacterial vaginosis. *N Engl J Med*. 2000:342:534–540.

Fredricks D, Fiedler T, Marrazzo J. Molecular ID of bacteria associated with bacterial vaginosis. *N Engl J Med*. 2005:353:1899–1911.

Gibbs R, Sweet R, eds. *Infectious Diseases of the Female Genital Tract*. 4th ed. Philadelphia, PA: Lippincott Williams & Wilkins; 2002.

Norwitz E, Robinson J, Challis J. The control of labor. *N Engl J Med*. 1999:341:660–666.

15

CHRONIC HYPERTENSION AND SUPERIMPOSED PREECLAMPSIA

PATRICIA LEE SCOTT, MD AND B. DENISE RAYNOR, MD

The key to the diagnosis of preeclampsia is early establishment of prenatal care. The diagnosis of chronic hypertension is made at 12 weeks of gestation when her blood pressure (BP) is >140/90. Baseline laboratory tests including complete blood count (CBC) with platelets, serum chemistries, and 24-hour urine protein and creatinine clearance should be performed at that time to determine if there is any hypertensive renal disease. Additionally, an ECG should be obtained, and if abnormal or if symptoms indicate, a cardiac echocardiogram may be indicated.

As the pregnancy progresses, the provider can use the baseline labs and blood pressures for comparison. Patients who begin pregnancy already on antihypertensive medications for chronic hypertension may need to discontinue them during the physiologic decrease in BP in second trimester, since hypotension may impair uterine blood flow. However, medications may need to be restarted with the normal third trimester rise in BP. If BP remains well controlled (≤140/90) on an antihypertensive regimen, and the patient remains without symptoms or fetal compromise or inappropriate fetal growth, the pregnancy may continue with fetal reassurance until term.

The diagnosis of superimposed preeclampsia should be considered under the following circumstances: (1) if the patient develops symptoms of preeclampsia, such as visual disturbance (double vision, spots in front of the eyes) or persistent headache, which reflects CNS disturbance, or epigastric pain, which reflects liver dysfunction, (2) blood pressures escalate and cannot be controlled with relatively minor adjustments in her antihypertensive regimen (especially if antihypertensive IV medications are necessary), and/or (3) worsening proteinuria or renal function is compromised.

Diagnosis of preeclampsia in this setting can be challenging, since it is based on worsening blood pressure and/or proteinuria, not the strict criteria used in the absence of chronic hypertension. As the diagnosis of superimposed preeclampsia on chronic hypertension carries more risk than either of the diagnoses alone, the patient should be hospitalized and prepared for delivery. Seizure prophylaxis with magnesium sulfate should be initiated, with appropriate adjustments made to account for any renal insufficiency. Prior to 35 weeks of gestation, antenatal corticosteroids should be given prior to delivery, either dexamethasone or betamethasone over a 48-hour period. If severe preeclampsia occurs at an extremely early gestational age (24 to 28 weeks), expectant management for a limited period of time is acceptable to allow for further fetal and maternal evaluation. Expectant management requires observation in an acute care unit with adequate monitoring to detect acute changes since both the mother and the fetus can deteriorate rapidly. Ideally, management should include consultation with perinatologists.

TAKE HOME POINTS

- Obtain baseline laboratory studies (CBC, platelets, urinalysis (UA), 24-hour urine protein collection, serum chemistries), ECG, and other appropriate evaluations such as ophthalmologic and renal evaluations when indicated.
- Initiate interval fetal growth assessments after 24 weeks of gestation.
- All pregnancies complicated by hypertensive disorders should be monitored with antepartum fetal surveillance at the appropriate gestational age.
- Closely monitor BP and renal function during the pregnancy.

SUGGESTED READINGS

Dunlop JC. Chronic hypertension and perinatal mortality. *Proc R Soc Med.* 1966;59:838.
Sibai BM, Abdella TN, Anderson GD. Pregnancy outcome in 211 patients with mild chronic hypertension. *Obstet Gyecol.* 1983;61:571.
Sibai BM, Anderson GD. Intensive management of severe hypertension in the first trimester. *Obstet Gynecol.* 1986;67:517.

16

DIAGNOSIS OF PREECLAMPSIA PRIOR TO 34 WEEKS OF GESTATION

PATRICIA LEE SCOTT, MD AND B. DENISE RAYNOR, MD

A 37-year-old G1 female at 27 weeks of gestation presents for her routine prenatal visit and is found to have blood pressure (BP) of 152/98. Upon repeat, BP is still elevated, at times >160/110. She reports an occasional headache that resolves with rest. Her husband has noticed that her face appears swollen. Prior to this point, her BPs have been normal. How is this situation managed?

Once the diagnosis of preeclampsia is made and the gestation is <34 weeks, it is important to balance the risks of prematurity against the risks of maternal and fetal morbidity and mortality. Hospitalization in labor and delivery and prompt evaluation of both the mother and the fetus are necessary. Preterm preeclampsia is more likely to be severe. Patients diagnosed with severe disease prior to 24 weeks should be offered immediate delivery, since the likelihood of fetal survival is close to zero and maternal morbidity is very high. Between 24 and 33 weeks, expectant management can be attempted. After 33 weeks, antenatal steroids should be administered prior to delivery in 48 hours. Criteria for severe disease include systolic blood pressure (SBP) ≥160 or diastolic blood pressure (DBP) ≥110, proteinuria of ≥3+ on random dipstick or 5,000 mg per 24 hours, oliguria, pulmonary edema, elevated aspartate aminotransferase (AST)/ alanine transaminase (ALT), or thrombocytopenia (platelet <100,000).

Consultation with the neonatology team is extremely important, as the patient will have many questions regarding the risks of prematurity. If the patient's BPs can be controlled with moderate doses of antihypertensive medications, then the pregnancy can be managed in an inpatient setting while continued maternal and fetal evaluation occurs to allow time for steroid administration for fetal benefit. Fetal assessment with antepartum testing and ultrasound of fetal growth and amniotic fluid level should be obtained. Additionally, umbilical artery Doppler may be useful. The testing regimen should include daily non–stress test (NST), weekly ultrasound for amniotic fluid index, and umbilical artery Doppler. Serial ultrasound for growth every 2 to 3 weeks should also be performed.

Patients with preeclampsia are at risk for placental abruption and fetal demise. The presence of growth restriction or oligohydramnios suggests fetal compromise, should prompt more intensive fetal surveillance, and may be an indication for delivery particularly when accompanied by abnormal fetal testing and/or absent or reverse umbilical artery diastolic flow. Maternal complications such as worsening BP control, renal compromise, development of HELLP syndrome, and cardiopulmonary compromise are associated with preeclampsia and should prompt consideration for delivery.

When delivery is indicated, mode of delivery may be an issue. Since preterm infants are more likely to have malpresentation, particularly with intrauterine growth restriction, and have low birth weight, cesarean may be indicated. Additionally, fetal intolerance of labor can often occur in the setting of preeclampsia due to possible uteroplacental insufficiency. Preterm labor inductions are more likely to be prolonged and subsequently fail to progress. Cesarean would again be indicated. Cesareans performed for early preterm infants are more likely via a classical (vertical) uterine incision, which have a higher risk of rupture in subsequent pregnancies and require repeat cesarean. Patients should be counseled concerning the risks of multiple repeat cesareans, which include injury to other abdominal organs and bladder, placenta previa, and placenta accreta.

HELLP syndrome is considered a variant of severe preeclampsia, which includes elevated AST or ALT (less than twice the upper limits of normal) and thrombocytopenia (platelet count <100,000/μL). Some clinicians include elevated indirect bilirubin, hemolysis detected on peripheral smear, or low serum haptoglobin. Women who develop HELLP syndrome should be delivered, regardless of gestational age, if possible after 48 hours for steroid administration. Expectant management of HELLP syndrome carries significant maternal and fetal morbidity, including pulmonary edema, renal failure, disseminated intravascular coagulation (DIC), subcapsular hematoma, and liver rupture.

TAKE HOME POINTS

- Preterm preeclampsia is more likely to be severe.
- Patients diagnosed with severe disease prior to 24 weeks should be offered immediate delivery, since the likelihood of fetal survival is close to zero and maternal morbidity is very high.
- Between 24 and 33 weeks, expectant management can be attempted.
- After 33 weeks, antenatal steroids should be administered prior to delivery in 48 hours.

SUGGESTED READINGS

Gonzalez-Ruiz AR, Sibai BM. Glucocorticoids for lung maturation in preeclampsia. *Contemp Obstet Gynecol.* 1987;29:147.

Martin TR, Tupper WRC. The management of severe toxemia in patients less than 36 weeks gestation. *Obstet Gynecol.* 1979;54:602.

Odendaal JH, Pattinson RC, Dutoit R. Fetal and neonatal outcome in patients with severe preeclampsia before 34 weeks. *S Afr Med J.* 1987;71:555.

Sibai BM. Definitive therapy for pregnancy induced hypertension. *Contemp Obstet Gynecol.* 1988;31:51.

17

PREMATURE RUPTURE OF MEMBRANE

EZEKIEL OSUNTOGUN, MD AND DIANA BROOMFIELD, MD, MBA, FACOG, FACS

A 16-year-old primigravida was brought to the Emergency Room with spontaneous rupture of membranes (SROM). Her LMP was unknown and she had no prenatal care. She was sent for transabdominal and transvaginal sonogram to estimate gestational age. She was then found to be at 27 weeks of estimated gestational age with oligohydramnios, and the diagnosis of preterm premature rupture of membranes (PPROM) was made.

Preterm delivery occurs in 11% of all births in the United States, and this constitutes a major factor in prenatal morbidity and mortality. Premature rupture of membranes complicates one fourth to one third of all preterm births. Management depends on risk of infection, cord accident, operative delivery, and gestational age. PROM refers to premature rupture of membrane before the onset of labor, while preterm rupture of membranes before 37 weeks of gestation is PPROM. A common error is not distinguishing between the two.

Among the etiological factors are weakening of the membranes secondary to physiologic changes combined with shearing forces created by uterine contractions, intrauterine infection, lower socioeconomic status, sexually transmitted disease (STD), prior preterm birth, vaginal bleeding, cervical conization, and cigarette smoking during pregnancy. Other factors include uterine distension (hydramnios, twins), emergency cervical cerclage, and preterm labor.

Term PROM complicates 8% of pregnancies and is usually followed by onset of labor and delivery. Ninety-five percent of patients deliver within 28 hours of rupture of membrane. The most significant maternal risk of term PROM is interuterine infection, and fetal risks include umbilical cord compression and ascending infection. Delivery within 1 week is the most likely outcome in PPROM, but the earlier in gestation, the greater the potential for pregnancy prolongation. Digital vaginal examination in earlier pregnancy increases the risk of infection; fetal malpresentation and placenta abruption are notable complications of PPROM.

The most significant risk to the fetus is prematurity, and the most common complication is respiratory distress. Other morbidities include necrotizing enterocolitis, intraventricular hemorrhage, and neonatal infection. Fetal demise in PPROM is usually caused by abruption, cord prolapse, or infection.

The diagnosis of PPROM is clinical and is generally based on a combination of characteristic history and visualization of amniotic fluid on physical examination. If the diagnosis is not obvious after direct visualization, the diagnosis can be confirmed by testing the pH of the vaginal fluid using the nitrazine paper. Amniotic fluid has a pH of 7.0 to 7.7 compared to the normal acidic pH of 3.8 to 4.2. False-negative and false-positive results occur in up to 5% of the cases. False-negative results can occur when leaking is intermittent or the amniotic fluid is diluted by other vaginal fluids. False-positive results can be due to the presence of alkaline fluids in the vagina, such as blood, seminal fluid, soap, or some infections.

A secondary confirmation test is the presence of arborization (ferning) as seen under the microscope. Amniotic fluid produces a delicate ferning pattern in contrast to the thick and wide arborization pattern of dried cervical mucus. Well-estrogenized cervical mucus or a finger print in the microscope slide may cause a false-positive fern test; false negative can be due to inadequate amniotic fluid on the swab or heavy contamination with vaginal discharge or blood. Fifty to seventy percent of women with PPROM have low amniotic fluid volume on initial sonography. A history suggestive of rupture of membranes and a finding of anhydramnios or severe oligohydramnios are further helpful. Instillation of indigo carmine into the amniotic cavity can be considered and usually leads to definitive diagnosis. AmniSure is a rapid slide test that uses immunochromatographic method to detect even trace of placenta α_1 protein in vaginal fluid.

MANAGEMENT

Expedition delivery in women with PPROM is indicated for interuterine infection, abruptio placentae, repetitive fetal heart rate deceleration, or cord prolapse (*Fig. 17.1*).

Where neonatal care is available, pregnancy >32 weeks of gestation with documented fetal lung maturity achieves better maternal and neonatal outcome with delivery than expected achievement.

ANTENATAL GLUCOCORTICOIDS

A course of glucocorticoids is given to pregnancies <32 weeks of gestation. This has been found to improve neonatal outcome in pregnancies completed by PPROM. Tocolytics are given to non-laboring, PPROM patients for

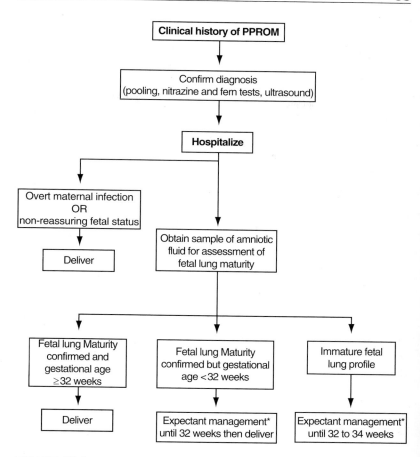

FIGURE 17.1

48 hours to allow the administration of antenatal corticosteroids. The goal of antibiotic therapy is to reduce the frequency of maternal and fetal infections and delay the onset of preterm labor. A single course of antibiotic is all that is necessary. Hospitalization for bed rest and pelvic rest is indicated after PPROM and maternal and fetal surveillance confirmed with non–stress test (NST) and biophysical profile. No evidence exists that any specific form of frequency of fetal surveillance directly improves perinatal outcome. Evidence of infection includes maternal fever, uterine tenderness, and maternal and fetal tachycardia. Leukocyte count alone is nonspecific especially following steroids administration. Amniocentesis to confirm infection usually reveals glucose <14 positive Gram stains, positive amniotic fluid culture, and positive interleukin-6 (IL-6) (*Table 17.1*).

TABLE 17.1	CORTICOSTEROID AND ANTIBIOTIC TREATMENT WITH PPROM IN THE ABSENCE OF LABOR

Week of gestation when PPROM occurs: 24–32 wk

Plan: Expectant management if no evidence of chorioamnionitis or fetal compromise

Corticosteroids[a]: Yes

Antibiotics: Yes,[b] and Group B Streptococcus (GBS) prophylaxis at delivery if indicated

Week of gestation when PPROM occurs: >32 but <34 wk

Plan: Deliver immediately if fetal lung maturity can be documented or there is evidence of an intraamniotic infection clinically or on amniocentesis; otherwise deliver at 34 wk

Corticosteroids[a]: Yes, if there is evidence of fetal lung immaturity or fetal lung status is unknown

Antibiotics: Yes, if expectant management[b] and GBS prophylaxis at delivery if indicated

Week of gestation when PPROM occurs: ≥34 wk

Plan: Deliver

Corticosteroids[a]: No

Antibiotics: GBS prophylaxis begun on admission and continued until delivery

[a]A single course of corticosteroids is given. If contractions begin and there are no contraindications to tocolytics, tocolytics can be given for 48 h during which time a course of corticosteroids is also administered.
[b]Broad-spectrum GBS prophylaxis is given at delivery if indicated because of positive or unknown GBS culture results.

TAKE HOME POINTS

- Antibiotics should be administered to patients with PPROM because they prolong the latent period and improve outcome.
- Corticosteroids should be given to patients with PPROM between 24 and 32 weeks of gestation to decrease the risk of intraventricular hemorrhage, respiratory distress syndrome, and necrotizing enterocolitis.
- Physicians should not perform digital cervical examinations on patients with PPROM because they decrease the latent period. Speculum examination is preferred.
- Long-term tocolytics are not indicated for patients with PPROM, although short-term tocolytics may be considered to facilitate maternal transport and the administration of corticosteroids and antibiotics.
- Multiple courses of corticosteroids and the use of corticosteroids after 34 weeks of gestation are not recommended.

SUGGESTED READINGS

American College of Obstetricians and Gynecologists. ACOG Committee Opinion No. 402: antenatal corticosteroid therapy for fetal maturation. *Obstet Gynecol.* 2008;111:805.

American College of Obstetricians and Gynecologists. Clinical Management Guidelines for Obstetrician-Gynecologists. ACOG Practice Bulletin No. 80: premature rupture of membranes. *Obstet Gynecol.* 2007;109:1007.

Cunningham FG, Leveno KL, Bloom SL. *Williams Obstetrics.* 22nd ed. New York, NY: McGraw-Hill; 2005.

Preterm premature rupture of membranes. UpToDate. www.uptodate.com

Preterm premature rupture of membranes. In *Prolog Obstetrics.* 6th ed. American College of Obstetrics and Gynecology, Washington, DC: pages 156–7.

U.S. Department of Health and Human Services, Public Health Service. Report on the Consensus Development Conference on the Effect of Corticosteroids for Fetal Maturation on Perinatal Outcomes. NIH Pub No. 95-3784, November 1994.

18

"HONEY, IT IS TIME!!!": WHEN PRETERM LABOR STRIKES

HOLLY SHEN, MD

How many times have we seen the classic scenario of the pregnant woman waking her husband in the middle of the night yelling "Honey, it is TIME!!," shortly followed by the husband running to get the car in a frantic daze? But, what happens when the run to the hospital happens before the suitcase is even packed and waiting by the front door? Preterm birth is the leading cause of neonatal mortality in the United States, with 40% to 50% of cases preceded by preterm labor. It accounts for 35% of all U.S. health care spending for infants and 10% for children. In 2006, March of Dimes reported the rate of preterm birth at 12.7% of all births, accounting for three quarters of neonatal mortality and one half of all long-term neurological impairments in children. Therefore, it is imperative to distinguish those patients suffering with preterm labor from those experiencing false labor or Braxton Hicks contractions in order to proceed accordingly. Further complicating matters, many patients present with late or no prenatal care, making the distinction of preterm or term difficult.

For instance, an 18-year-old primigravida presents to triage with complaints of lower abdominal pain and pressure for the past 8 hours. She rates her pain as 7/10, intermittent at every 5 minutes, with radiation to her back and pressure that increases with the pain. She denies vaginal bleeding, leakage of fluid, or vaginal discharge and says the baby is moving well. Fetal heart tones are overall reassuring. Upon questioning, she admits that she has only been to one prenatal visit at a clinic in another state and is unsure of what gestational age the visit took place. She reports irregular menses before the pregnancy and is unsure of her last menstrual period. The patient thinks that she is around 7 months pregnant.

This scenario should activate a cascade of "to do's" in the practitioner's mind. At this point, we become investigators trying to piece together the puzzle of what is currently going on in this patient's uterus. Is she really in labor or is she experiencing Braxton Hicks contractions? Is she really only 7 months pregnant? History is very helpful in identifying those patients who may be at an increased risk for preterm labor. Specific points to cover include history of prior preterm birth or preterm labor, history of induced abortion or other cervical procedures, and asymptomatic cervical dilation after midpregnancy in the absence of rupture of membranes, bleeding, or infection.

A bedside ultrasound can be performed to assess or confirm gestational age. If found to be <37 weeks of gestation, proceed with evaluation for preterm labor. The next step should be a sterile speculum exam to note visual dilation of the cervix. At this point, a fetal fibronectin test should be collected in cases of 34 weeks of gestational age or less. A positive assay at 22 to 34 weeks has a positive predictive value for delivery within 1 to 2 weeks of 30% and 41%, respectively. Conversely, a negative assay was associated with a negative predictive value of 98% and 96%, respectively. False-positive results can be obtained if the patient has had intercourse or a cervical exam in the past 24 hours, in the presence of vaginal bleeding and copious vaginal discharge, or if membranes are ruptured, so sample should be discarded or not collected in these instances. These circumstances account for the low positive predictive value. Because lower genital tract infection can be associated with preterm labor, cultures for gonorrhea and chlamydia and a wet prep should be collected, as well as swabs for Group B *Streptococcus* colonization. Urine specimens should be collected to dip and send for culture to rule out urinary tract infection.

Following the speculum exam, intravenous fluids should be started, as dehydration is common and can lead to uterine irritability. The patient should be placed on continuous fetal heart monitoring and tocometer. With rupture of membranes ruled out, a digital cervical exam can be performed to determine cervical dilation and effacement. The American College of Obstetricians and Gynecologists (ACOG; 1997) proposed the following criteria to document preterm labor:

1. Contractions of four in 20 minutes or eight in 60 minutes plus progressive cervical change
2. Cervical dilation of >1 cm
3. Cervical effacement of 80% or greater

After confirmation of labor, the following considerations should be made:

1. For pregnancies <34 weeks and no maternal or fetal indications for delivery, close observation with fetal heart tone monitoring and tocometer, along with serial cervical exams, is appropriate.
2. For pregnancies <34 weeks, administer glucocorticoids for fetal lung enhancement.
3. For pregnancies <34 weeks, consider tocolytics while glucocorticoids and group B streptococcal prophylaxis are given.
4. Pregnancies 34 weeks and beyond are monitored for labor progression and fetal well-being.

For active labor, group B *Streptococcus* prophylaxis is administered.

With respect to management of diagnosed preterm labor, the ACOG makes the following level A recommendations:

- Tocolytic drugs should be chosen based on clinical situation; there is no first-line choice.
- Antibiotic treatment does not prolong gestation and should be reserved for group B streptococcal prophylaxis in patients in whom delivery is imminent.
- Neither maintenance nor repeated use of tocolytic drugs improves perinatal outcome.
- Tocolytic drugs may prolong pregnancy for 2 to 7 days, which may allow for administration of steroids to improve fetal lung maturity or maternal transport to a tertiary care facility.
- Bed rest, hydration, and pelvic rest are not shown to improve outcome and should not be routinely recommended.
- In conclusion, strict adherence to the management recommendations for preterm labor may allow for early identification and diagnosis and can ultimately improve outcome. The before mentioned criteria give clear guidelines for practitioners to follow when the question of preterm labor arises. This allows time to administer glucocorticoids in those patients <34 weeks of gestation to decrease risk of fetal respiratory distress upon delivery, intraventricular hemorrhage, and necrotizing enterocolitis.

TAKE HOME POINTS

- Possible preterm labor needs immediate attention and evaluation!!
- Assess accuracy of dating.
- Get a good history (past preterm delivery, previous abortions, or other cervical procedures).
- Perform sterile speculum exam at once and ALWAYS collect a fetal fibronectin.
- DO NOT PERFORM DIGITAL CERVICAL EXAM IF A PATIENT HAS RUPTURED MEMBRANES.
- Perform digital cervical exam and monitor with tocometer; assess according to ACOG guidelines.
- If <34 weeks of gestation, ensure initiation of glucocorticoids ASAP and consider tocolytics.

SUGGESTED READINGS

American College of Obstetricians and Gynecologists. ACOG Practice Bulletin No. 31: assessment of risk factors for preterm birth. October 2001.

American College of Obstetricians and Gynecologists. ACOG Practice Bulletin No. 43: management of preterm labor. May 2003.

Cunningham FG, Leveno KJ, Bloom SL, et al., eds. Preterm birth. In: *Williams Obstetrics*. 22nd ed. New York, NY: McGraw-Hill; 2005:855–873.

19

PRETERM LABOR, IS IT TIME YET?

EZEKIEL OSUNTOGUN, MD AND DIANA BROOMFIELD, MD, MBA, FACOG, FACS

A 26-year-old G2P1001 female at 35 weeks of pregnancy by last menstrual period was seen at Labor and Delivery for preterm labor. The intern ordered group B Streptococcus (GBS) prophylaxis, tocolytics, and betamethasone. The patient asks the doctor to explain the risks and benefits for each of the medications ordered.

Preterm labor leading to preterm birth occurs in approximately 6% of pregnancies in the United States and accounts for 50% of cases of preterm births. Preterm labor is defined by the presence of uterine contractions—four or more in 20 minutes or eight or more in an hour—and documented cervical changes with intact membranes or advanced cervical dilatation between 20 and 36 and 6/7 weeks of gestation.

The neonatal morbidity and mortality associated with preterm birth occur in women who deliver before 34 weeks of gestation, especially before 32 weeks. At 34 weeks of gestation and beyond, the neonate has <1% risk of death and <1% risk of intraventricular hemorrhage or of necrotizing enterocolitis. Infants born preterm are more likely to develop visual and hearing impairment, chronic lung disease, cerebral palsy, and delayed development in childhood.

The risk in preterm births has been attributed to increased use of advanced reproductive technologies (ART) and increased willingness to choose delivery when medical or obstetric complications threaten the health of the mother or the fetus. Preterm births are either spontaneous or induced. Spontaneous preterm labor follows preterm rupture of membranes or related diagnoses such as incompetent cervix or amnionitis.

Indicated (or induced) preterm birth accounts for 15% of all preterm births following medical or obstetric conditions that create undue risk for the mother should the pregnancy be continued. Examples are poorly controlled chronic diseases with or without intrauterine growth restriction (IUGR), maternal hypertension, placenta previa, or placental abruption. The most common diagnoses that precede an indicated preterm birth are preeclampsia (40%), IUGR (10%), abruption (7%), and fetal demise (7%). Illicit drug use in pregnancy, especially cocaine ingestion, has been associated with both spontaneous and indicated preterm births.

RISK FACTORS FOR PRETERM BIRTH

A history of preterm birth confers twofold increase in the risk of early subsequent pregnancy. Infection not only includes that of the lower genital tract but also includes that of periodontal disease. Preterm birth occurs in black women nearly twice the rate observed in women from other ethnic groups. Other factors contributing to preterm birth are bleeding, uterine anomalies, multiple gestations, ART, and lifestyle–related risks.

DETECTION OF PRETERM BIRTH

Uterine contractions through maternal self-perception and electronic tocodynamometry have been studied to predict preterm delivery. Measurement of cervical length by transvaginal ultrasonography is currently being used with an increased risk of preterm labor in patients with a cervical length of <25 mm. Fetal fibronectin, a glycoprotein of fetal origin, is used to predict preterm birth. A positive test in asymptomatic women at 24 weeks of gestation has a sensitivity for spontaneous preterm birth before 34 weeks of 20% to 30%. The clinical usefulness is the negative predictive value.

INTERVENTIONS

Interventions have aimed at reducing the risk factors that cause preterm birth. These include

- Patient education
- Detection and pharmacologic suppression of uterine contractions
- Antimicrobial therapy of vaginal microorganisms
- Cerclage sutures to bolster the cervix
- Reduction of maternal stress
- Improvement of nutrition including hydration and access to perinatal care and reduced physical activity

All women before 24 to 34 weeks of gestation are candidates for corticosteroid therapy, and tocolytics may prolong gestation 2 to 7 days, allowing steroid therapy.

Contraindications to tocolytics include severe preeclampsia, placenta abruption, intrauterine infection, fetal congenital or chromosomal abnormalities, advanced cervical dilatation, evidence of fetal compromise, or placental insufficiency.

ADVERSE EFFECTS OF TOCOLYTICS

All tocolytics are associated with increased risk of pulmonary edema. Side effects of betamimetics are myocardial ischemia, hyperglycemia, hypokalemia, and fetal cardiac effects.

Magnesium sulfate causes maternal lethargy, drowsiness, double vision, and nausea and vomiting. Calcium channel blockers combined with magnesium sulfate can cause cardiovascular collapse, while NSAIDs cause oligohydramnios and premature closure of ductus arteriosus. Antibiotics do not appear to prolong gestation and should be reserved for GBS prophylaxis in patients in whom delivery is imminent.

Most recently, 17-α-hydroxyprogesterone has been approved by the FDA for the prevention of preterm labor. The usual dose is 250 mg IM starting between 16 and 20 weeks of gestation, especially in patients with a previous history of preterm labor.

TAKE HOME POINTS

Goals for management of patients in preterm labor are

- Early identification of risk factors associated with preterm labor
- Timely diagnosis of preterm labor
- Identifying the etiology of preterm labor
- Evaluating fetal well-being
- Providing prophylactic pharmacologic therapy to prolong gestation and reduce the incidence of respiratory distress syndrome and intraamniotic infection
- Initiating tocolytic therapy when indicated
- Establishing a plan of maternal and fetal surveillance with the patient and providing education to improve maternal and fetal outcomes

SUGGESTED READINGS

American College of Obstetricians and Gynecologists. ACOG Practice Bulletin No. 43. May 2003.

Cunningham FG, Leveno KL, Bloom SL, et al. Obstetrical complications: preterm birth. In: *Williams Obstetrics*. 22nd ed. New York, NY: McGraw-Hill; 2005.

Gabbe SG, Niebyl JR, Joe Leigh Simpson, et al. Preterm Labor. In Gabbe SG (ed.). *Obstetrics: Normal and Problem Pregnancies*. 5th ed., 2007, New York, NY, Elsevier.

Martin JA, Hamilton BE, Sutton PD, et al. Births: final data for 2004. *Natl Vital Stat Rep.* 2006;55(1):1-101.

20

POSTDATES PREGNANCY: WHAT IS IT AND WHAT TO DO WITH IT? DEFINITION AND MANAGEMENT

ELIZABETH COLLINS, MD

A G1P0 female presents to OB triage with contractions at 40.4 weeks of estimated gestational age (EGA) dated by a 25-week ultrasound (unknown last menstrual period [LMP]). Her cervix is 1 cm dilated and unchanged after two checks, 1 hour apart. Her contractions are every 10 to 15 minutes. Should she be admitted for augmentation of labor because she is "postterm"?

PROBLEM: DEFINING POSTTERM PREGNANCY

Defining postterm pregnancy is very important when planning an intervention after the estimated date of delivery (EDD). Postterm pregnancy is defined as gestation beyond 42 weeks. This definition *must* rely on accurate dating of the pregnancy. As such, the most common cause of postterm pregnancy is a dating error. Early assessment of gestational age with ultrasound, preferably in the first trimester, or use of accurate LMP consistent with uterine size on physical exam in a patient with regular menses can be used to accurately date a pregnancy. Other risk factors for postterm pregnancy include primigravity, anencephaly, male fetus, history of prior postterm pregnancy, and a possible association with placental sulfatase deficiency.

In this particular scenario, this patient has had her pregnancy dated by a late second-trimester scan. Second-trimester sonograms can have a margin of error for dating up to 2 weeks, meaning this patient could be 42.4 or 38.4 weeks pregnant. Because the dating is inaccurate, augmentation at this time would not be required and the patient could be managed expectantly.

A G3P2002 female presents to a clinic at 41.2 weeks of EGA dated by LMP consistent with a 20-week ultrasound with no signs or symptoms of labor. She wants to know if it is safe to continue the pregnancy because she passed her due date. She prefers to start labor on her own. What should you recommend?

PROBLEM: MANAGEMENT OF POSTTERM PREGNANCY

Data have shown that postterm pregnancy carries serious risk for the fetus (including mortality) due to uteroplacental insufficiency, meconium aspiration, and intrauterine infection. The risk of death at 42 weeks is two times greater than for fetuses at 40 weeks. Many providers have opted to offer induction by 42 weeks, with antenatal surveillance between 41 and 42 weeks, to reduce these risks. Due to ethical concerns, there are no studies performed without providing antenatal testing to patients between 41 and 42 weeks, but this intervention has not previously been shown to improve perinatal morbidity or mortality. Furthermore, there is wide variation on what constitutes appropriate antenatal surveillance. Options include nonstress test (NST), biophysical profile (BPP), modified BPP (NST plus measurement of amniotic fluid index), contraction stress test, or a combination of these tests. Of note, estimation of amniotic fluid volume is important because oligohydramnios is associated with adverse pregnancy outcomes. Delivery should be pursued if testing is nonreassuring or oligohydramnios is present (amniotic fluid index <5).

In this case, the patient may be offered an induction, antenatal testing, or expectant management with the ultimate goal of delivery by 42 weeks.

TAKE HOME POINTS

- You must have accurate dating when defining a postterm pregnancy.
- Risk factors for postterm pregnancy include primigravity, anencephaly, male fetus, history of prior postterm pregnancy, and a possible association with placental sulfatase deficiency.
- Postterm risks to the fetus include uteroplacental insufficiency, meconium aspiration, and intrauterine infection.

SUGGESTED READINGS

American College of Obstetricians and Gynecologists. AOCG Practice Bulletin No. 55: management of postterm pregnancy. *Obstet Gynecol.* 2004;104:639.

Bochner CJ, Medearis AL, Davis J, et al. Antepartum predictors of fetal distress in postterm pregnancy. *Am J Obstet Gynecol.* 1987;157:353–358.

Bonner CJ, Williams J III, Castro L, et al. The efficacy of starting postterm antenatal testing at 41 weeks as compared to 42 weeks of gestational age. *Am J Obstet Gynecol.* 1988;159:550–554.

Crowley P. Interventions for preventing or improving the outcome of delivery at or beyond term (Cochrane review). In: *The Cochrane Library,* Issue 2, Chicester, UK: John Wiley & Sons; 2004.

Crowley P, O'Herlihy C, Boylan P. The value of ultrasound measurement of amniotic fluid volume in the management of the prolonged pregnancies. *Br J Obstet Gynaecol.* 1984;91:444–448.

Feldman GB. Prospective risk of stillbirth. *Obstet Gynecol.* 1992;79:547–553.

Hilder L, Costeloe K, Thilaganathan B. Prolonged pregnancy: evaluating gestation-specific risks of fetal and infant mortality. *Br J Obstet Gynaecol.* 1998;105:169–173.

Oz AU, Holub B, Mendilcioglu I, et al. Renal artery Doppler investigation of the etiology of oligohydramnios in postterm pregnancy. *Obstet Gynecol.* 2002;100:715–718.

Phelan JP, Platt LD, Yeh SY, et al. The role of ultrasound assessment of amniotic fluid volume in the management of the postdate pregnancy. *Am J Obstet Gynecol.* 1985;151:304–308.

Smith GC. Life-table analysis of the risk of perinatal death at term and postterm in singleton pregnancies. *Am J Obstet Gynecol.* 2001;184:486–489.

Tongsong T, Srisomboon J. Amniotic fluid volume as a predictor of fetal distress in postterm pregnancy. *Int J Gynaecol Obstet.* 1993;40:213–217.

21

PLACENTA PREVIA, IS IT STILL THERE?

RICHARD ENCHILL, MD AND DIANA BROOMFIELD, MD, MBA, FACOG, FACS

A 41-year-old G5P4003 female at 35 weeks of gestation presented to L&D with profuse vaginal bleeding. She is a recent African immigrant, a person I will describe as an obstetric tourist (a person who migrates temporarily to another country just for obstetrical care and delivery). She has a history of having had C-sections for her first and third deliveries and no prenatal care for the current pregnancy. Upon probing, the patient admitted that she had occasional mild to moderate vaginal bleeding since 28 weeks of gestation but all spontaneously abated. The fetal monitor (confirmed by ultrasound) demonstrated sustained fetal bradycardia of 80 bpm (maternal pulse of 90). She underwent an emergency C-section. The procedure was complicated by uterine atony and heavy bleeding. The placenta was adherent to the myometrium—placenta accreta, resulting in a cesarean hysterectomy.

Placenta previa is the implantation of the placenta over or very near the internal os of the uterine cervix.

There are four degrees of this abnormal placentation:

1. Total placenta previa: Internal cervical os is completely covered by placenta
2. Partial placenta previa: Internal os is partially covered by placenta
3. Marginal placenta: The edge of the placenta is at the edge of the internal os
4. Low-lying placenta: The placenta is implanted in the lower segment such that the placenta's edge does not reach the internal os but is in close proximity.

Placenta previa is often associated with significant antepartum hemorrhage. It occurs in 0.3% to 0.5% of all pregnancies. This risk increases with a history of cesarean delivery. Placenta previa is also associated with preterm delivery. Salihu and associates in 2003 found that neonatal mortality rate was threefold higher in pregnancies complicated by placenta previa because of preterm delivery.

RISK FACTORS OF PLACENTA PREVIA

Prior C-section is known to predispose to the development of placenta previa. Getahun et al. conducted a retrospective study in 2006 and found that a cesarean first birth is associated with increased risk of placenta previa in the second pregnancy. There is a dose-response pattern in increasing risks of previa with increasing number of prior cesarean deliveries. A short interpregnancy interval is associated with increased risks of previa. In 2004, Gesteland et al., along with Gilliam et al. (2002), found that the risk of placenta previa increased progressively as parity and number of prior cesarean deliveries increased. Both groups calculated that the likelihood of placenta previa was increased more than eightfold in patients with greater than four previous pregnancies and greater than four prior cesarean sections.

Complications of Placenta Previa. Placenta previa may be associated with placenta accreta, increta, or percreta, which are increasing degrees of abnormal placentation and adherence to or onto the myometrium. Such abnormality results from poorly developed deciduas in the lower segment of the uterus causing abnormally firm attachment of the placenta. Other risk factors include

> Maternal age: Maternal age increases the risk of placenta previa.
> Multiparity: In 1997, Ananth et al. found that the rate of previa was 40% higher in multifetal gestations compared with that of singletons. Williams found that smoking has also been associated with increased placenta previa. These findings were confirmed by Ananth in 2003 and Handler in 1994.

Clinical Presentation. The typical symptomatology is consistent with painless bleeding, which begins at the end of the second trimester. This may be followed by many recurrences until it culminates in profound hemorrhage at onset of labor. The hemorrhage is caused by the tearing of placenta from its attachment during the formation of the lower uterine segment.

Diagnosis. A common error to avoid is not having a high index of suspicion for placenta previa. This diagnosis should be considered in any pregnant women who presents with painless vaginal bleeding in the second and third trimesters of pregnancy. Vaginal examination of such patients should be deferred until sonogram has clearly proved the absence of placenta previa. In the event that hemorrhage threatens the patient's or baby's hemodynamic stability, a STAT C-section should be considered even without a vaginal exam. In 2005, Cunningham demonstrated that a transabdominal ultrasound provides the safest, simplest, and most precise diagnosis.

Management of Placenta Previa. In preterm pregnancies with no active bleeding, conservative management is the key. The patient and family must be well educated to fully appreciate the problems of placenta previa, and the family must be prepared to transport her to the hospital should she start bleeding. In selected cases, some patients are best admitted to the antepartum unit for observation until delivery. If the fetal status is term or is expected to have lung maturity, and bleeding starts, then the safest management is to deliver her by C-section. In situations where hemorrhage is very severe and the patient is hemodynamically unstable, the delivery should be executed by an emergent C-section irrespective of fetal maturity.

TAKE HOME POINTS

- Placenta previa should be suspected in painless bleeding after 20 weeks of gestation.
- Transabdominal ultrasound is quick, safe, and precise in the diagnosis of placenta previa.
- Placenta previa may be complicated by placenta accreta.
- C-section increases the risk of placenta previa and accreta in subsequent pregnancies.

SUGGESTED READINGS

Ananth C, Smulian JC, Vintzileos AM. The effect of placenta previa on neonatal mortality: a population-based study in the United States, 1989 through 1997. *Am J Obstet Gynecol.* 2003;188(5):1299–304.

Cunningham KJ, Leveno KL, Bloom SL, et al. *Williams Obstetrics.* New York, NY: McGraw-Hill; 2005.

Getahun D, Oyelese Y, Salihu HM et al. Previous cesarean delivery and risks of placenta previa and placental abrubtion. *Obstet Gynecol.* 2006;107(4):771–8.

Gilliam M, Rosenberg D, Davis F. The likelihood of placenta previa with greater number of cesarean deliveries and higher parity. *Obstet Gynecol.* 2002;99(6):967–8.

Handler AS, Mason ED, Rosenberg DL, et al. The relationship between exposure during pregnancy to cigarette smoking and cocaine use and placenta previa. *Am J Obstet Gynecol.* 1994;170(3):884–9.

Saju J. *Placenta Previa Overview* (2008, August 12). Retrieved April 5, 2009, from eMedicine: http://www.emedicine.medscape.com/article/262065-overview

Salihu H, Li Q, Rouse DJ, et al. Placenta previa: neonatal death after live births in the United States. *Am J Obstet Gynecol.* 2003;188(5):1305–9.

Williams MA, Mittendorf R, Lieberman E, et al. Cigarette smoking during pregnancy in relation to placenta previa. *Am J Obstet Gynecol.* 1991;165(1):28–32.

22

AMNIOINFUSION

RICHARD ENCHILL, MD AND DIANA BROOMFIELD, MD, MBA, FACOG, FACS

A 35-year-old G3P2 woman being induced at 41 5/7 weeks of gestation has thick meconium and develops recurrent variable FHR decelerations at 6-cm dilatation. The patient was placed in left lateral decubitus position, oxytocin infusion was terminated, and transcervical infusion of warm saline was started. Variable deceleration eventually ceased, but the patient developed arrest of dilatation at 8-cm dilatation and subsequently underwent a C-section. The neonate was delivered with APGAR scores of 6 and 8 at 1 and 5 minutes, respectively. No meconium aspiration syndrome was noted.

Amnioinfusion is the instillation of a saline solution into pregnant uterine cavity before delivery to increase the amniotic volume. This helps to cushion the fetal umbilical cord from compression. It is a common procedure; one survey of American Teaching Hospitals published in 1995 revealed that amnioinfusion was used in 96% of the responding centers and that 3% to 4% of all women delivering at these institutions received amnioinfusion.

In 1976, Gabbe et al. demonstrated in a monkey that the removal of amniotic fluid produced variable decelerations, but restoration of the amniotic volume by infusing normal saline solution abolished the decelerations. They showed that variable deceleration related to oligohydramnios and cord compression was corrected by amnioinfusion. The conventional therapy of decelerations including variable decelerations has been maternal positional changes and oxygen therapy. When these fail, amnioinfusion is attempted. Miyazaki and Taylor in 1983 showed that amnioinfusion could abolish 68% of those with variable decelerations and 86% of those with prolonged decelerations.

In 1985, Miyazaki and Nevarex again in a randomized controlled trial (RCT) using 96 pregnant women in labor having repetitive variable decelerations not relieved by O_2 and maternal position changes showed that 51% of women randomized to amnioinfusion had the variable decelerations relieved, while only 4% of those in the noninfused control group had their decelerations relieved.

OLIGOHYDRAMNIOS

Oligohydramnios is associated with variable decelerations. Baron et al. in 1995 reported a 50% increase in variable deceleration during labor and a sevenfold increase in caesarian delivery rate in women with oligohydramnios. Some gynecologists, however, do not accept premise that amnioinfusion is beneficial in the management of variable deceleration.

Sponge et al. showed that variable decelerations are related to amniotic fluid index (AFI). They found high rate of 76% abnormal fetal heart rate pattern in women with AFI of less than or equal to 4 cm as against 33% in women with AFI > 8 cm.

Owens et al. in a randomized control trial in 1990 could not elicit any beneficial effect in management of variable deceleration.

MECONIUM-STAINED AMNIOTIC FLUID

The usefulness of amnioinfusion in meconium-stained amniotic fluid is rather controversial. Piece et al., in 1995, showed that neonates delivered with thick meconium-stained amniotic fluid had significant decrease in meconium below the cords and meconium aspiration syndrome as well as significant decrease in caesarean delivery rate.

In 12 studies done in 2002, Hofmeyer found amnioinfusion to be associated with decreased variable deceleration, caesarian deliveries, and meconium aspiration syndrome. On the other hand, Fraser et al. in a RCT concluded that amnioinfusion for thick meconium staining does not decrease the risk of meconium aspiration syndrome or perinatal death.

Contraindications of amnioinfusion include intraamniotic infection, placental abruption, late decelerations, flatline tracing, uterine anomaly, and multiple gestations. Complications of amnioinfusion comprise of prolonged FHR deceleration, cord prolapse, uterine rapture, placental abruption, and maternal death.

TAKE HOME POINTS

- Amnioinfusion appears to decrease the caesarian delivery rate for variable decelerations.
- It is safe and easy to perform.
- It can increase amniotic fluid volume and reduce repetitive variable FHR deceleration by alleviating pressure on the umbilical cord.
- It has been shown to decrease the rate of operative delivery for fetal distress.
- It may decrease the risk of meconium aspiration.

SUGGESTED READINGS

Fraser W. Hofmeyr J, Lede R, et al. Amnioinfusion for the prevention of the meconium aspiration syndrome. *N Eng J Med.* 2005;353(9):909–917.

Gabbe SG, Ettinger BB, Freeman RK, et al. Umbilical cord compression associated with amniotomy: laboratory observation. *Am J Obstet Gynecol.* 1976;353–355.

Hofmeyr G. *Aminoinfusion for econiumm–stained liquor in labour.* 2001. Retrieved April 5, 2009, from The Cochrane Collaboration: http://ww3.cochrane.org/reviews/en/ab000014.html

Miyazaki FS, Nevarez F. Saline Amnioinfusion for relief of repetitive variable deceleration: a perspective randomized study. *Am J Obstet Gynecol.* 1985;301–306.

Miyazaki FS, Taylor NS. Saline amnioinfusion for relief of variable or prolonged deceleration. *Am J Obstet.* 1983;670–678.

Owen J, Henson BV, Hauth JC. A prospective randomized study of saline solution amnioinfusion. *Am J Obstet Gynecol.* 1990;162(5):1146–9.

Pierce J, Gaudier FL, Sanchez-Ramos L. Intrapartum amnioinfusion for meconium-stained fluid; Meta analysis of prospective clinical trials. *Obstet Gynecol.* 2000;95:1051–6.

Sponge CY, Ogundipe OA, Ross MG. Prophylactic amnioinfusion for meconium stained amniotic fluid. *Am J Obstet Gynecol.* 1994;931–935.

Wenstrom K, Andrews WW, Maher JE. Amnioinfusion Survey: prevalence, protocols and complications. *Obstet Gynecol.* 1995;572–576.

23

IF IT IS STARING YOU IN THE FACE: FACE, BROW, AND COMPOUND PRESENTATIONS

FREZGHI GHEBREAB, MD AND DIANA BROOMFIELD, MD, FACOG, FACS

FACE PRESENTATION

You have just completed the delivery of a baby in face presentation. The patient presented in the first stage of labor with ruptured membranes. The pregnancy was at term, and the presentation was face with a mentoposterior position. She was expectantly managed until she reached and was arrested in the second stage. The baby was subsequently delivered by cesarean section. After delivery, the mother points to a blistering lesion on the cheek and asks you what has caused it.

In a face presentation, the head is hyperextended so that the occiput is in contact with the fetal back and the chin or mentum is presenting. This presentation occurs at a rate of 1 in 600 to 800 deliveries. The etiology is unknown, but it is presumed to occur because of factors that favor extension or prevent flexion of the fetal head. A common risk factor is a fetal anomaly such as anencephaly. Other predisposing factors include multiple nuchal cords, cephalopelvic disproportion/contracted pelvis, pendulous maternal abdomen seen with multiparity, and fetal macrosomia.

The diagnosis is made during pelvic examination by palpating the mouth, nose, malar bones, and orbital ridges, and it may be mistaken for a breech presentation. The mentum is the denominator and determines the position. In a term fetus, a mentum posterior position cannot be delivered vaginally. At the time of diagnosis, 60% are mentoanterior, 26% are mentoposterior, and 15% are mentotransverse, and almost half of those in mentoposterior and mentotransverse positions revert to mentoanterior.

In the absence of a contracted pelvis and with effective labor, successful vaginal delivery usually follows. Cesarean section is frequently required because pelvic contracture is a common cause. Attempts to convert a face presentation to a vertex presentation or a mentoposterior position to a mentoanterior are dangerous and should be avoided. Internal monitoring should be avoided and, if needed, should be cautiously applied over a bony structure. Neonates who were in a face presentation often have significant facial edema and skull molding. This usually resolves during the first 24 to 48 hours. However, difficulties in ventilation during resuscitation may occur due to laryngeal edema and trauma.

BROW PRESENTATION

You have just completed a cesarean section on a 25-year-old G2P1 female at 38 weeks of gestation for failed vacuum delivery, which was applied for prolonged second stage of labor. The patient had required augmentation with pitocin for dysfunctional labor. Following delivery, you note that the baby has caput succedaneum and the mark of the vacuum cup on the forehead.

In a brow presentation, the head is extended, but not to the degree seen in face presentation. The head is midway between full flexion and extension (*Fig. 23.1*). The presenting part is the sinciput and extends from the anterior fontanel to the orbital ridges but does not include the mouth.

A brow presentation occurs at a frequency of 1 in 1,400 deliveries. The etiology is the same as in a face presentation. It often is a transitional state and converts to either a vertex or a face presentation. The diagnosis is often made in labor. Persistent brow presentation is incompatible with vaginal birth unless the fetus is very small and the pelvis very capacious.

In the presence of adequate gynecoid pelvis, it is reasonable to allow labor to progress to see if the presentation converts to a more favorable presentation. In the presence of a narrow or contracted pelvis, cesarean section is recommended. Augmentation and instrumental delivery are contraindicated.

COMPOUND PRESENTATION

You are evaluating a 29-year-old G4P3 pregnant woman of 37 weeks of gestation who had presented in labor with ruptured membranes. She is contracting regularly and the fetal heart tracing is reassuring. On pelvic examination, you note that the cervix is fully effaced, dilated to 6 cm, with vertex presenting alongside a fetal

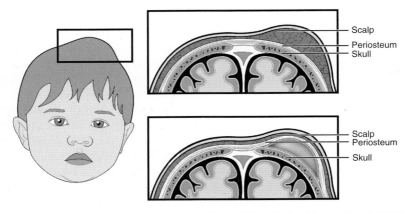

FIGURE 23.1 Caput succedaneum. (From Pillitteri, A. *Maternal and Child Nursing.* 4th ed. Philadelphia, PA: Lippincott Williams & Wilkins; 2003.)

hand and a station of 0. You attempt to replace the hand by pushing it up into the uterus and then you note that the cord has prolapsed and the patient is taken for a STAT C-section.

In a compound presentation, an extremity prolapses alongside the presenting part, with both presenting in the pelvis simultaneously. It occurs at a frequency of 1 in 700 to 1 in 1,500 deliveries. A hand or arm presenting alongside the head is the commonest presentation and occurs at a rate of 1 in 700 to 1 in 1,000 deliveries. One or both lower extremities presenting alongside a cephalic presentation or a hand presenting alongside a breech is much rarer.

The etiology is believed to be any condition that prevents complete occlusion of the inlet by the fetal head including preterm birth. The perinatal morbidity and mortality are increased due to concomitant preterm delivery, prolapsed cord, and traumatic obstetric procedures.

In most cases, the fetus should be left alone and as labor progresses the extremity will recede. If it fails to retract and appears to prevent descent of the presenting part, then it can be pushed gently upward while the head is, at the same time, pushed down from above.

TAKE HOME POINTS

- The mentum is the denominator and determines the position in a face presentation.
- Avoid internal monitoring in a face presentation.
- In most cases, an extremity that prolapses alongside the presenting part should be left alone and generally recedes back as labor progresses.

SUGGESTED READINGS

Bowes WA Jr, Lockwood CJ, Barss VA. Management of the fetus in transverse lie. UpToDate. July 11, 2008.

Cunningham FG, Leveno KL, Bloom SL, et al. *Williams Obstetrics*. 22nd ed. New York, NY: McGraw-Hill; 2005.

Hankins GD, Hammond TL, Snyder RR, et al. Transverse lie. *Am J Perinatol*. 1990;7:66.

Phelan JP, Stine LE, Edwards NB, et al. The role of external version in the intrapartum management of the transverse lie presentation. *Am J Obstet Gynecol*. 1985;151:724.

24

THE BOTTOM LINE: OPERATIVE DELIVERY

LONG NGUYEN, MD AND DIANA BROOMFIELD, MD, FACOG, FACS

A 28-year-old G1P1 patient is 2 weeks postpartum from a forceps-assisted vaginal delivery due to a prolonged second stage of labor and maternal exhaustion. The patient also underwent a repair of a fourth-degree perineal laceration complicated from the procedure. She reports severe perineal pain and purulent discharge for 3 days. The patient denies fever or change in perineal sensation. Examination shows an infected and broken down repair with moderate induration. The patient is concerned about the next steps of management and her risk of laceration in subsequent deliveries.

The rate of births by forceps-assisted or vacuum-assisted vaginal delivery in the United States has declined over the last decade from approximately 10% to 5% respectively, while the rate of cesarean deliveries has increased from approximately 20% to 30% during the same time. The rate of vacuum-assisted vaginal delivery is approximately four times higher than that of forceps-assisted vaginal delivery. The indications, complications, and individual provider experience may explain the current trend of operative vaginal delivery.

Prerequisites for forceps-assisted vaginal delivery include the following:

- The head must be engaged.
- The cervix must be fully dilated and retracted.
- The position of the head must be known.
- Pelvimetry: Clinical assessment of pelvic capacity should be performed. No evidence of disproportion should be suspected between the size of the head and the size of the pelvic inlet and midpelvis.
- The membranes must be ruptured.
- The patient must have adequate analgesia.
- Adequate staff, facilities, and supportive elements should be readily available.
- The operator should be competent in the use of the instruments and the recognition and management of potential complications. The operator should also know the amount of needed traction and when to stop.
- Asynclitism must be determined.

INDICATIONS

There is no absolute indication for an operative vaginal delivery as long as all of the above prerequisite criteria are met. An operative vaginal delivery can be considered when there is a prolonged second stage (nulliparous women: lack of continuing progress for 2 or 3 hours with regional anesthesia; multiparous women: lack of progress for 2 hours or 1 hour without regional anesthesia); suspicion of immediate or potential fetal compromise in the second stage of labor; shortening of the second stage for maternal benefits such as exhaustion, bleeding, and cardiac or pulmonary disease; and history of a spontaneous pneumothorax and fetal malpositions, including the after-coming head in a breech vaginal delivery. Indications of forceps- and vacuum-assisted vaginal deliveries are generally similar except that forceps can be used in cases <34 weeks of gestation and when there is a need of head rotation.

Forceps delivery is reclassified as outlet, low, and mid forceps. In an outlet forceps–assisted vaginal delivery, the scalp is visible at the introitus, the skull is at the pelvic floor, the sagittal suture is in the anterior-posterior plane, the fetal head is at or on perineum, and the rotation is <45 degrees. In a low forceps–assisted vaginal delivery, the station is at or below +2 cm but not on the pelvic floor and the rotation is less or greater than 45 degrees. In a midforceps–assisted vaginal delivery, the station is above +2 cm and the head is engaged.

COMPLICATIONS

Vacuum-assisted vaginal birth is more often associated with cephalohematoma and shoulder dystocia. Forceps delivery is more often associated with third- and fourth-degree peritoneal lacerations. The complication ratios of forceps over vacuum are 0.25 for cephalohematoma, 0.34 for shoulder dystocia, and 1.79 for third- or fourth-degree laceration. Other complications more often associated with forceps are urinary and rectal incontinence.

EPISIOTOMY REPAIR

There are four levels of episiotomy lacerations associated with vaginal deliveries with or without operative intervention. A first-degree laceration involves the vaginal mucosa and perineal skin. A second-degree laceration involves the fascia and muscle of the perineal body and the tissues included in a first-degree laceration. A third-degree laceration involves the anal sphincter and the tissues included in a second-degree laceration. A fourth-degree laceration involves the rectal mucosa and the tissue damaged with a third-degree laceration.

Hemostasis and anatomical restoration without excessive suturing are essential for any repair. A two-layered closure has been shown to decrease postpartum pain and healing complication compared with a three-layered closure. Polyglycolic acid suture may be preferable to chromic catgut because there are less perineal pain and dyspareunia. For fourth-degree lacerations, it is essential to approximate the torn edges of the rectal mucosa with sutures placed in the muscularis approximately 0.5 cm apart. The muscular layer should be covered with a layer of fascia. The cut ends of the anal sphincter are isolated and sutured together with four interrupted stitches.

Bleeding can be conservatively controlled with compression. Localized infection may resolve with perineal wound care; however, an abscess needs evacuation. A breakdown or dehiscence of an episiotomy repair should be closed early instead of by secondary intention healing. In rare cases, inadequately repaired episiotomy lacerations may lead to rectovaginal fistula formation, which should be repaired by a physician familiar with fistula repair techniques. There is an increased risk of spontaneous obstetric laceration in subsequent deliveries in women with a history of an episiotomy.

TAKE HOME POINTS

- Indications for forceps- and vacuum-assisted vaginal deliveries are generally similar; however, forceps have more indications in cases <34 weeks of gestation and in cases that require rotation.
- It is essential to know the position, presentation, lie, engagement, clinical pelvimetry, and asynclitism before the application of either forceps or a vacuum.
- Meticulous exploration of lacerations is necessary to identify tears of the anal sphincter and rectal mucosa in cases of episiotomy lacerations.
- A two-layered closure with polyglycolic acid suture is preferable.
- Early closure is recommended for an episiotomy dehiscence.
- There is an increased risk of spontaneous obstetric laceration in subsequent deliveries in women with a history of an episiotomy.

SUGGESTED READINGS

American College of Obstetricians and Gynecologists. ACOG Practice Bulletin No. 17. June 2000.

American College of Obstetricians and Gynecologists. ACOG Practice Bulletin No. 71. April 2006.

Alperin M, Krohn MA, Parviainen K. Episiotomy and Increase in the risk of obstetric laceration in a subsequent vaginal delivery. *Obstet Gynecol.* 2008;111(6):1274–8.

Caughley AB, Sandberg PL, Zlatnik MG, et al. Forceps compared with vacuum. *Obstet Gynecol.* 2005;106(5 Pt 1):1908–12.

Cunningham FG, Leveno KJ, Bloom SL, et al. *Williams Obstetrics.* 22nd ed. New York, NY: Mc Graw Hill; 2005.

Hankins GDV, Hauth JC, Gilstrap LC, et al. Early repair of episiotomy dehiscence. *Obstet Gynecol.* 1990;75(1):48–51.

Mackrodt C, Grant A, Fern E, et al. A randomized comparison of polyglactin 910 with chromic catgut for postpartum perineal repair. *Br J Obstet Gynaecol.* 1998;105:441–445.

Martin JA. National Vital Statistics Report, vol. 56, December 2007. http://www.cdc.gov/nchs/data/nvsr56/nvsr56_06.pdf

Oboro VO, Tabowei TO, Loto OM, et al. A multicenter evaluation of the two-layered repair of postpartum perineal trauma. *J Obstet Gynaecol.* 2003;23:5–8.

Ventura SJ, Martin JA, Curtin SC, et al. Births: final data for 1997. *Natl Vital Stat Rep.* 1999;47(18):1–96.

25

WHEN IS IT TOO LONG? DELIVERING THE PLACENTA

FREZGHI GHEBREAB, MD AND DIANA BROOMFIELD, MD, FACOG, FACS

You are supervising a 1st-year OB/GYN resident deliver the placenta in a primigravida who had an uncomplicated normal vaginal delivery at term. Fifteen minutes have elapsed since the baby was delivered. The patient does not have any unusual bleeding and no signs of placental separation were noted. The intern is trying to facilitate the delivery of the placenta by massaging and squeezing the uterus. He is also pulling on the umbilical cord in an attempt to express the placenta.

There are no universally agreed upon or acceptable criteria for the normal length of the third stage. Sometimes the placenta separates within 1 minute of the delivery of the baby and usually within 5 minutes. The median duration of the third stage is 6 minutes, and 97% of placentas are delivered within 30 minutes. Several measures of hemorrhage including curettage or transfusion increase when the third stage is prolonged to 30 minutes or more. A retained placenta is variably defined as a placenta that has not been expelled by 30 to 60 minutes after delivery of the baby.

If the uterus remains firm and there is no unusual bleeding, watchful waiting until the placenta separates is the usual practice. The signs of placental separation include the following:

1. The uterus becomes globular and rises in the abdomen.
2. Rush of blood occurs.
3. Lengthening of the cord.

Unnecessary kneading and squeezing of the fundus in an attempt to hasten the delivery of the placenta is dangerous and must be avoided. Once the signs of placental separation are noted, the mother may be instructed to bear down and the intra-abdominal pressure may be adequate to expel the placenta. If this fails, apply firm pressure on the fundus and try to propel the detached placenta. This is called physiological management of the third stage. Traction on the umbilical cord must never be used to pull the placenta out of the uterus.

Alternatively, active management of the third stage may be employed. It consists of early cord clamping, use of uterotonic agents, such as ergometrine-oxytocin, and controlled cord traction. The drugs used and the timing of administration of the drugs are variable. Active management is associated with a decreased risk of maternal blood loss and prolonged third stage. If active management is undertaken, uterotonic drugs should not be given until after delivery of the anterior shoulder.

A retained or partially detached placenta interferes with normal myometrial contraction and retraction, which leads to bleeding. A retained placenta should be removed manually, in the operating room, under anesthesia or conscious sedation.

Sonographic examination is appropriate when the third stage of labor is prolonged and the etiology is uncertain. If the placenta is already detached, further traction on the umbilical cord is warranted. If the placenta is still partially or totally attached, one may attempt manual removal or try pharmacologic interventions such as intravascular nitroglycerine or intraumbilical oxytocin. An intravascular injection of nitroglycerine relaxes the uterus and often facilitates removal of the placenta without manual exploration or anesthesia. As a drop in blood pressure almost always occurs, the blood pressure should be monitored carefully.

TAKE HOME POINTS

- The third stage is prolonged if it exceeds 30 minutes.
- Avoid constant kneading and squeezing on the fundus as well as traction on the cord to effect delivery.
- Active management of the third stage is associated with decreased blood loss and prolonged third stage.

SUGGESTED READINGS

Combs CA, Laros RK Jr. Prolonged third stage of labor: morbidity and risk factors. *Obstet Gynecol*. 1991;77:863.

Cunningham FG, Leveno KL, Bloom SL, et al. *Williams Obstetrics*. 22nd ed. New York, NY: McGraw-Hill; 2005.

Dombrowski MP, Bottoms SF, Saleh AA, et al. Third stage of labor: analysis of duration and clinical practice. *Am J Obstet Gynecol*. 1995;172:1279.

Silverman F, Bornstein E, Lockwood CJ, et al. Management of third stage of labor. UpToDate. July 31, 2008.

World Health Organization. Maternal and Child Health and Family Planning. The prevention and management of postpartum hemorrhage. Report of a technical working group. WHO/ MCH 1990;90.7:3.

26

WHAT DOES UMBILICAL ARTERY CORD GAS MEAN?

FREZGHI GHEBREAB, MD AND DIANA BROOMFIELD, MD, FACOG, FACS

A 35-year-old G3P0202 laboring mother who is on induction of labor with pitocin for superimposed severe preeclampsia at a gestational age of 37 weeks was noted to have repetitive late decelerations. Intrapartum resuscitation was then started and the pitocin drip discontinued. The pelvic examination showed that the cervix was fully dilated and effaced with the vertex at (+3) station. The baby was delivered with a vacuum with two pulls and "no pop off." The Apgar scores were 4 and 8 in the 1st and 5th minutes, respectively, and the umbilical artery cord gas analysis revealed a pH, PCO_2, PO_2, HCO_3, and base excess of 7.0, 60, 20, 18, and −6, respectively. The mother asks you about the possibility of long-term neurological impairment in the baby.

Normal blood gas values for the newborn are given below:

pH: 7.27 to 7.28
PCO_2 (mm Hg): 49.2 to 50.3
HCO_3^- (mEq/L): 22.0 to 23.1
Base excess (mEq/L): −2.7 to −3.6

Normal metabolism in the fetus results in the production of both carbonic acid (formed by oxidative metabolism of CO_2) and organic acids (formed by anaerobic metabolism and include lactic and hydroxybutyric acids). Accumulation of H_2CO_3 in fetal blood without an increase in organic acids results in *respiratory acidemia*. Accumulation of organic acids without an increase in H_2CO_3 results in *metabolic acidemia*. A decrease in bicarbonate (HCO_3^-) accompanies metabolic academia, since it is used to buffer the organic acid. An increase in H_2CO_3 accompanied by an increase in organic acid (manifested as a decrease in HCO_3^-) is known as a *mixed respiratory-metabolic acidemia*.

Umbilical artery pH <7.20 has traditionally been used to define newborn acidemia. Most clinicians define acidemia as 2 SD below the mean umbilical artery pH (7.10 to 7.18). Most fetuses will tolerate intrapartum acidemia with a pH as low as 7.00 without neurological sequelae. Neonatal mortality and the birth of infants with neurological impairment are significantly increased if a pH cutoff value of <7.00 is used to define newborn acidemia.

Almost all newborns are hypoxic at the time of delivery, and umbilical artery PO_2 is not predictive of any adverse neonatal outcome. The criteria used to establish the diagnosis of acute neurological injury related to hypoxia proximate to delivery are

- Umbilical artery blood pH <7.00 with a metabolic component
- Apgar scores of ≤3 for >5 minutes
- Neurological manifestations such as seizures, coma, hypotonia
- Evidence of multisystem organ dysfunction

In contrast to adult pathophysiology, in which distinct conditions result in either respiratory or metabolic acidemia, in the fetus, respiratory acidemia and metabolic acidemia, and ultimately tissue acidosis, are part of a progressively worsening continuum. One principal cause of fetal acidemia is a decrease in uteroplacental perfusion, which results in the retention of CO_2 (respiratory acidemia) and, if protracted and severe enough, leads to a mixed or metabolic acidemia.

Respiratory acidemia results from increased CO_2 tension and, in the fetus, is usually associated with a decrease in PO_2 as well. The most common cause of acute respiratory acidosis in the fetus is a sudden decrease in placental/umbilical perfusion. This includes umbilical cord compression, uterine hyperstimulation, and placental abruption. Conditions associated with maternal hypoventilation or hypoxia can also result in fetal respiratory acidosis.

Metabolic acidosis is characterized by a loss of bicarbonate, high base deficit (increased negative base excess), and a subsequent fall in pH. It results from protracted periods of O_2 deficit to a degree that results in anaerobic metabolism and usually implies the existence of a chronic metabolic derangement. The causes include intrauterine growth restriction resulting from chronic uteroplacental hypoperfusion, maternal metabolic acidosis, and prolonged fetal respiratory acidosis.

To obtain a cord blood sample immediately after birth, isolate and clamp a 10- to 20-cm segment of cord. *Arterial blood* is drawn from the isolated segment of cord into a 1- to 2-mL syringe. The sample is then transported, on ice, to the laboratory. Although it is generally recommended that the blood be transported to the laboratory promptly, studies have shown that neither the pH nor the PCO_2 changes significantly in blood kept at room temperature for up to 1 hour.

TAKE HOME POINTS

- Fetal acid base disturbance occurs as a continuum, with respiratory acidemia progressing to metabolic acidemia if protracted and severe.

- A pH cutoff value of 7.20 is generally used to define acidemia, but significant neurological impairment or mortality is unlikely unless the pH falls below 7.00.
- Umbilical artery PO_2 is not useful in evaluating fetal acid base status.
- Metabolic acidemia defines and predicts acute neurological injury related to hypoxia proximate to delivery.
- A segment of cord should be isolated and clamped immediately for cord gas analysis. Although it is desirable to send the specimen to the lab immediately, a specimen kept at room temperature for up to 1 hour may still be used.

SUGGESTED READINGS

American Academy of Pediatrics and the American College of Obstetricians and Gynecologists. Care of the neonate. In: *Guidelines for Perinatal Care.* 5th ed. Washington, DC: AAP and ACOG; 2002.

American Academy of Pediatrics and the American College of Obstetricians and Gynecologists. *Neonatal Encephalopathy and Cerebral Palsy: Defining the Pathogenesis and Pathophysiology.* Elk Grove Village, IL: Washington, DC: AAP and ACOG; 2003.

Creasy RK, Resnik R, Iams JD. *Maternal–Fetal Medicine. Principles and Practice.* 5th ed. New York, NY, Elsevier; 2003.

Cunningham FG, Leveno KL, Bloom SL, et al. *Williams Obstetrics.* 22nd ed. New York, NY: McGraw-Hill; 2005.

Freeman JM, Nelson KB. Intrapartum asphyxia and cerebral palsy. *Pediatrics.* 1988;82:240.

Gilstrap LC III, Leveno KJ, Burris J, et al. Diagnosis of birth asphyxia on the basis of fetal pH, Apgar score, and newborn cerebral dysfunction. *Am J Obstet Gynecol.* 1989;161:825.

Goldaber KG, Gilstrap LC III, Leveno KJ, et al. Pathologic fetal acidemia. *Obstet Gynecol.* 1991;78:1103.

Riley RJ, Johnson JW. Collecting and analyzing cord blood gases. *Clin Obstet Gynecol.* 1993;36:13.

Yeomans ER, Hauth JC, Gilstrap LC III, et al. Umbilical cord pH, PCO_2, and bicarbonate following uncomplicated term vaginal deliveries. *Am J Obstet Gynecol.* 1985;151:798.

27

IF IT IS GOT TO GO, IT IS GOT TO GO: PERIPARTUM HYSTERECTOMY AND OTHER TECHNIQUES TO STOP THE BLEEDING

FREZGHI GHEBREAB, MD AND DIANA BROOMFIELD, MD, FACOG, FACS

A 32-year-old gravida 2 para 2 mother who had delivered an hour previously by an outlet forceps delivery following a prolonged induction of labor for postterm pregnancy is taken to the operating room for intractable postpartum hemorrhage (PPH) secondary to uterine atony. She is hemodynamically stable with continuous ooze. At laparotomy, the attending physician asks you to discuss your initial surgical management plan.

Traditionally, postpartum hemorrhage has been defined as the loss of 500 mL of blood or more after completion of the third stage of labor. PPH is best defined and diagnosed clinically as excessive bleeding that makes the patient symptomatic and/or results in signs of hypovolemia. Whether postpartum bleeding begins before or after placental delivery, or at both times, there may be no sudden massive hemorrhage but rather steady bleeding that, at any given instant, appears to be moderate but persists until serious hypovolemia develops. Especially with hemorrhage after placental delivery, the constant seepage may lead to enormous blood loss. The effects of hemorrhage depend to a considerable degree on the nonpregnant blood volume, magnitude of pregnancy-induced hypervolemia, and degree of anemia at the time of delivery. Except possibly when intrauterine and intravaginal accumulations of blood are not recognized, or in some instances of uterine rupture with intraperitoneal bleeding, the diagnosis of postpartum hemorrhage should be obvious. The differentiation between bleeding from uterine atony and from lacerations is tentatively made on predisposing risk factors and the condition of the uterus. If bleeding persists despite a firm, well-contracted uterus, the cause of the hemorrhage most likely is from lacerations. Bright red blood also suggests lacerations.

Once PPH is diagnosed, initiate a sequence of nonoperative and operative interventions and promptly assess the success or failure of each measure. If an intervention does not succeed, the next treatment in the sequence must be swiftly initiated. Indecisiveness delays treatment and results in excessive hemorrhage, which eventually causes dilutional coagulopathy, severe hypovolemia, tissue hypoxia, hypothermia, and acidosis. Management is generally initiated with the assumption that the cause is uterine atony until proven otherwise.

Initial management includes (1) calling for help; (2) fundal massage and bimanual compression; (3) intravenous access with two large-bore catheters; (4) uterotonic drugs such as oxytocin, methylergonovine, Hemabate, misoprostol, and dinoprostone; and (5) fluid replacement and blood transfusion when abdominal uterine massage and oxytocin fail to control bleeding.

Subsequent intervention should include a thorough inspection of the birth canal with a repair of any lacerations. The uterus should then be explored and removal of retained products should be done either manually or with ring forceps or a banjo curette. Although intractable hemorrhage from uterine atony may require a hysterectomy as a lifesaving measure, other medical and less radical measures are undertaken before that decision is made, which include tamponade with a Bakri tamponade balloon. If a balloon is not available, you can use a No. 24 Foley catheter with a 30-mL balloon inflated to 60 to 80 mL or a uterine pack. Arterial embolization is extremely effective if interventional radiology personnel and facilities are readily available and the patient is hemodynamically stable. A laparotomy can be performed through a vertical incision to pursue bilateral ligation of uterine vessels such as with an O'Leary stitch, uterine compression sutures, and internal iliac artery ligation, and a hysterectomy is the last resort but should not be delayed in women who require prompt control of uterine hemorrhage to prevent death.

TAKE HOME POINTS

- Always call for help first.
- Once PPH is diagnosed, initiate the above sequence of events and assess the success or failure of each measure, and if not successful, institute the next step in the management.
- Treatment is generally initiated with the assumption that uterine atony is the cause of the PPH.
- Hysterectomy is the last resort but should not be delayed when it is required to control bleeding and prevent death.

SUGGESTED READINGS

Cunningham FG, Leveno KL, Bloom SL, et al. *Williams Obstetrics*, 22nd ed. New York, NY: McGraw-Hill; 2005.

Jacobs AJ, Lockwood CJ, Barss VA. Causes and treatment of postpartum hemorrhage. UpToDate. Feb 10, 2009.

28

Postpartum care

John-Charles Akoda, MD and Diana Broomfield, MD, MBA, FACOG, FACS

Anna, a 26-year-old G1P1, is 4 days status postnormal spontaneous vaginal delivery. She calls her obstetrician and reports breast tenderness, uterine cramping, and dysuria and wonders if these symptoms are normal. The patient is advised to report to office for urine C&S.

This period usually lasts about 6 to 12 weeks, a time when physiologic and anatomic changes of pregnancy reverse to the nonpregnant state. It includes a period of involution of the genital organs and return of menses, which is usually about 6 weeks in nonlactating women, and the return of cardiovascular and psychological functions, which may take longer.

Uterine Changes

Uterine vessels: After delivery, the size of the extrauterine vessels decreases to about the size of the prepregnant state. Cervix and lower uterine segment: The cervical opening contracts postpartum. By the end of the 1st week, it has narrowed significantly. As the opening narrows, the cervix thickens and a canal reforms. By the end of this involution, the external os does not completely resume its pregravid appearance. It remains wider with bilateral depressions at the site of laceration. Involution of the uterine corpus: Immediately following delivery of the placenta, the uterus contracts with the fundus slightly below the umbilicus. About 2 days after delivery, the uterus begins to shrink, and within 2 weeks, it descends into the true pelvic cavity. It regains its nonpregnant size about 4 weeks postpartum. The total number of uterine muscle cells does not decrease appreciably, but the cells decrease markedly in size.

Afterpains: The postpartum uterus in primiparous patients tends to remain tonically contracted, whereas it contracts vigorously and intermittently at intervals in multiparous patients. It worsens with increasing parity and with breast-feeding likely due to oxytocin release. The intensity usually decreases by day 3.

Lochia: Sloughing of the decidual tissues leading to vaginal discharge. It consists of RBCs, shredded deciduae, epithelial cells, and bacterial cells. The color is red for the first few days postpartum secondary to blood; it is known as lochia rubra. After 3 or 4 days, it becomes progressively pale—lochia serosa, but about the 10th day, it assumes a white or yellowish-white color—rubra alba. In 1986, Oppenheimer and colleagues noted that lochia persists for up to 4 weeks and may stop and resume up to 8 weeks postpartum. Maternal age, parity, infant weight, and breast-feeding do not influence the duration of lochia.

Endometrial regeneration: Within 2 or 3 days postpartum, the decidua differentiates into the superficial necrotic layer and the basalis layer, which remains intact and is the source of the new endometrium.

Subinvolution: Arrest or slowing of involution accompanied by prolongation of lochia and irregular or excessive uterine bleeding. On bimanual exam, the uterus is larger and softer than expected. This may be secondary to placental fragment retention or pelvic infection. Ergonovine and antimicrobial therapy may be effective.

Placental site involution: Complete extension of the placental site takes up to 6 weeks. If defective, it may lead to postpartum hemorrhage. It is brought about by sloughing of infracted and necrotic superficial tissues followed by a reparative process.

Late postpartum hemorrhage: It may develop 1 to 2 weeks postpartum. It is usually due to involution of the placental site. It used to be treated with prompt curettage. Now found to actually worsen the hemorrhage thus initial treatment may be medical use of IV oxytocin, ergonovine, or prostaglandins. In general, curettage is done if there is appreciable bleeding or medical management has failed.

Urinary tract changes: Pregnancy is associated with increase in extra-cellular water. The diuresis that occurs postpartum is the physiological reversal of this process. This usually occurs by the 2nd to 5th day postpartum, especially in preeclampsia. The postpartum urinary bladder has an increased capacity and a relative insensitivity to intrarenal fluid press leading to overdistention, incomplete emptying, and excessive residual urine. Intrapartum analgesics, especially epidural and spinal blocks, are often contributory. The dilated ureters and renal pelves return to their prepregnant state over 2 to 8 weeks postpartum. Urinary tract infection is a concern at this time due to residual urine and bacteriuria in a traumatized bladder.

Incontinence: Farrell and colleagues in 2001 found that 3% to 26% of women report episodes of incontinence in the 3 to 6 months postpartum. This is usually secondary to obstetrical factors such as a prolonged second stage of labor, fetal macrosomia, and episiotomy. Seventy percent of women whose deliveries were all vaginal had a higher risk of incontinence compared to those whose deliveries were all by cesarean section.

Caution: For an individual woman, a decision to deliver all her infants by cesarean section would decrease her risk of moderate to severe incontinence from 10% to only 5% and that there was no evidence that this effect would persist past 50 years of age.

Uterine prolapsed: The vagina postpartum rarely returns to its nulliparous state. The vaginal outlet becomes extremely relaxed in addition to the pelvic support resulting in uterine prolapse and urinary stress incontinence. Surgical correction is usually deferred after childbearing years.

Abdominal wall: The abdominal wall is soft and flaccid postpartum. Recovery is aided by exercise.

Weight loss: It is mainly due to evacuation of the uterus, blood loss, and diuresis. Most women approach their self-reported prepregnancy weight 6 months after delivery but still retain an average surplus of 3 lb.

Breast-feeding: Postpartum breasts secrete colostrums by the 2nd day, which persist for about 5 days with gradual conversion to mature milk in the following 4 weeks or so, and colostrums contain IgA antibodies that protect against enteric pathogens.

Milk production: Nursing mothers make at least 600 mL of milk per day. Most milk proteins are unique and not found elsewhere. Thirty to forty hours postpartum, there is a sudden increase of lactose concentration. Some lactose enters maternal circulation and is excreted by the kidneys, which may sometimes be misread as glucosuria unless specific glucose oxidase is used in testing.

All vitamins except vitamin K are found in human milk. Hence, vitamin K is administered to the infant soon after delivery to prevent hemorrhagic disease of the newborn. Milk production is complex. Progesterone, prolactin, estrogen, and human placental lactogen (HPL) all play a role. Postpartum progesterone withdrawal leads to formation of lactalbumin and also frees prolactin to act unopposed in stimulation of α-lactalbumin to increase milk production. Women with Sheehan syndrome do not lactate due to little or no production of prolactin secondary to extensive pituitary necrosis.

Women who breast-feed have a lower risk of breast cancer, and their children have increased adult intelligence independent of a wide range of other factors.

Most women (~65%) who underwent augmentation mammoplasty have lactation insufficiency especially if incision was periareolar.

Aerobic exercises—four to five times per week between 6 and 8 weeks postpartum—have been found to have no adverse effects on milk content or production.

Lactation inhibition: About 35% to 45% of American females elect not to breast-feed leading to considerable pain and engorgement, which peaks at 3 to 5 days postpartum. In 1989, the FDA advised against pharmacologic agent of milk suppression because bromocriptine was found to be associated with strokes, myocardial infarction, seizures, and psychiatric disturbances.

Contraception: Ovulation may resume 3 weeks postpartum even in lactating women. Progestin-only contraceptives—mini pills and Depo-Provera—do not affect quality or decrease milk volume.

Contraindications to breast-feeding: These include street drugs, excessive ethanol use, HIV, certain anticancer medications, and infants with galactosemia. Breast-feeding is not contraindicated in mothers with CMV, in mothers who are Hep B positive or Hep C positive, or in patients on methadone.

Breast fever: Transient elevation up to 37.8°C to 39°C seldom persisted longer than 4 to 16 hours. Other causes of fever especially due to infection must be excluded.

Mastitis: It occurs in approximately 2% to 33% of breast-feeding women. Symptoms seldom appear before the end of the 1st postpartum week and as a rule around the 3rd or 4th week. It is usually unilateral. The first sign is chills followed by fever and tachycardia with severe pain. About 10% of females with mastitis lead to breast abscesses. The most common organism isolated is *Staphylococcus aureus*. The treatment is to express milk from affected breast for culture prior to commencing antibiotic. Dicloxacillin may be started empirically and she may continue breast-feeding. Traditional treatment for abscess is drainage.

Hospital care: For the first postpartum hour, vital signs should be checked every 15 minutes, the amount of bleeding is monitored, and the fundus is checked for contraction. If regional analgesia or general anesthesia is used, the mother should be observed accordingly.

Care of the vulva: Instruct the patient to clean the vulva toward the anus; the patient may apply ice pack to perineum to reduce edema and discomfort immediately postpartum. Encourage early ambulation.

Bladder function: Due to infused fluid and the sudden withdrawal of the anti-diuretic hormone (ADH) effect of oxytocin, rapid bladder filling is common. The bladder sensation and ability to empty spontaneously may be diminished by anesthesia as well as by episiotomy, lacerations, or hematomas leading to overdistension and urinary retention. If the woman has not voided after 4 hours, catheterize and search for cause.

Depression: It is fairly common to exhibit some postpartum blues due to the discomfort of early puerperium, fatigue from insomnia during labor and immediate postpartum, anxiety over infant care, or fear of losing sexual or physical attraction to spouse. Treatment in most cases is anticipation and reassurance usually self-limited to 2 to 3 days.

Abdominal wall relaxation: The patient may wear girdle if the abdomen is pendulous. Abdominal exercises may be started anytime after vaginal delivery and as soon as the patient can tolerate after cesarean birth.

TAKE HOME POINTS

- *Diet*: No restrictions if normal spontaneous vaginal delivery (NSVD). If breast-feeding, increase protein and calories.
- *Obstetric neuropathies*: Most common is lateral femoral cutaneous nerve damage. Nulliparity and prolonged second stage of labor are independent risk factors.
- *Pelvic joint separation*: Usually painful locomotion. Treatment is generally conservative with rest in the lateral decubitus position and use of pelvic binder.
- *Immunizations*: RhoGAM, if indicated.
- Rubella vaccination if not immune.
- *Contraceptions*: If not breast-feeding, menses usually returns in 6 to 8 weeks; therefore, start contraception as soon as sexual activities resume.
- *Coitus*: No definite time after delivery for coitus to resume. After 2 weeks, coitus may be resumed based on the patient's comfort and desires.

SUGGESTED READINGS

ACOG Committee Opinion 361. Breastfeeding: maternal and infant aspects. American College of Obstetricians and Gynecologists. *Obstet Gynecol.* 2007;109:479–80.

Anderson WR and Davis J. Placental Site Involution. *Am J Obstet Gynecol.* 1968;102(1): 23–33.

Cunningham FG, Leveno KL, Bloom SL, et al. *Williams Obstetrics.* 22nd ed. New York, NY: McGraw-Hill; 2005.

Dewey KG, Lovelady CA, Nommsey-Rivers LA, et al. A randomized study of the effects of aerobic exercise by lactating women on breast milk volume and composition. *N Engl J Med.* 1994;330(7):449–53.

Farrell SA, Allen VM, Baskett TF. Parturition and urinary incontinence in primiparas. *Obstet Gynecol.* 2001;97(3):350–6.

Oppenheimer LW, Sherriff EA, Goodman JD, et al. The duration of lochia. *Br J Obstet Gynaecol.* 1986;93(7):754–7.

29

WOW! THAT IS A LOT OF BLOOD

TIA M. GUSTER, MD

The postpartum period is very dynamic and starts from the moment the placenta is delivered up to 6 to 12 weeks postpartum. Anyone who has spent time on a busy L&D floor can fully appreciate the term "all hands on deck." Because the stakes are just as high in the postpartum period, not recognizing problems and not mobilizing help can lead to your postpartum ship sinking faster than you can say TITANIC. Bleeding, infection, thrombosis, and hypertension are a few key items that you should keep in mind in order to stay afloat.

Hemorrhage is the third leading cause of maternal mortality. Uterine atony is the most common cause of hemorrhage followed by laceration, retained placental tissue, and finally coagulation defects. Get help, find the source of the bleeding, and get large-bore IVs in place for resuscitation and administration of drugs.

If the patient needs blood products replaced, the following criteria are helpful:

- Hematocrit >21%
- Platelet count >50,000/μL
- Fibrinogen >100 mg/dL
- Prothrombin and partial thromboplastin time <1.5 times

Bimanual compression and massage is the first step in controlling atonic postpartum hemorrhage. This bolsters contraction and compression of uterine vessels. Emptying the bladder greatly increases the success rate. Uterine massage can also assess if retained products of conception (POC) are present until an ultrasound can be brought to the bedside. If the uterus remains tonic, use uterotonic agents. Intravenous fluids with pitocin should be "running wide open." Methergine, Hemabate, and Cytotec are additional agents to have at the bedside. Operative management needs to be considered immediately if hemostasis cannot be achieved by the above measures.

An inspection of the birth canal should be done to locate any cervical and vaginal lacerations. Risk factors for significant cervical lacerations include precipitous labor, operative vaginal delivery, and cerclage. Repair sutures should not be placed superior to the fornix, as this can result in ureteral ligation. When such extension exists, laparotomy should be performed with the patient's thighs abducted in stirrups, thus allowing surgery to proceed simultaneously through abdominal and vaginal routes to facilitate identification of the bladder and ureters.

Vaginal hematomas should not be drained unless they are expanding. Attempts at operative drainage can result in significant additional blood loss because it is often difficult to identify and ligate bleeding vessels in a fresh vaginal sulcus hematoma. A stable hematoma may be drained if it becomes infected or pain is not relieved adequately with analgesics. Continuous expansion of a hematoma leading to hypovolemia may necessitate drainage and packing.

Uterine tamponade such as a balloon or a pack is effective in many patients with atony or lower segment bleeding. Arterial embolization by an interventional radiologist is an option if the woman is hemodynamically stable and personnel and facilities are readily available. A selective procedure is done when a single bleeding vessel is identified and can be occluded. Alternatively, if the area of bleeding is diffuse or a single bleeding vessel cannot be identified, then a large artery that feeds multiple smaller vessels in the area that is bleeding can be occluded.

Laparotomy to assess and treat bleeding in the pelvis should be performed through a vertical midline incision. If a discrete vessel is responsible for hemorrhage, it is clamped and ligated with appropriate suture material. Bilateral ligation of the uterine vessels (O'Leary stitch) has become the first-line procedure for controlling uterine bleeding in the postpartum patient at laparotomy. The B–Lynch suture envelops and compresses the uterus, similar to the result achieved with manual uterine compression. Bilateral ligation of the internal iliac arteries (hypogastric arteries) has been used to control uterine hemorrhage by reducing pulse pressure of blood flowing to the uterus. The technique is difficult, especially with a large uterus, a small transverse incision, a pelvis full of blood, and a surgeon who rarely operates in the pelvic retroperitoneal space. For these reasons, uterine artery ligation has largely replaced this procedure. It is possible to mistakenly ligate the external iliac instead of the internal iliac artery, which usually leads to loss of the ipsilateral lower limb if not promptly corrected. Another area of concern is the large, dilated and fragile internal iliac vein that lies just behind and slightly medial to the artery and is often not visualized during isolation of the artery. Laceration of this vein can lead to rapid exsanguination. Finally, a hysterectomy should be performed if all other operative options are unsuccessful in stopping the loss of blood.

TAKE HOME POINTS

- Bimanual compression and massage is the first action to take with an atonic uterus.
- Empty the bladder.
- Use uterotonic agents and have two large-bore 18-gauge IVs.
- Operative techniques to consider are balloon tamponade or packing, sutures to ligate the uterine or internal iliac vessels, and hysterectomy as a final option.

SUGGESTED READINGS

American Society of Anesthesiologists. Practice guidelines for perioperative blood transfusion and adjuvant therapies: an updated report by the American Society of Anesthesiologists Task Force on Perioperative Blood Transfusion and Adjuvant Therapies. *Anesthesiology*. 2006;105:198.

Bakri YN, Amri A, Abdul Jabbar F. Tamponade-balloon for obstetrical bleeding. *Int J Gynaecol Obstet*. 2001;74:139.

Combs CA, Murphy EL, Laros RK Jr. Factors associated with postpartum hemorrhage with vaginal birth. *Obstet Gynecol*. 1991;77:69.

Mousa HA, Alfirevic Z. Treatment for primary postpartum haemorrhage (Cochrane Review). *Cochrane Database Syst Rev*. 2003:CD003249.

Ornan D, White R, Pollak J, et al. Pelvic embolization for intractable postpartum hemorrhage: long-term follow-up and implications for fertility. *Obstet Gynecol*. 2003;102:904.

POSTPARTUM PREECLAMPSIA

PATRICIA LEE SCOTT, MD AND B. DENISE RAYNOR, MD

A 17-year-old G1 female delivered at 40 weeks after an uncomplicated pregnancy and uncomplicated vaginal delivery. On postpartum day 2, she has BP readings of 166/98 and 162/96, and she reports a significant headache since waking. How should this patient be managed?

Postpartum preeclampsia and eclampsia are rare but can occur after a completely uncomplicated pregnancy and delivery. Just as in an antepartum patient, a postpartum patient should be evaluated fully for preeclampsia as well as other complications related to labor and delivery that can present in a similar fashion. Laboratory studies including urinalysis for protein should be obtained. Magnesium sulfate for seizure prophylaxis should be initiated, and antihypertensive agents should be used to lower blood pressures to below stroke range, with careful avoidance of hypotensive episodes. If the patient's headache or other neurological symptoms do not resolve with BP control, the differential diagnosis must be broadened to include such diagnoses as postepidural puncture headache and intracranial abnormalities. Imaging of the head may be indicated, with CT used for detection of intracranial hemorrhage and MRI (and possibly magnetic resonance angiogram (MRA)/magnetic resonance venography (MRV) for assessment for thrombosis such as venous sinus thrombosis. Early consultation with anesthesiology and neurology is crucial in the management of these patients.

TAKE HOME POINTS

- Postpartum preeclampsia and eclampsia are rare but can occur after a completely uncomplicated pregnancy and delivery.
- Magnesium sulfate for seizure prophylaxis should be initiated.
- Antihypertensive agents should be used to lower blood pressures to below stroke range.
- Imaging of the head may be indicated for assessment for thrombosis such as venous sinus thrombosis.

SUGGESTED READING

Sibai BM. The HELLP syndrome—much ado about nothing? *Am J Obstet Gynecol.* 1990;162:311.

CHECK THE BLOOD: POSTPARTUM ENDOMYOMETRITIS

HEMANT SATPATHY, MD

Postpartum endomyometritis is the commonest infection seen in the postpartum period. Its incidence is 3% to 5% following normal vaginal delivery and 10% following cesarean. In the absence of antibiotics prophylaxis prior to cesarean delivery, this could be as high as 30%. That is why, irrespective of the type of cesarean delivery, elective or nonelective, preoperative antibiotics are recommended to reduce the incidence of postpartum endomyometritis.

This is a clinical diagnosis. These patients present with a temperature >100.4°F after the first 24 hours from the time of delivery. Rarely, they present after postpartum day 10. This fever is documented on at least two occasions 24 hours apart. Other signs and symptoms associated include lower abdominal pain, tender uterus and lower abdomen, foul smelling lochia, excessive vaginal bleeding, malaise, etc.

As postpartum endomyometritis is a clinical diagnosis, these patients need limited workup to exclude other common infections seen in the postpartum period. The workup normally includes urine analysis, urine culture, and CBC with differential count. Other tests are recommended only in presence of relevant history and physical findings. Endometrial culture is discouraged as it is hard to find a good sample without contamination. Even if one gets a good sample without contamination using a triple lumen catheter, its clinical utility is limited as majority of these patients have already responded to the empiric antibiotic regimen and ready to go home by the time the culture results are back. Similarly, the utility of blood culture is limited in most patients with this diagnosis. As with endometrial culture, the blood culture also takes minimum of 48 hours in most patients. By that time, 90% to 97% of these patients with endomyometritis have already responded to the first line of antibiotics (clindamycin with gentamicin). So, the blood culture is redundant and it should not be a routine part of the workup. There are certain exceptions to this rule. These include patients with rigor, those with failed response to conventional antibiotics given for 48 to 72 hours, or those with high clinical suspicion for bacteremia. In these patients, the blood culture helps identify the resistant organisms and their drug sensitivity. That will help change the antibiotics to the appropriate regimen. In general, endomyometritis patients need antibiotics till they are afebrile for at least 24 to 48 hours. In presence of bacteremia, these patients need to go home on a 7-day course of oral antibiotics following their initial treatment with intravenous antibiotics. Thus, the blood culture is useful and cost-effective only in special situations and should not be routinely ordered.

THINGS TO DO

1. Blood culture should be ordered only in endomyometritis patients with rigor, poor response to 48 to 72 hours of conventional antibiotics, or in patients with high suspicion for bacteremia.
2. Following the initial course of intravenous antibiotics, the patients with bacteremia should receive another 7-day course of oral antibiotics.

THINGS NOT TO DO

1. Routine blood culture and endometrial culture in postpartum endomyometritis patients are discouraged.
2. Intravenous antibiotics are only continued for 24 to 48 hours following last temperature spike.
3. In the absence of bacteremia, these patients are not sent home on oral antibiotics.

SUGGESTED READINGS

Creasy RK, Resnick R, Iams JD (eds). *Creasy & Resnik's Maternal-Fetal Medicine*. 6th ed. Philadelphia, PA: W.B. Saunders; 2009.
Cunningham FG, Leveno KL, Bloom SL, et al. *Williams Obstetrics*. 22nd ed. New York, NY: McGraw Hill; 2005.

32

POSTPARTUM CARE: HYPERTENSION

TIA M. GUSTER, MD

Hypertension during postpartum care needs to be assessed and managed quickly as the consequence could be seizure activity, stroke, or further cardiovascular damage. Hypertension is defined as a systolic blood pressure of 140 or diastolic blood pressure of 90. Headache, vision changes, and epigastric or RUQ pain with nausea or emesis are red flags. Once recognized, elevated blood pressure should begin to be reduced to avoid adverse events. In the immediate postpartum period, one should consider the use of hydralazine or labetalol. If this is a consequence of preeclampsia, the administration of magnesium sulfate will decrease the seizure threshold. Dilantin can also be used.

All postpartum patients should have their blood pressure monitored during the initial 6 weeks postpartum period. Blood pressure should be measured during the time of peak postpartum blood pressure, which is days 3 to 6 after delivery. If blood pressures are elevated, antihypertensive treatment should be started; the specific agent used should reflect whether the patient is breast-feeding. Antihypertensive agents acceptable for use in breast-feeding include the following: nifedipine XL, labetalol, methyldopa, captopril, and enalapril. There should be confirmation that end–organ dysfunction of preeclampsia has resolved. Nonsteroidal anti–inflammatory drugs (NSAIDs) should not be given postpartum if hypertension is difficult to control or if there is oliguria, an elevated creatinine, or low platelets. Postpartum thromboprophylaxis may be considered in women with preeclampsia, particularly following antenatal bed rest for >4 days or after cesarean section. Low–molecular-weight heparin should not be administered postpartum until at least 2 hours after epidural catheter removal.

Beyond 6 weeks postpartum, women with a history of severe preeclampsia, especially if they presented before 34 weeks' gestation, should be screened for preexisting hypertension, underlying renal disease, and thrombophilia. Women should be informed that intervals between pregnancies of <2 or ≥10 years are both associated with recurrent preeclampsia. Women with preexisting hypertension should undergo the following investigations: urinalysis; serum sodium, potassium, and creatinine; fasting glucose; fasting total cholesterol and high–density lipoprotein cholesterol, low–density lipoprotein cholesterol and triglycerides; and standard 12-lead electrocardiography. All women who have had an elevated blood pressure should pursue a healthy diet and lifestyle.

TAKE HOME POINTS

- Significant changes in blood pressure or a new elevation as well as signs and symptoms of preeclampsia should be thoroughly evaluated and treated.
- Concerning signs of elevated blood pressure are headache, vision changes, epigastric or RUQ pain with nausea or emesis.
- Antihypertensive agents used while breast-feeding are nifedipine XL, labetalol, methyldopa, captopril, and enalapril.
- Patients with preexisting hypertension should have the following testing: urinalysis; serum sodium, potassium, and creatinine; fasting glucose; fasting total cholesterol and high-density lipoprotein cholesterol, low-density lipoprotein cholesterol and triglycerides; and electrocardiography.

SUGGESTED READINGS

Ghuman N, Rheiner J, Tendler BE, et al. Hypertension in the postpartum woman: clinical update for the hypertension specialist. *J Clin Hypertens.* 2009;11(12):726–733.

Lindheimer MD, Taler SJ, Cunningham FG. Hypertension in pregnancy. *J Am Soc Hypertens.* 2008;2:484–494.

Magee L, Sadeghi S. Prevention and treatment of postpartum hypertension. *Cochrane Database Syst Rev.* 2005;(1):CD004351.

Sibai BM. Diagnosis, prevention, and management of eclampsia. *Obstet Gynecol.* 2005;105:402–410.

POSTPARTUM CARE: THROMBOEMBOLISM

TIA M. GUSTER, MD

Venous thromboembolism is promoted by hypercoagulation, vascular damage, and venous stasis. Risk factors include obesity, bed rest, preeclampsia, and cesarean delivery. The risk increases with a history significant for thrombophilia. If a patient complains of unilateral leg pain and edema, examine both legs and get a Doppler ultrasound to evaluate the presence of a deep venous thromboembolism (DVT). Pulmonary embolism is a serious complication of a DVT. It occurs more commonly during the postpartum period than during pregnancy. If clinical suspicion is high, order a spiral CT and start empiric anticoagulation therapy. It can always be stopped.

TAKE HOME POINTS

- Risk factors include obesity, bed rest, preeclampsia, history of thrombophilia, and cesarean delivery.
- If a patient complains of unilateral leg pain and edema, examine both legs and get a Doppler ultrasound to evaluate the presence of a DVT.

SUGGESTED READINGS

James A, Jamison M, Brancazio L, et al. Venous thromboembolism during pregnancy and the postpartum period: incidence, risk factors, and mortality. *Am J Obstet Gynecol.* 2006;194(5):1311–1315.

Toglia MR, Weg JG. Venous thrombolism during pregnancy. *N Engl J Med.* 1996;335(2): 108–114.

Postpartum care: Infection

Tia M. Guster, MD

An infection should be suspected if your patient has a temperature >38°C on two occasions at least 4 hours apart after the first 24 hours postpartum. The empiric diagnosis is usually endometritis. Endometritis is associated with cesarean section, operative management, premature rupture of membranes, and manual expulsion of the placenta. Antibiotic treatment covers the vaginal flora, aerobic and anaerobic, which has entered into the uterine cavity. Clindamycin and an aminoglycoside are standard first-line therapy. Manual expulsion of the placenta also requires prophylactic antibiotic treatment as well.

A good history and physical exam can never be over emphasized as other sequelae such as urinary tract infection (UTI), pyelonephritis, mastitis, atelectasis, pneumonia, wound infection, septic pelvic thrombophlebitis, hematoma, and abscess should be considered especially if signs and symptoms of infection persist despite treatment. A UTI is the second most common cause of postpartum fever. Mastitis is also common and is categorized as breast engorgement or infective. All wounds should be examined. If necessary, they should be opened and cleaned to promote formulation of granulation tissue. Abscesses and hematomas should be opened, drained, and hemostasis achieved if necessary. A septic pelvic thrombophlebitis can present as extreme illness during febrile spikes. Initiation of heparin therapy should resolve fevers within 24 to 48 hours.

TAKE HOME POINTS

- Fever that persists should be evaluated for other sources and/or consideration of an additional antibiotic agent.
- Evaluate the urine, breasts, lungs, skin, and the pelvic cavity if fevers are unresolved.

SUGGESTED READINGS

Cunningham G, Levano KJ, Gilstrap LC, et al. *Williams Obstetrics.* 22nd ed. New York, NY: McGraw-Hill; 2005.

Garcia J, Aboujaoude R, Apuzzio J, et al. Septic pelvic thrombophlebitis: diagnosis and management. *Infect Dis Obstet Gynecol.* 2006;2006:15614.

Maharaj D. Puerperal pyrexia: a review. Part II. *Obstet Gynecol Surv.* 2007;62(6):400–406.

Schwartz MA, Wang CC, Eckert LO, et al. Risk factors for urinary tract infection in the postpartum period. *Am J Obstet Gynecol.* 1999;181(3):547–553.

Sweet RL, Gibbs RS. Postpartum infection. In: *Infectious Diseases of the Female Genital Tract.* 3rd ed. Baltimore, MD: William and Wilkins, 1995:578–600.

Yokoe DS, Christiansen CL, Johnson R, et al. Epidemiology of and surveillance for postpartum infectious. *Emerg Infect Dis.* 2001;7(5):837–841.

35

POSTPARTUM DEPRESSION: SCREENING AND TREATMENT

AEVA GAYMON-DOOMES, MD, MONIQUE POWELL-DAVIS, MD AND DIANA BROOMFIELD, MD, MBA, FACOG, FACS

Ms. X, a 29-year-old African American woman G2P2003, presented for a 6-week follow-up after giving birth to a set of twins. She complained of fatigue and irritability over the past 2 weeks along with increased worry and anxiety about how she was managing her newborns and transition to work after maternity leave. She is not interested in having sex with her husband, and worries about how the babies will change her marriage. She complained that her family thinks she is "too sensitive" and cries over "everything." She denied any thoughts of wanting to hurt herself or anyone else. One week after her 6-week follow-up, she telephoned her OB/GYN to inquire about sleeping medication and asked if she could come in to pick up a prescription. When she came in to pick up her prescription, her physician administered the Postpartum Depression Screening Scale (Beck and Gable, 2000) and received a positive result. After assessing for immediate risk of suicidality or homicidality, Ms. X was then referred for an evaluation at the mental health clinic and given a 3-day supply of sleeping medication.

A common error to avoid is not assessing your postpartum patients for new onset or exacerbation of mental disease, namely depression. Postpartum depression (PPD) has the same diagnostic criteria as major depression, except that it specifically occurs during the postpartum period. Many women experience changes in mood during and after the course of pregnancy. During the postpartum period, symptoms of baby blues and PPD are very similar and both include changes in sleep, appetite, mood, changes in weight, and increased anxiety. Normal mood instability, due to hormonal changes of the postpartum period, can make distinguishing between baby blues and PPD difficult for a new mother and health care professionals. PPD affects up to 15% of women, yet each year physicians detect only 2% of cases.

SIGNS AND SYMPTOMS

PPD is not listed as a separate diagnosis in the *Diagnostic and Statistical Manual of Mental Disorders (DSM-IV TR)*, but rather with criteria of major depressive disorder and a postpartum "specifier." The *DSM-IV TR* criteria for major depressive episode consist of five or more of the following symptoms: depressed mood for most of the day, decreased interest in pleasure, significant weight loss, changes in sleep, agitation, fatigue, guilt or worthlessness, change in concentration, and recurrent thoughts of death or dying, all for at least 2 weeks with at least one of the symptoms being either depressed mood or loss of interest in pleasure. The "specifier" in the *DSM-IV TR* is that the symptoms of PPD arise within 4 weeks of the postpartum period; however, most experts agree that PPD can be clinically diagnosed anytime in the 12 months following delivery. The clinician must be careful to watch for poor bonding, lack of attachment, obsessive thoughts about the baby being harmed, feeling inadequate as a mother, and guilt about not being able to care for a new or additional child. There is no one single cause of PPD, but the disease may more likely affect women with the following risk factors.

RISK FACTORS
The prevalence of PPD is similar to major depression, with a lifetime risk of 10% to 15%. Women with "baby blues" or a previous history of depression are at higher risk for developing PPD. Other risk factors include discord with co-parent/partner, financial trouble, family history of mental illness, poor social and family supports, physical health trouble, or other life stressors.

SCREENING
Assessing a woman for PPD can include the use of scales such as the Edinburgh Postnatal Depression Scale (EPDS), the Postpartum Depression Screening Scale, or the Beck Depression Inventory (BDI) and should always include questions about safety of both the mother and the baby. Screening can be done on paper in the waiting room or incorporated into the postpartum visits up to 12 months postpartum. The most useful form of screening is proper communication with the patient. The CDC studied 52,000 mothers in 17 states to assess for PPD by asking two questions: "Since your new baby was born, how often have you felt down, depressed, or hopeless?" "Since your new baby was born, how often have you had little interest or little pleasure in doing things?" The possible responses were "always," "often," "sometimes," "rarely," and "never." When mothers responded with "often or always" to either of the two questions, they were classed as experiencing self-reported PPD. The most important aspect of screening is safety. If you suspect PPD, you must ensure that the mother and baby are safe by checking for suicidal or homicidal thoughts in the mother.

TREATMENT
Women with mild symptoms of PPD may benefit from therapy and support groups alone. However, women with moderate to severe symptoms will likely benefit most from pharmacologic intervention, therapy, and increased

community supports. Currently, the pharmacologic treatment of choice is selective serotonin reuptake inhibitors (SSRIs) antidepressants. Untreated PPD places the mother at risk for recurrent and treatment-resistant depression and disturbs the mother's ability to bond and establish attachment with her baby. Infants born to mothers with untreated mood disorders have shown difficulties with emotional regulation and affective stability. The best course of treatment is early detection, treatment, and appropriate follow-up.

TAKE HOME POINTS

- During the postpartum period, up to 85% of women experience some type of mood disturbance. Screening all patients for PPD, even when you have a low index of suspicion, is the best form of patient care.
- Around 10% to 15% of those women who experience a change in mood have a more severe form of mood change, either PPD or postpartum psychosis.
- Although women with a previous or family history of mood or psychiatric disorders are at higher risk for PPD, all women should be routinely screened.
- Commonly used and easy to interpret screening scales are the EPDS and BDI.
- Remember that women who have lost a pregnancy will still need to be screened for PPD.
- Any woman who expresses fear about having thoughts of wanting to harm herself or the baby will need an emergency evaluation by a mental health clinician.
- Patients with concerns of suicidality and/or safety should be co-treated with a psychiatrist. However, an obstetrician that feels comfortable with treating PPD should consider initiating treatment.
- When evaluating a woman for PPD symptoms, make sure to rule out any thyroid disturbances in the postpartum period.
- If clinically indicated the drug class of choice for treating PPD is the SSRIs. However, always be sure to carefully select a medication based on the symptoms of the patient and other factors such as breast-feeding and drug-drug interactions.

SUGGESTED READINGS

American Psychiatric Association. *Diagnostic and Statistical Manual of Mental Disorders.* 4th ed. Washington, DC: American Psychiatric Association; 1994.

Cohen LS and Ruta M. Nonacs. *Mood and Anxiety Disorders During Pregnancy and Postpartum.* Washington, DC: American Psychiatric Publishing, Inc.; 2005.

Kornstein SG, Clayton AH (eds). *Women's Mental Health: A Comprehensive Textbook*. New York, NY: Guilford Press; 2002.

Leigh H, Streltzer JM (eds). *Handbook of Consultation-Liaison Psychiatry*. New York, NY: Springer; 2008.

Mayes LC. *The Yale Child Study Center Guide to Understanding Your Child: Healthy Development from Birth to Adolescence*. UK: Little, Brown and Company; 2003.

Raffelock D. *A Natural Guide to Pregnancy and Postpartum Health*. New York, NY: Avery; 2003.

Sadock BJ, Sadock VA (eds). *Kaplan & Sadock's Synopsis of Psychiatry: Behavioral Sciences / Clinical Psychiatry*. Philadelphia, PA: Lippincott Williams & Wilkins; 2007.

Stein DJ. *Textbook of Mood Disorders*. Washington, DC: The American Psychiatric Publishing, Inc.; 2005.

U.S. Centers for Disease Control and Prevention (CDC). Prevalence of Self-Reported Postpartum Depressive Symptoms, 17 States, 2004–2005. *Morbid Mortal Weekly Rep*. 2008;57(14):361–366.

36

WHY IS THE BABY BLUE? CAUSES OF CYANOSIS IN THE NEWBORN

INEZ REEVES, MD

Baby Boy C is a 1,075-g preterm (gestational age = 28 weeks by early sonogram) born via spontaneous vaginal delivery (SVD). The Mother is a 25-year-old married G2P1 female who had adequate prenatal care since 8 weeks gestation. Her prenatal course was complicated by PPROM at 20 weeks of gestation requiring admission for bed rest and monitoring of amniotic fluid volume and fetal well-being. She has been on antibiotics and has received a complete course of antenatal steroids. She had no fever but failed tocolysis. All her lab results remained negative and she had been in good health with an unremarkable social history.

The amniotic fluid was clear and the infant initially had weak respirations, which progressed to apnea in the delivery room. He was suctioned, given positive pressure ventilation (PPV), intubated, and had intratracheal instillation of a surfactant. Apgar scores were 5 and 8 at 1 and 5 minutes, respectively. The infant was admitted to the neonatal intensive care unit (NICU) with PPV and oxygen via Neopuff infant resuscitator during transport.

On physical examination, he was noted to be mildly cyanotic despite surfactant therapy but otherwise healthy looking with no contractures. His skin was mildly bruised. He was placed on the high-frequency ventilator and his initial umbilical artery catheter arterial blood gas (ABG) was 7. 21/56/72/18/-4. Chest x-ray revealed a borderline small lung volume and minimal reticulogr anularity.

Newborn cyanosis commonly results from problems relating to the respiratory system. Respiratory disorders of the newborn can be managed medically and/or surgically. Medical conditions associated with newborn respiratory distress are discussed below.

RESPIRATORY DISTRESS SYNDROME

A developmental condition associated with premature birth is due to relative surfactant deficiency. Surfactant deficiency, which is inversely related to premature birth, is a major cause of morbidity and mortality. Progress in knowledge and effective treatment has improved survival at lower gestational ages, as low as 24 weeks. The combination of antenatal steroids and postnatal surfactant has shown to decrease morbidity and mortality in preterm infants. Antenatal steroids are used for preventing respiratory distress syndrome (RDS) in 24 to 34 weeks of gestations, with optimal effects if delivery occurs after completion of two doses.

Congenital Pneumonia

This is commonly caused by bacterial infection, especially group B streptococcal infection. It presents similarly but is difficult to distinguish from RDS especially in preterm newborns. In term newborns, it can be associated with pulmonary vasoconstriction during hypoxemia and acidosis, resulting in pulmonary hypertension. Pulmonary hypertension is a progressive form of respiratory failure that requires aggressive and progressive respiratory management in the intensive care nursery. The management of severe pulmonary hypertension may progress to high-frequency ventilator care, nitric oxide, or extracorporeal membrane oxygenation (ECMO).

SURFACTANT PROTEIN B DEFICIENCY

This is an autosomal recessive disorder due to a molecular genetic defect of surfactant protein B and its mRNA. Term infants with this defect present with preterm RDS. They often die from histological features of severe RDS by 1 to 6 months, and they do not respond to exogenous surfactant. Lung transplant is the treatment option for this familial condition.

TRANSIENT TACHYPNEA OF THE NEWBORN (WET LUNG)

This condition is a transient pulmonary edema caused by delayed clearance of fetal lung fluid by the lymphatic system. It is commonly seen in infants born under certain conditions: (1) cesarean delivery that lacks the "big squeeze" effect of vaginal delivery that assists in removal of lung fluid, (2) maternal antenatal management with hypotonic fluids, (3) perinatal distress, (4) infants of diabetic mothers, and (5) breech deliveries. These infants have marked tachypnea (respiratory rates at 80 to 120 breaths per minute), cyanosis, and hyperinflated chest walls from air trapping. The chest x-ray shows engorged pulmonary lymphatics and fluid in fissures. Resolution occurs in 1 to 5 days.

MECONIUM ASPIRATION SYNDROME

Meconium staining of the amniotic fluid complicates about 12% of term or postterm infants. It is indicative of fetal compromise as passage of meconium and gasping respirations occur in utero. Meconium is aspirated into the lungs and is associated with various lung pathologies such as pneumonitis, atelectasis, airway obstruction, gas trapping, ventilation/perfusion (V/Q) mismatch, and pulmonary hypertension. Meconium aspiration syndrome, which is associated with respiratory failure from pulmonary hypertension, complicates 4% of all deliveries. The management involves prevention of meconium aspiration via endotracheal suctioning of depressed infants in the delivery room.

ALVEOLAR CAPILLARY DYSPLASIA

This is a pathologic diagnosis of maldevelopment of pulmonary lobules with deficient capillary beds that do not support lung function.

PULMONARY HYPOPLASIA

This is a pathologic definition of low lung volume–to–body weight ratio. Clinically, it is seen as a relatively small-sized lung on chest x-ray. When lung growth is impaired, there is a small cross-sectional area of vascular bed that predisposes infants to developing pulmonary hypertension. Pulmonary hypoplasia is seen commonly with anatomical sources of hemithorax compression such as diaphragmatic hernias. The exposure of the fetal lungs to amniotic fluid of inadequate volume and appropriate protein composition during the time of branching morphogenesis through alveolar development is also associated with pulmonary hypoplasia.

CONGENITAL HEART LESION

Congenital cyanotic cardiac lesions can present in the peripartum period with the loss of placental support. The Hyperoxia Challenge Test is a common test to determining whether there is a fixed shunt (cardiac etiology) or a reversible shunt (most pulmonary etiology). Immediate cardiology consult and echocardiogram is warranted when suspected.

The surgical conditions associated with newborn respiratory distress are discussed below.

PULMONARY AIR LEAKS

These leaks result from alveolar rupture with dissection of air via vascular sheet into the perivascular sheet and cavities. Pneumothorax occurs when free air enters into the pleural cavity. Pneumopericardium occurs when free air enters into the pericardial space. This can be associated with profound cyanosis not responsive to conventional therapy. A transilluminator and/or chest x-ray can diagnose the free air for immediate evacuation (by needle aspiration and/or chest tube placement) and can be lifesaving to improve the profound hypoxemia and cardiovascular compromise.

DIAPHRAGMATIC HERNIA

Diaphragmatic hernia occurs when there is a failure of the pleuroperitoneal membrane to close the pericardioperitoneal canal at the 5th to 7th week of fetal development. Abdominal contents enter via the posterior lateral foramen of Bochdalek into the pleural space. Diaphragmatic hernia is seen in 1:2,000 to 4,000 deliveries, 80% occur on the left side, and it is associated with a high mortality (24% to 74%) due to severe pulmonary hypoplasia and associated complications. It is associated with maternal polyhydramnios. The infant will present with cyanosis with respiratory difficulties in the delivery room, bowel sounds will be heard in the chest, and the abdomen will be scaphoid. Mortality is high and depends on the degree of lung underdevelopment (pulmonary hypoplasia).

Congenital Cystic Adenomatoid Malformation

This is similar to pulmonary sequestration or bronchogenic cyst. The lesion is usually confined to a single lobe of the lung and it is mostly on the right side. It results from failure of the pulmonary mesenchyme to progress to normal bronchoalveolar development (terminal bronchioles). It is mostly asymptomatic but an enlarged cyst can cause compression symptoms, air trapping, mediastinal displacement, or rupture (pulmonary air leak). It is managed conservatively but intraoperative resection may be necessary if compression of lung tissue occurs. If congenital cystic adenomatoid malformation is not associated with fetal hydrops, there is a 100% survival rate.

Space-Occupying Lesions of the Thoracic Cavity

This can be in the form of a mediastinal mass, usually cystic, and represents congenital remnants or malformation. It can displace the trachea and cause airway narrowing and wheezes.

Disorders of the major airways (choanal atresia, laryngeal webs) that obstruct respirations, rib cage abnormalities that impair the support of respirations, or fulminant bacterial sepsis can also cause cyanosis in the delivery room.

TAKE HOME POINTS

- Maternal prenatal diagnosis of congenital lung defects can aid in anticipation and management of respiratory compromise at delivery.
- There are many etiologies of cyanosis in the newborn. They include disorders of the respiratory, cardiovascular, central nervous (impairing respiratory muscle function), and metabolic system. An organized approach in managing all newborns with the standard of neonatal resuscitation training can place all delivery personnel in readiness for maximal newborn support.

SUGGESTED READINGS

American College of Obstetricians and Gynecologists. ACOG Practice Bulletin No. 97: fetal lung maturity. *Obstet Gynecol.* 2008;112(3):717–726.

American Heart Association and American Academy of Pediatrics. American Heart Association, American Academy of Pediatrics: 2005 American Heart Association (AHA) guidelines for cardiopulmonary resuscitation (CPR) and emergency cardiovascular care (ECC) of pediatric and neonatal patients: neonatal resuscitation guidelines. *Pediatrics.* 2006;117:e1029–e1038.

Jobe AH. Prenatal corticosteroids: a neonatologist's perspective. *NeoReviews.* 2006;7(5): e259–e267.

Rosenberg A. The neonate. In: *Gabbe: Obstetrics: Normal and Problem Pregnancies.* 4th ed. Philadelphia, PA: Churchill Livingstone; 2002:653–699.

Stoll BJ and Adams-chapman I. In Kliegman RM, Behrman RE, Jenson HB et al. (eds.). *Nelson Textbook of Pediatrics, Delivery Room Emergencies.* 18th ed. Philadelphia, PA: Elsevier; 2007:723–728.

Taeusch HW, Ballard RA, Gleason CA (eds). *Avery's Diseases of the Newborn. Respiratory Distress in the Preterm Infant.* 8th ed. Philadelphia, PA: Elsevier Saunders Company; 2004:687–722.

Wert SE. Normal and abnormal structural development of the lung. In: Polin RA, Fox WW, Abman SH, eds. *Fetal and Neonatal Physiology.* 3rd ed. Philadelphia, PA: WB Saunders Company; 2004:783.

37

IT IS OKAY, MOM AND DAD: BENIGN SKIN LESIONS IN THE NEWBORN

MICHAL A. YOUNG, MD, FAAP

This 3,200-g male infant was an normal spontaneous vaginal delivery (NSVD) to an 18-year-old primagravida with Apgars of 8 and 9 at 1 and 5 minutes, respectively. On your morning rounds the day after delivery, the mother asks you about a pustular rash on the baby's face and a small amount on the chest. You tell her that it is probably a normal baby rash. Later in the evening, the baby is sent back to the nursery by the mother because she is concerned because the infant seems irritable and the rash appears more intense. The pediatrician notes that there are two different rashes on the infant, one vesiculopustular lesion on an erythematous base overlying the scalp and the other rash is a small pustular eruption on the cheeks, chest, and back. The pediatrician asks you to do a herpes culture on the mother and ask whether she gave any history of herpes.

Neonatal rashes can appear challenging although most of them are benign. It is important to note whether any of the rashes are over the presenting part. If a rash is noted on the presenting part, one must always consider herpes simplex infection and do the necessary testing to rule it out. In the scenario above, this infant's rash on the scalp was a pustular variation of erythema toxicum. The other rash was another one of the common neonatal rashes, transient neonatal pustular melanosis (TNPM).

SIGNS, SYMPTOMS, AND MANAGEMENT

The pustular lesions are the most common eruptions in the newborn period. Most are easily diagnosed once you know what you are looking for and stay mindful of the rash distribution.

TNPM occurs primarily in African Americans. TNPM has three phases and thus three types of lesions. All phases can be seen at one time. The first phase, superficial vesicopustules, ranging in size from 2 mm to as large as 10 mm, may be present in utero and are virtually always evident at or shortly after birth. The second phase is ruptured pustules manifesting as hyperpigmented macules surrounded by a fine collarette of scale. The third phase consists of hyperpigmented macules without a scale. The most common locations for TNPM are forehead, behind the ears, under the chin, on the neck and back, and on the hands and feet. Palms and soles can also be affected. Diagnosis is made clinically; a Gram stain usually demonstrates polymorphonuclear neutrophils (PMNs) but no bacteria. The lesions resolve spontaneously.

Erythema toxicum is a common condition of term infants, rarely seen in the preterm. Most cases occur between 24 and 48 hours of age. The rash manifests as erythematous macules and wheals of varying sizes with 1- to 2-mm papules and pustules superimposed. Occasionally, lesions appear as vesicles before becoming pustular. The rash often begins on the face, followed by the buttocks, torso, and proximal extremities. The palms and soles are virtually never involved. Diagnosis is usually made clinically; however, the diagnosis can be confirmed with Wright stain of a pustule, which demonstrates numerous eosinophils. The lesions resolve spontaneously over hours to 1 to 2 days. However, new lesions may continue to develop over several days.

Miliaria (prickly heat) is relatively common in newborns especially in warm climates. There are two types of miliaria seen, miliaria rubra and miliaria crystallina. Miliaria rubra is due to blockage of the sweat duct in the stratum corneum, but the obstruction leads to focal leakage of sweat into the dermis resulting in an inflammatory response that presents as erythematous papules and pustules. This rash is more common after the 1st week of life. Miliaria crystalline is due to blockage of the sweat duct at the level of the stratum corneum. Sweat accumulates beneath the stratum corneum, causing tiny flaccid vesicles resembling dewdrops. There is no specific treatment necessary for miliaria as the conditions will dissipate spontaneously if overheating is avoided.

Sebaceous hyperplasia is most prominent on the face, especially around the nose and mouth. It appears as follicular, regularly spaced smooth white-yellowish papules that may group into plaques. No erythema surrounds the lesions. These occur in nearly half of term newborns. It gradually involutes in the first few weeks of life.

Milia are common papules occurring primarily on the face and scalp. They are up to 2 mm, white, smooth-surfaced papules, which are usually discrete. They may be present at birth or occur later. Milia are tiny inclusion cysts within the epidermis that contain concentric layers of trapped, keratinized stratum corneum. The diagnosis is a clinical one. If confirmation is needed, a small incision with the tip of a No. 11 blade will release the contents, which appear either as a smooth white ball or keratinous debris. The lesions usually resolve spontaneously in several months without treatment.

TAKE HOME POINTS

- Rashes that occur over the presenting part should be called to the attention of the pediatrician for further review.
- Most newborn rashes are benign and resolve spontaneously.
- Parents are often concerned about rashes and blemishes on their infants. Reassure them but please refer them to their pediatricians to ensure patient satisfaction.

SUGGESTED READING

Eichenfield L, Frieden I, Esterly N. *Textbook of Neonatal Dermatology*. Philadelphia, PA: W.B. Saunders Company; 2001.

38

NO NEWS IS GOOD NEWS: REPEAT FIRST TRIMESTER PREGNANCY LOSS

NIKKIA HENDERSON WORRELL, MD

"Doctor, why do I keep having miscarriages?" This is a question that nearly all OB/GYN physicians have tried to answer on numerous occasions while starring into the eyes of a tearful patient who desperately wants to have a child. "I don't have a problem getting pregnant; I have a problem staying pregnant." A comment made all too often by women with recurrent pregnancy loss (RPL).

Why this P0030 female has had multiple pregnancy losses is usually not an easy question to answer. As her physician, you know that the differential is broad and requires a costly, long list of laboratory studies, imaging, and a considerable amount of counseling. You are also aware that the majority of the time there is no identifiable cause. Thirty to fifty percent of couples with RPL will still be seeking the answer to that question after sufficient diagnostic evaluation. The nebulous nature of this clinical dilemma is dissatisfying to the goal-oriented physician whose practice is focused on finding problems and solving them efficiently. This situation is often compounded by a patient who is emotionally charged, coping with the psychological challenges of multiple losses. She likely also shares the clinician's desire to quickly find the reason, fix it, and get on with the process of becoming a mother.

How do you effectively guide her through the diagnostic maze, while at the same time preparing her for the possibility that at the end of the day she may still be left wondering? Just remember the common saying, "No News Is Good News!"

RPL is defined as three or more consecutive spontaneous abortions that occur at or before 20 weeks of gestation. In some situations, physicians may choose to initiate an RPL workup with only two consecutive losses, particularly in the setting of advanced maternal age or couples with infertility.

There are many factors that predispose a couple to recurrent miscarriages. The most common factors listed in order of prevalence are

> *Uterine anatomic anomalies*: Septated uterus, Asherman syndrome, leiomyoma
>
> *Immunologic anomalies*: Antiphospholipid syndrome
>
> *Endocrine anomalies*: Thyroid dysfunction, luteal phase defect
>
> *Genetic anomalies*: Parental chromosomal abnormality, fetal chromosomal abnormality
>
> Infection
>
> Environmental

True, the risk of recurrent miscarriages increases with successive losses. However, there does seem to be a plateau effect. Even in the setting of six prior miscarriages, the risk of loss in the next pregnancy is a little over 50%. Jeng demonstrated through meta-analysis of randomized prospective studies that 60% to 70% of couples with unexplained RPL will have a successful next pregnancy. This is a fairly optimistic prognosis that is comparable to success rates of known causes of RPL postintervention.

Therefore, even in the light of a negative workup, the clinician may remain cautiously optimistic about this patient's chance to achieve a successful pregnancy. "No news is good news!" Often, unexplained RPL patients are successful without any intervention. Some clinicians recommend empiric exogenous progesterone or even low-dose aspirin therapy, despite the lack of clear evidence of their effectiveness. Many couples who fall into this category do well with timed intercourse, close follow-up, and supportive care. With time and effort nature usually finds a way.

TAKE HOME POINTS

- The most common etiology of RPL is idiopathic.
- RPL is defined as three or more consecutive spontaneous abortions that occur at or before 20 weeks of gestation.
- The majority of couples with RPL will successfully achieve a successful pregnancy without intervention.

SUGGESTED READINGS

American College of Obstetricians and Gynecologists. ACOG Practice Bulletin No. 24: management of recurrent early pregnancy loss. February 2001. Reaffirmed 2008.

Jeng GT, Scott JR, Burmeister LF. A comparison of meta-analytic results using literature vs. individual patient data. Paternal cell immunization for recurrent miscarriage. *JAMA.* 1995;274:830–836.

Speroff L, Fritz M (eds). Recurrent early pregnancy loss. In: *Clinical Gynecologic Endocrinology and Infertility.* 7th ed. Philadelphia, PA: Lippincott Williams & Wilkins; 2005:1070–1101.

39

"SO WHAT IF I HAVE TRIPLETS OR QUADRUPLETS? I SEE IT ALL THE TIME ON TV": THE RISKS ASSOCIATED WITH MULTIPLE GESTATION

JENNIFER FAY KAWWASS, MD

With the popularity of television shows such as "Jon and Kate Plus 8," a reality show chronicling the life of two parents and their twins and sextuplets, the media has normalized multiple gestation and subsequently minimized the public's perceived risk associated with carrying more than one fetus.

Between 1992 and 2002, there was a 65% increase in the frequency of twins and a 500% increase in triplet and high-order births. The majority of the increase resulted from increased use of ovulation induction and of assisted reproductive technology.

Most remarkable, however, is the fetal morbidity associated with multiple gestation. Multifetal births account for only 3% of all live births but are responsible for a disproportionate share of perinatal morbidity and mortality. They account for 17% of all preterm births (at <37 weeks of gestation), 23% of early preterm births (prior to 32 weeks of gestation), 24% of low-birth-weight infants (<2,500 g), and 26% of very-low-birth-weight infants (<1,500 g). Although twins do have an increased risk of morbidity and mortality, a far greater proportion of triplet and high-order multiple gestations have poor outcomes. neonatal intensive care unit (NICU) stays reflect this heightened morbidity; one fourth of twins, three fourth of triplets, and nearly 100% of quadruplets require hospitalization in the NICU, with an average length of stay of 18, 30, and 58 days, respectively. Moreover, all survivors of preterm multifetal births have a significantly increased risk of mental and physical handicap, such as cerebral palsy.

Multifetal gestations also increase maternal morbidity significantly. Women with multiple gestations are nearly six times more likely to be hospitalized with complications, including preeclampsia, preterm labor, preterm premature rupture of membranes, placental abruption (8.2 times more likely), pyelonephritis, postpartum hemorrhage, acute fatty liver of pregnancy, and thromboembolism. In addition, studies that controlled for other contributing factors such as age, weight, and parity found that each additional fetus increases the mother's risk of developing gestational diabetes mellitus (GDM) by 1.8-fold and that fetal reduction significantly decreases this risk. As with GDM, the risk of developing preeclampsia increases significantly (2.6 times higher in twin gestation) with increasing gestational number and is more likely to be more severe and to occur at an earlier gestation than that of a singleton pregnancy complicated by preeclampsia.

As a result of the increased maternal and fetal morbidity and mortality associated with multifetal gestations, high-order multiples merit both specialized care from a maternal fetal medicine specialist and increased antepartum surveillance. Specifically, serial ultrasounds in the 3rd trimester monitor growth, amniotic fluid volume, size discordance, and fetal biophysical profiles. Unfortunately, the ideal frequency and gestational age of initiation of these ultrasounds have not yet been determined by a randomized control trial, and current American College of Obstetrics and Gynecology (ACOG) recommendation suggests heightened monitoring only in the presence of another comorbid condition such as intrauterine growth restriction or maternal disease that would merit heightened screening in a singleton pregnancy.

TAKE HOME POINTS

- There has been a significant increase in the number of multifetal gestations in the past 10 years.
- Multifetal gestation is associated with significant increase in fetal mortality and morbidity including spontaneous abortion, preterm birth, preterm premature rupture of membranes, NICU hospitalization, and long-term motor and cerebral deficits.
- Multifetal gestation is also associated with significant increase in maternal morbidity—particularly preeclampsia, preterm labor, preterm premature rupture of membranes, placental abruption, pyelonephritis, postpartum hemorrhage, acute fatty liver of pregnancy, thromboembolism, and GDM.
- Multifetal gestations merit heightened antenatal testing; however, the specifics of such testing have not been agreed upon by the ACOG.

SUGGESTED READINGS

American College of Obstetricians and Gynecologists. ACOG Practice Bulletin No. 56: multiple gestation: complicated twin, triplet, and high-order multifetal pregnancy. October 2004.

Gabbe SG, Niebyl JR, Joe leigh simpson, et al. (eds). *Multifetal Gestation: Perinatal Morbidity and Mortality. Obstetrics: Normal and Problem Pregnancies.* 5th ed. 2007 New York, NY; Elsevier.

Martin JA, Hamilton BE, Sutton PD, et al. Births: final data for 2002. *Natl Vital Stat Rep.* 2003;52(10):1–102.

Roach VJ, Lau TK, Wilson D, et al. The incidence of gestational diabetes in multiple pregnancy. *Aust N Z J Obstet Gynaecol.* 1998;38:56–57.

40

"I AM PREGNANT WITH TRIPLETS: WHAT ARE MY OPTIONS?"

JENNIFER FAY KAWWASS, MD

Multifetal pregnancy reduction is defined as a first-trimester or early second-trimester procedure for termination of one or more fetuses in a multifetal pregnancy, performed to increase the chances of survival of the remaining fetuses and decrease long-term morbidity for the delivered infants. Selective reduction refers to early intervention, whereas selective termination occurs later usually in response to a documented fetal anomaly and thus incurs greater risk and is rarely performed. With the advent of reproductive technology and the increase in multifetal gestation, more and more couples and physicians face the ethically charged decision of whether or not to pursue selective reduction.

The ideal solution to the question of selective reduction is prevention. It is the responsibility of the physician, particularly the reproductive endo-crinologist, to inform his or her patient of the risk of multifetal gestation, to discontinue cycles if an exceptionally high risk is present, and to diligently monitor such risk throughout an induction cycle. However, no randomized control trial has demonstrated criteria that can reliably determine risk of multifetal pregnancy. Trials have focused on number of ultrasonographi-cally documented follicles (>6) and on serum estrogen levels (>1,500 pg/mL); however, neither reliably predicts risk of multifetal gestation. However, when many follicles are present, the physician possesses the power to pursue alternative approaches and to counsel his or her patient as such. Possibilities include conversion of a gonadotropin cycle to an in vitro fertil-ization (IVF) cycle, selective aspiration of the supernumerary follicles, and limiting the number of embryos transferred in an IVF cycle.

Selective reduction is not without risk—specifically pregnancy loss and lower birth weight of remaining fetuses. Randomized controlled trials suggest pregnancy loss rates of between 4.5% and 15% and are a function of the performing physician's skill and experience. Additional risks include abortion of the remaining fetuses, abortion of the wrong (normal) fetus, retention of a genetically abnormal fetus after reduction, damage without death to a fetus, perterm labor, development of discordancy or growth restriction, maternal infection, hemorrhage, or possible disseminated intra-vascular coagulopathy because of retained products of conception.

The procedure can be performed transcervically, transvaginally, or transabdominally; however, the transabdominal approach is usually the easiest and is performed at 10 to 13 weeks at which time spontaneous abortions have likely occurred and the remaining fetuses can be evaluated ultrasonographically. The smallest or anomalous fetus is chosen for reduction and injected with potassium chloride under ultrasound guidance.

Pregnancy outcomes appear to improve significantly after selective reduction. This trend has been demonstrated in several large trials. Miscarriage rates, delivery prior to 28 weeks, delivery prior to 32 weeks, and perinatal morality have all been shown to decrease significantly. Likewise, take-home baby rates significantly increase in pregnancy managed with selective reduction rather than conservative measures.

TAKE HOME POINTS

- It is the responsibility of the physician to inform his or her patient of the risk of multifetal gestation, to discontinue cycles if an exceptionally high risk is present, and to diligently monitor such risk throughout an induction cycle.
- Selective reduction is not without risk—specifically pregnancy loss, 4.5% to 15%, depending on physician expertise.
- The procedure is most often performed transabdominally under ultrasound guidance at 10 to 13 weeks of gestation.
- Pregnancy outcomes appear to improve significantly after selective reduction.

SUGGESTED READINGS

American College of Obstetricians and Gynecologists. ACOG Committee Opinion No. 369: multifetal pregnancy reduction. June 2007.

Berkowitz RL, Lynch L. Selective reduction: an unfortunate misnomer. *Obstet Gynecol.* 1990;75:873–874.

Gabbe SG, Niebyl JR, Joe Leigh Simpson, et al. (eds). *Multifetal gestation: perinatal morbidity and mortality. Obstetrics: Normal and Problem Pregnancies.* 5th ed. 2007, New York, NY; Elservier.

Gleicher N, Oleske DM, Tur-Kaspa I, et al. Reducing the risk of high-order multiple pregnancy after ovarian stimulation with gonadotropins. *N Engl J Med.* 2000;343:2–7.

Cunningham FG, Leveno KJ, Bloom SL, et al. Multifetal gestation. *Williams Obstetrics.* 22nd ed. 2005, New York, NY McGraw Hill.

41

PHYSIOLOGY OF REPRODUCTIVE ENDOCRINOLOGY: DO NOT FORGET HOW YOU GOT HERE!

PAVNA BRAHMA, MD

Understanding the underlying physiology of reproductive endocrinology provides the foundation for obstetrics and gynecology. The following section reviews key concepts of neuroendocrinology, regulation of the menstrual cycle, and ovarian physiology.

NEUROENDOCRINOLOGY AND REPRODUCTIVE HORMONES

Hypothalamus. The hypothalamus contains neurons that are responsible for the release of several different hormones into the circulation. All of the below hormones are released into the bloodstream and capillaries and travel immediately, via the portal veins, to a second capillary bed in the anterior pituitary where they exert their effects.

> *Thyrotropin-releasing hormone* (TRH): a tripeptide that stimulates the release of thyroid-stimulating hormone (TSH) and prolactin (PRL) when it reaches the anterior pituitary.
>
> *Gonadotropin-releasing hormone* (GnRH): a peptide of ten amino acids, the initiation of pulsatile secretion is essential for the onset of puberty in both males and females. At the level of the anterior pituitary, GnRH triggers the release of luteinizing hormone (LH) and follicle-stimulating hormone (FSH).
>
> *Growth hormone–releasing hormone* (GHRH): a mixture of two peptides, one containing 40 amino acids and the other containing 44. GHRH stimulates cells in the anterior pituitary to secrete growth hormone (GH).

Corticotropin–releasing hormone (CRH): a peptide of 41 amino acids, CRH acts at the level of the anterior pituitary to trigger the release of adrenocorticotropic hormone (ACTH).

Somatostatin: a mixture of two peptides, one of 14 amino acids and the other of 28. The main action of somatostatin is on the anterior pituitary, where it inhibits the release of GH and TSH. Somatostatin is also secreted by the pancreas and the intestine where it inhibits the secretion of many other hormones.

Dopamine: a derivative of the amino acid tyrosine whose main function is to inhibit the release of PRL from the anterior pituitary.

Anterior Pituitary. The anterior lobe of the pituitary contains six types of secretory cells that are specialized to secrete the below hormones in response to hormones from the hypothalamus.

Thyroid-stimulating hormone (TSH): TSH is also known as thyrotropin and is a glycoprotein that consists of an alpha chain and a beta chain. The alpha chain contains 89 amino acids and is identical to the alpha chain in LH, FSH, and human chorionic gonadotropin (HCG). The beta chain contains 112 amino acids and gives TSH its unique properties. *TSH stimulates* the thyroid gland to secrete thyroxine (T_4) by binding to transmembrane G-protein–coupled receptors on the surface of cells of the thyroid.

Follicle-stimulating hormone (FSH): FSH is a heterodimeric glycoprotein that consists of the same alpha chain as in TSH and a beta chain of 115 amino acids that gives it unique properties. The synthesis and release of FSH occur in response to GnRH release from the hypothalamus. FSH controls follicular development and the number of follicles that mature to the preovulatory stage. It also regulates aromatization of androgenic precursors to estradiol in the granulosa cell.

Luteinizing hormone (LH): LH is also a heterodimeric glycoprotein consisting of the same alpha chain as TSH and FSH and a unique beta chain of 115 amino acids. GnRH release from the pituitary is also responsible for the synthesis and release of LH. LH is essential for ovulation and formation of corpus luteum and the LH surge triggers the completion of meiosis I. LH is required for androgen synthesis from cholesterol within theca cells.

Prolactin (PRL): PRL contains 198 amino acids and is responsible for promoting the production of milk. The release of PRL is stimulated by TRH and suppressed by estrogens and dopamine.

Growth Hormone (GH): GH, a protein of 191 amino acids, is also called somatotropin. The release of GHRH from the hypothalamus stimulates the synthesis and release of GH. GH promotes the release of insulin-like growth factor (IGF-1) from the liver.

Adrenocorticotropic hormone (ACTH): ACTH is a peptide of 39 amino acids that works on the cells of the adrenal cortex, stimulating them to produce glucocorticoids, mineralocorticoids, and androgens. The release of CRH from the hypothalamus stimulates the production of glucocorticoids by stimulating the conversion of cholesterol to pregnenolone, a precursor of cortisol.

Posterior Pituitary. *Oxytocin*: Circulating as a free peptide with a short half-life, oxytocin is involved in parturition and milk letdown. It stimulates muscular contractions in the uterus and myoepithelial contractions in the breast. By stimulating prostaglandin synthesis, oxytocin stimulates cervical dilation during labor.

Vasopressin: Vasopressin's main function is the regulation of osmolality and blood volume. It is released when plasma osmolality rises and it is a powerful vasoconstrictor. Angiotensin II stimulates the release of vasopressin in response to osmoreceptors in the hypothalamus and volume receptors in the left atrium, aortic arch, and carotid sinus.

OTHER HORMONES

Inhibin: Inhibin belongs to the TGF-B subfamily and contains an alpha and beta subunit linked by disulfide bonds. Its main action is to inhibit FSH. Inhibin is produced in the gonads, pituitary gland, and placenta. There are two forms of inhibin that differ in their beta subunits (A or B), while their alpha subunits are identical. Inhibin A reaches its peak in the midluteal phase, while inhibin B reaches its peak in early follicular phase and a second peak at ovulation. FSH stimulates the secretion of inhibin from the granulosa cells. In turn, inhibin suppresses FSH. Inhibin secretion is diminished by GnRH and enhanced by IGF-1.

Antimüllerian hormone (AMH): AMH is also known as müllerian-inhibiting substance and belongs to the TGF-B subfamily. It is secreted by granulosa cells and has an inhibitory effect on primordial follicle recruitment. AMH has two main functions: it inhibits initial follicle recruitment and inhibits FSH-dependent growth and selection of pre-antral and small antral follicles. AMH levels decrease with age, making it a possible ideal marker for the size of the ovarian follicle pool.

THE MENSTRUAL CYCLE

The menstrual cycle can be divided into two phases, the follicular or proliferative phase and the luteal or secretory phase.

Follicular Phase. The follicular phase of the menstrual cycle begins with the day of menstruation and continues until ovulation. Development of ovarian follicles occurs in this phase, beginning during the last few days of the preceding menstrual cycle. FSH levels rise during the last few days of the menstrual cycle, as inhibin A and B levels decline dramatically. The rise in FSH activates aromatase activity in granulosa cells, therefore increasing conversion of androgens to estrogens. These granulosa cells also secrete peptides that work in an autocrine and paracrine fashion to rescue a cohort of follicles from apoptosis, pushing them to the preantral stage. The increased FSH and estrogen levels increase FSH receptors and further stimulate the proliferation of granulosa cells. Selection of a dominant follicle is the process by which a single follicle is destined for ovulation. The development of the dominant follicle begins on days 1 through 4 of the menstrual cycle in response to rising FSH. Multiple factors, including withdrawal of gonadotropin support, local growth factors, and autocrine-paracrine interactions, contribute to atresia of the less developed follicles. Apoptosis, or programmed cell death, is thought to be responsible for diminishing the remaining follicle cohort.

Ovulation. The preovulatory follicle produces large amounts of estradiol, which leads to an LH surge. Ovulation typically occurs 10 to 12 hours after the LH peak and 34 to 36 hours after the LH surge begins. The LH surge induces luteinization of granulosa cells and stimulates synthesis of progesterone. It also stimulates the resumption of meiosis and the division of the oocyte leading to release of the first polar body.

Luteal Phase. Following ovulation, the granulosa cells continue to enlarge and accumulate lutein, a yellow pigment. The corpus luteum is formed by luteinized granulosa cells, theca lutein cells, and surrounding stroma. Its main function is to secrete progesterone and prepare the endometrium for implantation. Active angiogenesis occuring in the early luteal phase is mediated by vascular endothelial growth factor (VEGF). Eight or nine days after ovulation, the endometrium peaks in vascularization, correlating with peak levels of estradiol and progesterone. During the luteal phase, new follicular growth is inhibited by the central feedback of estradiol, progesterone, and inhibin A levels. Approximately 9 to 11 days after ovulation, corpus luteum function begins to decline. Unless pregnancy occurs and HCG is produced, the corpus luteum undergoes luteolysis and becomes scar tissue, otherwise known as the corpus albicans.

THE TWO-CELL, TWO-GONADOTROPIN HYPOTHESIS

This important two-cell system describes the interaction between the granulosa and theca cell compartments. It describes activation by LH and

FSH that results in the ultimate conversion of cholesterol to androgens and estrogens. LH stimulates androstenedione and testosterone production in theca cells. Androstenedione is then transported to the granulosa cells where it is aromatized to estrone. It is finally converted to estradiol by 17-β-hydroxysteriod dehydrogenase type I. This concept is known as the two–cell, two–gonadotropin hypothesis of regulation of estrogen production in the human ovary.

UNDERSTANDING OOGENESIS

During fetal and early postnatal life, oogonia (immature germ cells) undergo mitosis. They become arrested in prophase of meiosis I, where they continue to grow in size, accumulate cytoplasm, and begin to form a zona pellucida. The preovulatory surge of LH initiates the resumption of meiosis I at the onset of puberty and at each ovulatory cycle. Near the time of ovulation, meiosis I ends, and the primary oocyte divides into a secondary oocyte and the first polar body. Meiosis is then arrested again in metaphase II until penetration of the ooctye by spermatozoa occurs.

TAKE HOME POINTS

- Hormones released by the hypothalamus travel via the portal veins to a capillary bed in the anterior pituitary where they exert their effects.
- The alpha chain in TSH, LH, FSH, and HCG is an identical chain of 89 amino acids. The beta chains of these hormones give them their distinguishing properties.
- During the follicular phase of menstruation, the rise in FSH stimulates a rise in estradiol and proliferation of granulosa cells. During the luteal phase, the corpus luteum secretes progesterone which prepares the endometrium for implantation and may later sustain a pregnancy.
- AMH is secreted by granulosa cells, decreases with age, and may be an ideal marker for ovarian reserve.
- Activation by LH and FSH results in the ultimate conversion of cholesterol to androgens and estrogens.
- Oogonia are arrested in prophase of meiosis I until the LH surge occurs at puberty.

SUGGESTED READINGS

Bauer-Dantoin AC, Wess J, Jameson JL. Roles of estrogen, progesterone, and gonadotropin-releasing hormone (GnRH) in the control of pituitary GnRH receptor gene expression at the time of the preovulatory gonadotropin surges. *Endocrinology*. 1995;136:1014.

De Koning J. Gonadotropin surge-inhibiting/attenuating factor governs luteinizing hormones secretion during the ovarian cycle: physiology and pathology. *Hum Reprod*. 1995;10:2854.

Durlinger AL, Visser JA, Themmen APN. Regulation of ovarian function: the role of anti-Mullerian hormone. *Reproduction.* 2002;124:601.

Erickson GF, Magoffin DA, Dyer CA, et al. The ovarian androgen producing cells: a review of structure/function relationships. *Endocr Rev.* 1985;6:371.

Evans JJ. Modulation of gonadotropin levels by peptides acting at the anterior pituitary gland. *Endocr Rev.* 1999;20:46.

Fillicori M. The role of luteinizing hormone in folliculogenesis and ovulation induction. *Fertil Steril.* 1999;71:405.

Magoffin DA, Jakimiuk AJ. Inhibin A, inhibin B, and activin A in the follicular fluid of regularly cycling women. *Hum Reprod.* 1997;12:1714.

42

DO NOT FORGET ALL THE SIGNS OF OVULATION

TARA P. CLEARY, MD

After counseling a patient on the several methods of contraception, she states that she and her partner do not want to use any contraception or they wish to only use condoms. You affirm that they are not actively trying to conceive, they just do not wish to use contraception. Is there any further information you can provide to prevent an unplanned pregnancy? The answer is yes—you can educate her on the several methods of contraception that come under the umbrella of Fertility Awareness.

In order to consider a fertility awareness method (FAM), the couple should be counseled that 25% of women practicing FAM become pregnant. They should also be aware that FAM does not protect against sexually transmitted diseases. To be most effective, the female ought to have regular menstrual cycles and the specific method needs to be practiced consistently. FAMs include the calendar rhythm method (CRM), standard days method (SDM), basal body temperature (BBT) method, ovulation/cervical mucus method, symptothermal method, and lactational mmenorrhea method, which is discussed in another chapter.

Besides the lactational amenorrhea method, all of these methods identify the fertile window and promote abstinence or barrier methods during this window to prevent conception. Most educated women know that ovulation occurs in the middle of their menstrual cycle. Day 1 of the cycle marks the 1st day of menses, and ovulation usually occurs 2 weeks prior to menses or around day 14 in a 28-day cycle. From the time of ovulation, a female egg can survive 24 hours, while sperm survive for 3 days; thus, unprotected intercourse 3 days prior to and up until ovulation can impregnate a woman. These are basic principles; however, the methods of Fertility Awareness follow more precise guidelines.

According to the SDM, approximately 80% of cycles last 26 to 32 days; thus, the majority of cycles have a fertile window between days 8 and 19. Therefore, patients are able to have unprotected intercourse from day 1 through day 7 and day 20 through the end of the cycle while abstaining from days 8 to 19 or using a barrier method. SDM is most appropriate for women with regular cycles. If the patient has greater than one cycle in 1 year of <26 days or >32 days, she should be encouraged to use another method. The CRM focuses on an individual patient's cycle pattern, identifying the shortest and longest cycles and calculating the probable days of fertility for the current cycle. Patients are to keep record of the past 6 to 12 cycle lengths. Once the patient identifies the longest and shortest cycles, the patient should subtract 18 from the number of days in the shortest cycle to identify the first fertile day in the current cycle. To identify the last fertile day, the patient should subtract 11 from the number of days in the longest cycle. The patient must update the calculation for each cycle and avoid unprotected intercourse during the fertile window.

The ovulation, or Billings, method involves the observation of cervical mucus. This method requires the assistance of a trained instructor to teach the patient how to "look, touch, and feel" for changes indicating fertility. Patients must check mucus before and after every urination; they must look at the color and consistency, touch to determine stretch and slipperiness, and feel how wet is the vulvar sensation. Highly fertile mucus is abundant, clear, stretchy, wet, and slippery. The fertile window is when this highly fertile mucus is first observed till 4 days past the peak day or last day of wetness. Patients are advised not to douche and to avoid any intercourse or lubrication during the first cycle to avoid contamination. Unlike the SDM or CRM, this method can be used by women who have slightly irregular cycles.

The symptothermal approach combines the Billings method with BBT monitoring. BBT is lower in the first part of the cycle, rises around ovulation, and remains elevated for the rest of the cycle. The patient is to check and record her temperature upon waking in the morning, either orally, rectally, or vaginally. This allows her to retrospectively identify whether she has ovulated and can then identify the end of her fertile window. A patient following BBT alone must abstain from day 1 of menses until the postovulatory period or until the 3rd consecutive day of temperature rise. By combining BBT with the ovulation method—the symptothermal approach—a patient can use cervical secretion changes to identify the beginning of the fertile window and use BBT to identify the end of the window.

The effectiveness of the FAM depends on the accuracy of the method in identifying the fertile window. The couple must thus be able to identify that time period, and they must be able to follow instructions for the method. In the 1st year of use, perfect users of the method experienced an unintended pregnancy rate of 2% to 5%, while SDM typical use is 12% and condom use 15%.

Advantages of the FAMs are that their teaching not only affords patients the knowledge of when they should abstain from unprotected sex but also lets them know when they can best attempt conception. There are times when these methods are difficult to use such as recent childbirth, current breast-feeding, recent menarche, recent discontinuation from hormonal contraceptive methods, and the perimenopause period. Poor male cooperation also makes these methods difficult. These methods are not recommended for irregular cycles—especially the SDM, the inability to interpret fertility signs correctly, or persistent reproductive tract infections that affect signs of fertility.

TAKE HOME POINTS

- SDM is an easy method for women with regular cycles between 26 and 32 days and must abstain or use a barrier method from days 8 to 19.
- CRM requires active documentation of a patient's menstrual history to identify the patient's fertile window.
- The Billings method requires a trained instructor to teach the patient how to "look, touch, and feel" for fertile mucus, which is abundant, clear, stretchy, wet, and slippery. The fertile window is when this highly fertile mucus is first observed till 4 days past the peak day or last day of wetness.
- The end of the fertility window can be identified with BBT as the 3rd consecutive day of temperature rise.

SUGGESTED READINGS

Gribble J, Lundgren RI, Velasquez C, et al. Being strategic about contraceptive introduction: the experience of the Standard Days Method. *Contraception*. 2008;77:147–154.

Grimes D, Gallo MF, Grigorieva V, et al. Fertility awareness-based methods for contraception: systematic review of randomized controlled trials. *Contraception*. 2005;72:85–90.

Hatcher R, Trussell J, Nelson AL, et al. *Contraceptive Technology*. New York, NY: Ardent Media; 2004.

ABNORMAL BLEEDING

43

ABNORMAL UTERINE BLEEDING: BLOOD IS NORMAL, ISN'T IT?

OSUEBI OKECHUKWU, MD AND DIANA BROOMFIELD, MD

A 27-year-old nulliparous sales executive presents with a history of prolonged heavy menstrual flow. Symptoms started about a year ago and she admits to using about eight pads per day with associated clots. Her menstrual cycle occurs every 30 days with duration of about 10 days. She reports a history of having had two blood transfusions for symptomatic anemia. She is sexually active and uses condoms occasionally and denies any history of sexually transmitted infections (STIs). She was initially placed on oral contraceptive pills (OCPs) and reports noncompliance. She is a known asthmatic for which she uses albuterol. She is allergic to penicillin. She smoked occasionally in the past but stated that she quit about 6 years ago. Her mother is a diabetic and suffered a cardiovascular accident (CVA) about 4 years ago. Apart from mild pallor, physical examination was unremarkable. Her hematocrit was 28% with a low serum ferritin level. All other laboratory and radiologic investigations were unremarkable.

Abnormal uterine bleeding (AUB), which can have varied presentations, affects women in all age groups and can present as frequent bleeding episodes, excessive menstrual loss, prolonged bleeding and intermenstrual bleeding. It is a known cause of discomfort, reduced quality of life, lost time from work, and anxiety and depression among affected women with increased cost on the health care system.

ETIOLOGY
The etiology of AUB is varied and is broadly classified into two groups:

1. Organic
2. Dysfunctional

Identified organic etiologies can range from blood coagulation disorders (Von Willebrand disease, prothrombin disorder), hypothyroidism, liver cirrhosis, accidents of pregnancy, malignancy of the female genital tract, endometriosis, leiomyomas, foreign bodies to structural anomalies. Dysfunctional uterine bleeding (DUB) categories include both anovulatory and ovulatory causes.

DIAGNOSIS

A complete history and physical examination with laboratory and radiologic workup are indicated in a woman presenting with AUB to elicit the cause of the bleeding. After the organic and iatrogenic causes have been ruled out, a diagnosis of DUB can be made. DUB can be ovulatory or anovulatory, including estrogen breakthrough bleeding, estrogen withdrawal bleeding, and progestin breakthrough bleeding. Ovulatory DUB is common in adolescent years and before perimenopause, while anovulatory DUB occurs in the extremes of reproductive life. DUB has been described as

- Amenorrhea: No uterine bleeding for 6 months or longer
- Intermenstrual bleeding (spotting): Uterine bleeding of variable amounts occurring between regular menstrual periods
- Menorrhagia: Prolonged (>7 day) or excessive (>80 mL daily) uterine bleeding occurring at regular intervals
- Metrorrhagia: Uterine bleeding occurring at irregular and more frequent than normal intervals
- Menometrorrhagia: Prolonged or excessive uterine bleeding occurring at irregular and more frequent than normal intervals
- Oligomenorrhea: Uterine bleeding occurring at intervals of 35 days to 6 months
- Polymenorrhea: Uterine bleeding occurring at regular intervals of <21 days

TREATMENT OPTIONS

The management of AUB should be tailored toward the etiology of the symptom and the reproductive needs of the patients. In the absence of an anatomic etiology, medical treatment is preferred over surgical treatment especially in a woman of reproductive age group who desires the preservation of fertility.

Treatment options include the use of progestins, estrogen, NSAIDs, antifibrinolytics, danazol, and GnRH agonists.

When long-term treatment of abnormal bleeding by hormonal management has failed due to continued symptoms, poor compliance, or side effects, an endometrial ablation is an effective alternative, but this treatment option is unsuitable for women who desire to preserve their fertility. Hysterectomy, though the definitive treatment for AUB, is also not indicated for women who wish to preserve fertility.

PROGESTIN INTRAUTERINE DEVICES

There is a strong evidence to suggest that the levonorgestrel-containing intrauterine device (IUD) may be considered as first line in the treatment of AUB since it is easy to insert, cost-effective, and has minimal side effects. Levonorgestrel causes decidualization of endometrial stroma and atrophy of endometrial glands, thus the levonorgestrel-containing IUD compares favorably to oral progesterone, NSAIDs, and endometrial ablation at reducing menstrual loss. The levonorgestrel-containing IUD has no effect on blood pressure, lipid profile, and glucose control in well-controlled diabetics and poses no additional risk of thromboembolism.

TAKE HOME POINTS

- AUB is a great source of discomfort and reduced quality of life compared with women in the general population within the same age group.
- Treatment of AUB should be tailored toward the identified cause and desire for future fertility.
- The levonorgestrel-containing IUD has been shown to be a highly effective, cost-effective, and acceptable modality of treatment of menorrhagia especially in women of reproductive age group and can be considered as a first line of treatment.
- The purported risks associated with IUD use have at best not been confirmed by controlled clinical researches.
- Adequate patient counseling and selection are important in achieving the desirable effect in the management of AUB with progestin IUD.

SUGGESTED READINGS

American College of Obstetricians and Gynecologists. ACOG Committee Opinion No. 392. 110(6), 2007.

Andersson JK, Rybo G. Levonorgestrel-releasing intrauterine device in the treatment of menorrhagia. *Br J Obstet Gynaecol*. 1990;97:690–694.

Barrington JW, Bowen-Simpkins P. The levonorgestrel intrauterine system in the management of menorrhagia. *Br J Obstet Gynecol*. 1997;104:614–616. (Level II-2).

Busfield RA, Farquliar CM, Sowter MC, et al. A randomized Trial comparing the Levonorgestrel Intrauterine System and Thermal balloon ablation for heavy menstrual bleeding. *Obstet Gynecol Surv*. 2006;61(7):257–263.

Fedele L, Bianchi S, Raffaelli R, et al. Treatment of adenomyosis-associated menorrhagia with a levonorgestrel-releasing intrauterine device. *Fertil Steril*. 1997;68:426–429.

Graff-Iversen S, Tonstad S. Use of progestogen-only contraceptives/medications and lipid parameters in women age 40 to 42 years: results of a population-based cross-sectional Norwegian Survey. *Contraception*. 2002;66:7.

Hurskainen R, Paavonen J. Levonorgestrel releasing intrauterine system in the treatment of heavy menstrual bleeding. *Curr Opin Obstet Gynecol*. 2004;16:487–490.

Hurskainen R, Teperi J, Rissanen P, et al. Quality of life and cost-effectiveness of levonorgestrel- releasing intrauterine system versus hysterectomy for treatment of menor-rhagia: a randomized trial. *Lancet.* 2001;357:273–277.

Katz LK, Lentz GM, Lobo RA, et al. *Comprehensive Gynecology.* 5th ed. Philadelphia, PA: Elsevier; 2007.

Lethaby AE, Cooke I, Rees M. Progesterone or progestogen-releasing intrauterine systems for heavy menstrual bleeding. *Cochrane Database Syst Rev.* 2005:CD002126.

Lukkainen T, Allonen H, Haukkamaa M, et al. Effective contraception with the levonorg-estrel- releasing intrauterine device: 12-month report of a European multicenter study. *Contraception.* 1987;36:169–179.

Mercorio F, Simone RD, Sardo ADS, et al. The effect of a levonorgestrel-releasing intrauterine device in the treatment of myoma related menorrhagia. *Contraception.* 2003;67:277–280.

Mosher WD, Martinez GM, Chandra A, et al. Use of contraception and use of family plan-ning services in the United States: 1982–2002. *Adv Data* 2004;350:1–36.

Phillips V, Graham CT, Manek S, et al. The effects of the levonorgestrel intrauterine system (Mirena Coil) on endometrial morphology. *J Clin Pathol.* 2003;56:305–307.

Rogovskaya S, Rivera R, Grimes DA, et al. Effect of a levonorgestrel intrauterine system on women with type 1 diabetes: a randomized trial. *Obstet Gynecol.* 2005;105:811–815.

Sheppard BL. Endometrial morphological changes in IUD users: a review. *Contraception.* 1987;36:1–10.

Speroff L, Fritz M. *Clinical Gynecologic Endocrinology and Infertility.* 7th ed. Philadelphia: Lippincott Williams & Wilkins; 2005.

Tang GW, Lo SS. Levonorgestrel intrauterine device in the treatment of menorrhagia in Chinese women: efficacy versus acceptability. *Contraception.* 1995;51:231–235 (Level III).

World Health Organization. *Medical Eligibility Criteria for Contraceptive Use.* Geneva, Swit-zerland: World Health Organization; 2004.

44

ACUTE HEAVY BLEEDING SHOULD BE TREATED WITH ESTROGEN OR DILATION AND CURETTAGE

MARTINA BADELL, MD

If a patient presents to the emergency room complaining of heavy vaginal bleeding and she has evidence of significant blood loss such as anemia, tachycardia, or hypotension, she requires admission to the hospital and acute treatment. If the patient is hemorrhaging and hemodynamically unstable, she requires resuscitation with two large-bore IVs, rapid fluid infusion, possible blood transfusion, placement of a Foley catheter with a 30-mL balloon in the uterus for tamponade, and to be taken to the OR for evaluation and treatment with likely dilation and curettage (D&C) or possible hysterectomy if the bleeding cannot be controlled and the patient remains unstable. However, it is much more common for patients to present with heavy vaginal bleeding, anemia, and hemodynamic stability.

A detailed history is crucial, and information such as the volume and duration of bleeding, gynecologic, obstetric, and medical history, medications, prior episodes of bleeding, possibility of pregnancy, and associated symptoms needs to be obtained. Physical exam must be performed noting vitals, as well as general exam and then a thorough gynecological exam. Some basic laboratory exams that should be ordered include pregnancy test, complete blood count, and type and screen. In addition, a pelvic ultrasound is helpful in evaluating the endometrial lining once the patient is stabilized.

Most cases of acute bleeding can be treated with medical therapy and do not require surgical intervention. Estrogen is used to treat acute vaginal bleeding as it causes rapid endometrial growth. In addition, it is thought that large doses of estrogen may potentially lead to helping platelet adhesiveness. Estrogen therapy can be given intravenously or orally to treat acute bleeding. Conjugated equine estrogen (Premarin) dosing is 25 mg IV every 3 to 4 hours or 2.5 mg orally every 4 hours. It takes at least a couple of hours to see bleeding improvement or cessation as it takes time for the required mitotic activity and endometrial growth. Combination oral contraceptive pills (OCPs) at high doses can also be used to treat acute bleeding. Four 35-μm OCPs can be taken in divided doses every 24 hours. This usually provides adequate estrogen to stop bleeding. However, as OCPs have a progestin component, they may not work as effectively or quickly as estrogen alone as progestin inhibits estrogen receptors and therefore delays endometrial proliferation. Overall, an oral estrogen regimen is generally more practical than an intravenous regimen. High-dose estrogen is often associated with significant nausea and sometimes vomiting and therefore an antiemetic should be concomitantly prescribed while treating these patients.

Although a D&C is more invasive, it is the best choice for women who are hemodynamically unstable, severely anemic, do not respond with a significant decrease in bleeding in the first 24 hours of estrogen therapy, or have a contraindication to estrogen therapy. Also if the pelvic ultrasound reveals the endometrium is >10 mm or if any anatomic pathology is seen, it may be more beneficial to perform a D&C.

After the acute bleeding has resolved, amenorrhea should be maintained for several weeks to allow improvement of anemia. The best method of therapy is usually combination oral contraceptives. Iron therapy should also be prescribed to all anemic patients. Once the patient is stabilized and her anemia improved, it is important to determine the underlying disorder that lead to the acute bleed and treat appropriately.

It is important that high-dose estrogen be prescribed with caution given the increased risk of thromboemoblic events. Women with history of prior thrombosis, cardiac disease, estrogen-responsive cancers, and smokers over 35 years old are not candidates for estrogen therapy.

TAKE HOME POINTS

- High-dose estrogen given either orally or intravenously usually stops acute bleeding. Oral estrogen is less expensive and easier to give.
- A D&C should be strongly considered to stop acute bleeding in patients who are hemodynamically unstable, older than 35 years old, severely anemic, do not respond to estrogen therapy within the first 24 hours, or those who have a contraindication to estrogen therapy.
- Always do a pregnancy test when a woman of reproductive age presents with abnormal bleeding.
- Prescribe antiemetic medication when giving high-dose estrogen to patients.

SUGGESTED READINGS

American College of Obstetricians and Gynecologists. Clinical Management Guidelines for Obstetrician-Gynecologist. ACOG Practice Bulletin No. 14: management of anovulatory bleeding. March 2000.

Jurema M, Zacur HA. Menorrhagia. In: Rose BD, ed. *UpToDate*. Wellesley, MA. 2008.

Lobo RA. In: Katz VL, ed. *Comprehensive Gynecology*. 5th ed. Philadelphia, PA: Mosby Elsevier; 2007:915–931.

45

WHEN IN DOUBT: BIOPSY, BIOPSY, BIOPSY

RUSSELL HILL, MD

A 55-year-old female G1P0010 complains of vaginal spotting. She has not had menses since 4 years ago and she thought everything was over. She is interested in knowing what should be done. She denies use of any hormone replacement and she has an occasional hot flash, which is not bothersome.

Postmenopausal bleeding can be initially evaluated by endometrial sampling or transvaginal ultrasound. Sometimes, office endometrial sampling is inadequate and transvaginal ultrasound is nonreassuring. Further endometrial sampling is recommended to evaluate the endometrial lining. Office sampling is less likely to identify focal lesions such as submucous myomas, focal hyperplasias, and polyps. Unenhanced endovaginal ultrasonography followed by saline infusion sonohysterography can be used to decide if no endometrial sampling, nondirected sampling, or directed sampling should be done depending on if anatomic abnormalities, globally thickened endometrial tissue, or focal abnormalities were detected. When compared with endometrial biopsy and saline infusion sonography, endometrial sampling provided a diagnosis 52% of the time compared with 89% of the time for the former method.

Three-dimensional (3D) transvaginal ultrasound when compared with two-dimensional (2D) ultrasound in tissue confirmed diagnosis was better at determining negative cases of endometrial cancer than 2D ultrasound. Endometrial volume cutoff was 2.7 mL, and the mean endometrial thickness for endometrial cancer was 16.6 mm.

Hysteroscopy can be performed as an inpatient and as an office procedure. In 1996, the number of women to have the outpatient hysteroscopy was estimated at 232,000 and 20% had operative procedures. Hysteroscopy is superior in detecting focal abnormalities and also in diagnosing cases with endometrial thickness <4 mm.

TAKE HOME POINTS

- Office sampling may misdiagnose endometrial pathology.
- Patients with postmenopausal bleeding may be triaged by utilizing unenhanced sonohysterography.

- If available, 3D ultrasonography, endometrial volume measurement, is superior to 2D ultrasonography.
- Hysteroscopy is useful in detecting focal lesions and in diagnosing lesions with endometrium <4 mm.

SUGGESTED READINGS

American College of Obstetricians and Gynecologists. ACOG Committee Opinion No. 426: the role of transvaginal ultrasonography in the evaluation of postmenopausal bleeding. *Obstet Gynecol.* 2009:113:462–464.

Goldstein SR, Zeltser I, Horan CK, et al. Ultrasonography-based triage for perimenopausal patients with abnormal uterine bleeding. *Am J Obstet Gynecol.* 1997;177(1):102–108.

Moschos E, Ashfaq R, McIntire DD, et al. Saline-infusion sonography endometrial sampling compared with endometrial biopsy in diagnosing endometrial pathology. *Obstet Gynecol.* 2009;113(4):881–887.

Van Doorn HC, Opmeer BC, Burger CW, et al. Inadequate office endometrial sample requires further evaluation in women with postmenopausal bleeding and abnormal ultrasound results. *Int J Gynaecol Obstet.* 2007;99(2):100–104.

Yaman C, Habelsberger A, Tews G, et al. The role of three-dimensional volume measurement in diagnosing endometrial cancer in patients with postmenopausal bleeding. *Gynecol Oncol.* 2008;110(3):390–395.

46

TO PAP OR NOT TO PAP, THAT IS THE QUESTION: PREVENTIVE CARE FOR THE GYNECOLOGIC PATIENT

LYDIA MAYIDA, MD AND DIANA BROOMFIELD, MD, MBA, FACOG, FACS

A 17-year-old female patient comes to see you for her first annual exam; she admits early first sexual intercourse at age 16. To Pap or not to Pap, that is the question?

The Papanicolaou (Pap) smear is a screening test that identifies abnormal cells sampled from the transitional zone, the junction of the ectocervix and the endocervix where cervical dysplasia and cancers arise. There are different ways of performing the Pap smear:

- The conventional Pap that is taken with a spatula and spread with fixative onto a slide.
- The liquid-based cytology only recently available that can take the same specimen and perform HPV testing, GC, and *Chlamydia*.

The Pap smear gives cytology results and for actual diagnosis a biopsy is needed. HPV testing has been proposed as a primary screening modality and also as a method to triage equivocal or low-grade Pap smear abnormalities such as ASCUS. It is positive in approximately 35% of young women between ages 15 and 19 and about 6% of women between ages 50 and 65. Reflex HPV testing is recommended for women over age 30 because of the higher sensitivity of the combination of tests to detect cervical dysplasia. Most HPV infections in women under age 30 are transient and do not confer benefit to Pap smear screening or triage.

Increased risk for cervical cancer is associated with smoking, early coitarche, having multiple sex partners or having a sexual partner who has multiple sex partners too, high parity, sexual exposure to high-risk HPV infection, and the prolonged use of combined oral contraceptive pills.

Partners who are circumcised have reduced risk of carrying HPV infection and hence reduce risk of HPV infection.

With the advent of Pap smear testing, the incidence of cervical cancer has been significantly reduced so that it is no longer the seventh leading cause of death in America; however, it remains the second leading cause of cancer death in the developing world due to inadequate cancer prevention programs worldwide.

There are three major organizations that issue guidelines for cervical cancer screening; they are the U.S. Preventive Services Task Force (USPSTF), the American Cancer Society (ACS), and the American College of Obstetricians and Gynecologists (ACOG).

All the three organizations recommend initial screening 3 years after patients become sexually active or by age 21 whichever comes first because it is admittedly difficult to obtain accurate sexual histories, realizing at the same time most American adolescents are sexually active by age 18.

Patients can be offered the HPV vaccine per ACOG recommendations. The HPV vaccine is for girls and young women between ages 9 and 26. The quadrivalent vaccine targets HPV types 6, 11, 16, and 18 (Gardasil) administered in three doses at 0, 2, and 6 months. Duration of protection is not known at this time and hence does not replace cervical screening, which would be appropriate 3 years after coitarche or at age 21.

At the time of Pap, it may be important to consider testing for sexually transmitted infections such as hepatitis, gonorrhea, Chlamydia, and HIV. At this time, the CDC guidelines recommend the opt-out approach whereby the patient is voluntarily screened as long as she does not specifically elect not to be screened.

No data are available about screening after age 65, but discontinuing screening may be recommended for women over 65 years old who have been receiving adequate Pap smear screening with normal Pap smears over the last 10 years, who remain with the same partner as per the USPSTF, or by age 70 per ACS guidelines. Patients who have not had adequate screening benefit the most from Pap smears especially if they have never had one. ACOG recommends individual cervical cancer screening incorporating age, life expectancy, prior Pap results, HPV status, current sex activity, and history of hysterectomy. By these guidelines, it is reasonable to screen a 65-year-old with a new partner.

The USPSTF recommends Pap smear screening at least every 3 years. According to ACS and ACOG, frequency of Pap smears may be 2 to 3 yearly after three annual consecutive negative Pap smears for women over 30 years and when a combination of both negative Pap smear and negative HPV test, the recommendation is to repeat testing every 3 years. For women under 30 years, ACS and ACOG recommend annual Pap smears;

however, two yearly Pap smears if using liquid-based testing is used per ACS guidelines. However, more frequent testing is recommended for HIV positive, immunosuppressed women, and patients with history of in utero DES exposure.

For women who have undergone total hysterectomy for benign indications, cervical cancer screening may be discontinued according to all three organizations. For those women who had cervical intraepithelial neoplasia (CIN) 2 or 3 at hysterectomy, then three negative annual Pap smears are required before discontinuing Pap smear testing according to guidelines issued by ACS and ACOG. ACS notably recommends continued screening for women with in utero DES exposure. ACOG recommends yearly screening for women who have had cervical cancer.

Smoking is always discouraged especially in patients at high risk for cervical cancer.

All patients are encouraged to exercise regularly and eat a balanced diet and maintain a healthy weight.

In addition to Pap smear screening, screening for hypertension is important. Hypertension is defined when BP is >140/90 on two different occasions in the office and the treatment of hypertension reduces incidence of cardiovascular disease. Patients at moderate to high risk of cardiovascular disease, who are obese, age >35 years, and who are relatively inactive may benefit from an antihypertensive drug along with statin therapy and low-dose aspirin. Patients who are diabetics also benefit from strict control of their blood pressure.

All patients are encouraged to have a colonoscopy performed at age 50 and then every 10 years thereafter or sigmoidoscopy every 5 years unless they have a family history or abnormal findings that indicate a need to screen specific individuals more frequently.

Mammograms are recommended in women annually from age 40 along with clinical breast exams, and this may be discontinued when predicted life expectancy is <10 years. Women with a family history of breast cancer may need genetic testing and more intensive screening.

TAKE HOME POINTS

- Initial Pap smear is recommended at age 21 or 3 after coitarche whichever comes first.
- Frequency of Pap smears is annually while under 30 years of age and may be every 2 years if using the liquid-based Pap smear.

- Frequency of Pap smears over 30 years of age with three prior normal Paps may be reduced to every 3 years. Use of the liquid-based Pap smear in combination with HPV testing as long as both tests are negative may also be every 3 years.
- Discontinuation of screening is based on individual risk factors per ACOG Guidelines.

SUGGESTED READINGS

American College of Obstetricians and Gynecologists. *Compendium of Selected Publications.* ACOG; Washington, DC; 2007.

Stenchever MA, Droegemueller W, Herbst AL, et al. (eds). *Comprehensive Gynecology.* 4th ed. 2002, New York, NY, Elsevier.

Gordon JD, et al. *Obstetrics and Gynecology and Infertility Handbook.* 6th ed. uptodate.com

47

VAGINITIS: DIAGNOSTIC PROCEDURES

FRANCIS KWARTENG, MD AND DIANA BROOMFIELD, MD, MBA, FACOG, FACS

A 28-year-old G3P2012 female, last menstrual period 3 weeks ago, called her physician's office with a complaint of recurrent vulvovaginal itching with discharge characterized as whitish without much odor. She describes her predominant symptoms as itching especially after intercourse. This symptom began 3 months ago and has been recurrent and refractory to self-prescribe over-the-counter (OTC) antifungal agents. Her past medical history is noncontributory but has a significant family history of type II diabetes mellitus. Upon further inquiry, her physician calls in a prescription for Diflucan 150 mg single dose for treatment of presumed vaginal candidiasis.

Most common vaginal infections include bacterial vaginosis, vaginal candidiasis, and trichomoniasis. These infections constitute over 92% of all vaginal infections with bacterial vaginosis being the most common. Other infections of the cervicovaginal milieu include HPV, *Chlamydia*, gonorrhea, and herpetic infections. Common complaints include vaginal discharge, vulvovaginal pruritus or itching, and vaginal odor. Bacterial vaginosis, candidiasis, and trichomoniasis are common presentation in most gynecologic offices. It is estimated that over 10 to 12 million gynecologic visits are documented annually contributing to over a half a billion dollar burden on the health care budget.

Approximately 20% to 60% of healthy women harbor *Candida* species in the vagina and remain asymptomatic. The vaginal colonization of *Trichomonas vaginalis* is estimated at 20% to 50% with facultative and obligate anaerobes considered by some as "normal" vaginal flora. Normally, the healthy ecosystem of the vagina is preserved by *Lactobacillus acidophilus*. This organism metabolizes glycogen into lactic acid in preserving the vaginal milieu with a pH between 3.8 and 4.2.

Symptoms of vaginitis arise with a fall in colony counts of *Lactobacillus*, usually to $<10^3$ bacteria/mL. This creates a less acidic vaginal ecosystem that favors growth of pathogenic organism, which eventually causes various forms of vaginitis.

A common error to avoid is to consider all vaginal discharge as infectious. It is essential for women health care providers to appreciate that not all forms of vaginal discharge are infectious. Features of a normal or healthy discharge include white to gray thin or slightly thick discharge without odor, abundant lactobacillus, WBC count <4/hpf, bacteria 3.8 to 4.2 pH, and normal squamous epithelial cells. Specific features of some infections are seen in *Table 47.1*.

The purpose of this chapter is to outline common mistakes persistently made by patients and women health care providers in accurately diagnosing and treating complaints of vaginitis. It is not uncommon to discover that patients have self-diagnosed and treated themselves for several weeks or months for vaginal discharge with OTC medications (most commonly antifungal agents) before presenting to the physician's office as seen in the illustrated patient above. There are television commercials now that advise women that if they "know" that they have a yeast infection they may go to their local pharmacy and purchase an OTC medication to treat themselves. In fact, in our office at Howard University Hospital as seen in many gynecologic centers, patients present for office visits only when self-prescribed treatment has failed. It is even more worrisome to find women health care providers assuming that every pruritic vaginal discharge is candidiasis and calling in antifungal prescriptions for patients without proper diagnostic criteria and testing. Such practices only result in wrong diagnosis, delayed treatment, or mistreatment with a huge cost differential and burden on society and the patient. There is also an added risk of persistent or recurrent vaginitis.

Clinical presentations of the common forms of vaginitis are illustrated in Table 47.1. Review of this table shows pruritus as a symptom is not pathognomonic for the diagnosis of vaginal candida infections. In fact, a good proportion of patients with trichomoniasis have itching as well, with both conditions requiring different therapeutic modalities.

Ferris and colleagues found <34% of women who have self-diagnosed and treated themselves with OTC agents to have candidiasis. In addition, there is often coexistence of more than one infection, one of which may be left untreated with symptoms-based therapy alone without proper diagnostic testing.

Efficient and cost-effective treatment of any complaint of vaginitis includes review of the characteristic discharge, presence or absence of odor, the presence of specific signs on clinical examination such as erythema of vulvovaginitis, petechial hemorrhages as with Trichomoniasis, thick or chessy discharge usually associated with candidiasis, vaginal pH, and the characteristic findings seen on wet mount or KOH testing of the discharge. In spite of these findings, the likelihood of detecting the cause of vaginitis may be elusive or enigmatic. Such situation requires Gram stain, culture, and other diagnostic modalities such as DNA hybridization. Gram stain has been found useful in diagnosis of bacterial vaginosis but has yet to gain prominence in clinical practice.

TABLE 47.1 FEATURES OF VARIOUS FORMS OF VAGINITIS

	NORMAL PHYSIOLOGIC DISCHARGE	CANDIDIASIS	BACTERIAL VAGINOSIS	TRICHOMONIASIS
APPEARANCE	White gray and thin	White cheesy or thick	Usually grayish white	Thick to thin grayish to greenish discharge
MICROSCOPY	Normal epithelial cell	Pseudohyphae on KOH/saline wet mount	Clue cells and WBC	Flagellated organism
WHIFF TEST	–	–	+++	–
pH	3.8–4.2	<4.5	>4.5	>4.5
COMMON ORGANISM	Normal vaginal flora (*Lactobacillus* predominant) >106	*Candida albicans* *C. glabrata* *C. tropicalis*	*Gardnerella vaginalis* Bacteroides *Provetella* spp., Ureolyticus	*Trichomonas vaginalis*
CULTURE RESULTS	–	With Sabouraud agar	Gram stain	Using Diamond media
TESTING AVAILABLE	–	–	DNA hybridization	DNA hybridization
PRURITUS	None	Yes (+++)	Yes (++)	Yes (++)
ODOR	None	None (typically)	Fishy odor	Yes

Comparison of hybridization (DNA) studies versus Gram stain in detecting bacterial vaginosis in asymptomatic women resulted in superior detective rate with hybridization methods. If such studies become clinically acceptable, the cost-related factors may have to be considered for patients to be able to afford them. However, they may be considered in cases of unyielding diagnosis from routine diagnostic testing and disease refractory to medications.

TAKE HOME POINTS

- Diagnosis and treatment of vaginitis requires integration of symptoms, examination of the patient, and wet mount/KOH testing.
- If diagnosis is still elusive, Gram stain, cultures, and DNA studies are available.
- Women health care providers should aim at treating diagnosis and not symptoms as symptom overlap for various vaginal infections is common.
- Symptom-based treatment of vaginitis is highly ineffective and leaves the patient with huge cost burden.

SUGGESTED READINGS

Allsworth JE, Peiper JF. Prevalence of bacterial vaginosis: 2001–2004 National Health and Nutrition Examination Survey data. *Obstet Gynecol*. 2007;109:114.

American College of Obstetricians and Gynecologists. Technical Bulletin No. 26: vaginitis. 1996.

Brown HL, Fuller DD, Jasper Lt, et al. Clinical evaluation of Affirm VPIII in the detection and identification of *Trichomonas vaginalis, Gardnerella vaginalis*, and *Candida* species in vaginitis/vaginosis. *Inf Dis Obstet Gynecol*. 2004;12(1):17–21.

Ekgren J, Norling BK, Degre M, et al. Comparison of tinidazole given as a single dose and on 2 consecutive days for the treatment of nonspecific bacterial vaginosis. *Gynecol Obstet Invest*. 1988:26:313.

Ferris DG, Litaker MS, Woodward L, et al. Treatment of bacterial vaginosis: a comparison of oral metronidazole, metronidazole vaginal gel, and clindamycin vaginal cream. *J Fam Pract*. 1995;41:443.

Klebanoff MA, Hauth JC, Macpherson CA, et al. Time course of the regression of asymptomatic bacterial vaginosis in pregnancy with and without treatment. *Am J Obstet Gynecol*. 2004;190:363.

Landers DV, Wiesenfeld HD, Heine RP, et al. Predictive value of the clinical diagnosis of lower genital tract infection in women. *Am J Obstet Gynecol*. 2004;190:1004.

Martin HL, Richardson BA, Nyange PM, et al. Vaginal lactobacilli, microbial flora and the risk of human immunodeficiency virus type I and sexually transmitted disease acquisition. *J Infect Dis*. 1999;180(6):1863–1868

Morris M, Nicoll A, Simms I, et al. Bacterial vaginosis: a public health review. *Br J Obstet Gynecol*. 2001;108:439–450.

Ness RB, Hillier SL, Richter HE, et al. Douching in relation to bacterial vaginosis, lactobacilli, and facultative bacteria in the vagina. *Obstet Gyynecol*. 2002;100:765.

Robinson SC, Mirchandani G. Observations on vaginal trichomoniasis. IV. Significance of vaginal flora under various conditions. *Am J Obstet Gynecol*. 1965;91:1005–1012

Sexually transmitted diseases treatment guidelines 2002. Centers for Disease Control and Prevention. *MMWR Recomm Rep*. 2002;51(RR-6):1–78.

Smart S, Singal A, Mindel A. Social and sexual risk factors for bacterial vaginosis. *Sex Transm Infect*. 2004;80:58.

Sobel JD. Vaginitis. *N Eng J Med*. 1997;337:1896–1903.

Spiegel CA. Bacterial vaginosis. *Clin Microbiol Rev*. 1991;4:485.

Stenchever MA, Droegemueller W, Herbs AL, et al., eds. *Comprehensive Gynecology*. 4th ed. St. Louis, MO: Mosby; 2001.

Wathne B, Holst E, Hovelius B, et al. Erythromycin versus metronidazole in the treatment of bacterial vaginosis. *Acta Obstet Gynecol Scan*. 1993;72:470.

Yen S, Shafer MA, Moncada J, et al. Bacterial vaginosis in sexually experienced and non-sexually experienced young women entering the military. *Obstet Gynecol*. 2003;102:927.

48

DELAYED DIAGNOSIS: WORKUP ANY BREAST ABNORMALITY

VICTORIA GREEN, MD, MHSA, MBA, JD

Breast cancer is a significant public health problem that affects >180,000 women and results in nearly 41,500 female deaths annually. Although more prevalent in the female population, breast cancer is diagnosed in nearly 2,000 men (accounting for about 1% of all breast cancers) and results in 450 deaths per year. As women continually seek a full spectrum of primary and preventive care from primary care practitioners, specifically obstetrician gynecologists, we are increasingly involved not only in the diagnosis of breast disease but also often in the management and treatment. Thus, delayed diagnosis of breast cancer has become an ever important source of concern, consternation, and medicolegal liability within the specialty. According to the most recent ACOG Professional Liability Survey, delayed diagnosis of cancer and specifically breast cancer was the most frequent gynecologic allegation against obstetricians/gynecologists. Of the top three errors in diagnosis resulting in claims for medical malpractice, breast cancer was number one. Breast cancer was also number one for general surgery and radiology. Moreover, it was second for family practice and third for internal medicine. In terms of all diagnostic errors among providers of primary health care to women, the delayed diagnosis of breast cancer is also the most prevalent condition resulting in claims of medical malpractice, surpassing the brain-damaged infant, pregnancy, and acute myocardial infarction for all specialties combined with the volume of claims increasing by nearly 10% over the last decade. Additionally, it is the second most expensive area of claims to indemnify (second only to brain-damaged infant) by liability carriers with indemnity payments approaching $200 million or approximately 30% of payments of paid out liability claims for medical misadventures.

Several common themes combine to result in this error including skepticism about the possibility of breast cancer in young women, a complete reliance on negative mammograms, "system failures" in which the abnormal mammogram was not brought to the attention of the provider, inattention to medical history and a delay in offering chemopreventive initiatives in high-risk women, and, finally, failure to diagnose recurrent disease partially due to lack of acceptance of the "captain of the ship" mentality for the primary care practitioner.

Although breast cancer most commonly occurs in women over 50 years of age, the obstetrician gynecologist must realize that nearly 5% to 10% of breast cancer occurs in women under the age of 45 and 3% in women under the age of 35. Moreover, although incidence rates have been declining in women aged 50 and older, incidence rates have remained stable since 1986 among women younger than age 50. Importantly, although incidence rates are about 12% lower in African American than in white women, among African American women under the age of 40, the incidence of breast cancer is higher than in white women. Changes in the breast exam are often dismissed as fibrocystic condition and not evaluated further. Moreover, in many cases, further evaluation of an atypical breast exam is pursued but halted in the fact of a seemingly negative mammogram/ultrasound, even in the face of a mass. As mammograms are known to have a false-negative rate of nearly 15%, this may be even greater in women with dense breasts, implants, fibrocystic condition, prior breast surgery, and those on hormone replacement therapy (HRT). Although digital mammography and other advances in imaging modalities including MRI may improve our ability to detect abnormalities in this limited group, their ability to decrease the likelihood of litigation remains to be seen.

Practitioners must ensure a thorough evaluation in spite of contradictory imaging studies. The triad of a young patient with a self-detected breast mass and a negative mammogram is the most frequent scenario preceding the delayed diagnosis of breast cancer. Average length of delay is 15 months with a median of 11 months. The delay can be divided between physician-associated delays and patient-associated delays. Thirty-five to fifty percent of patients delayed seeking medical consultation for >3 months and 15.6% delayed for over 1 year. Given the large number of new cases of breast cancer expected to be diagnosed in American women in 2003 (211,000), it has been estimated that >70,000 American women will sustain patient-associated diagnostic delays exceeding 3 months.

Importantly, in many cases, an imaging result indicating the need for further follow-up is misplaced and thus not acted upon by the medical personnel. This may be due to a lack of a tickler file (or similar follow-up system) as is often in place for an abnormal Pap smear triage. Genomic or hereditary cancer liability may evolve into the next forefront for litigation in the field of medicine. Practitioners are being warned to thoroughly review the cancer history in the pregnant state in order to assess the individual's risk of the development of cancer and institute (or offer) important chemopreventive options or genetic testing and counseling as appropriate. Allegations include failure to diagnose, failure to consider the patient's genealogy, failure to inform other family members (one must be cognizant of HIPAA considerations), and failure to offer testing. This has already occurred in obstetrics with Tay–Sachs testing. Physicians should familiarize themselves with the Gail model, which is the only clinically validated model that derives an individual's risk for development of breast cancer; however, counseling must stress these figures are estimates and not absolute risks and thus balance the magnitude of risk for the individual patient. Clinicians must also become familiar with the eligibility criteria for breast cancer susceptibility gene testing, the principles of genetic counseling, options available to those at high risk, and follow-up of patients at high risk.

Additional diagnostic errors occur in failing to examine a breast containing an obvious tumor while treating the patient for an unrelated disease; failing to find the tumor of concern during palpation of the breast, failing to recommend a referral, biopsy/excision, failing to follow-up actions of non-physician providers, failing to determine the cause of a nipple discharge, mistaking a carcinomatous tumor for a breast infection/benign lesion, and disregarding a definite retraction sign or history of acute or sharp pain.

The most common reason underlying delay in diagnosis was physical examination findings that did not impress the physician (35%). Other reasons included failure to follow-up in a timely fashion (31%), negative/misread mammogram (26%/23%), failure to perform a biopsy (23%), delayed/failure to consult (16%), failure to order/react to mammogram (11%/12%), communication failure (11%), and poor clinical examination (10%). Because mammography has a 15% to 20% false-negative rate, the practitioner should not rely on a "negative" mammogram in the face of a dominant lesion or suspicious examination. However, because mammography may not detect neoplastic changes in the breast until the cancer has been developing for 6 years, some lesions will not be seen on mammography in retrospect, some should be considered as subthreshold, and some are appropriately classified as missed.

Perpetual/sustained vigilance will easily reduce the likelihood of a delay in diagnosis. Practitioners should develop systems for follow-up to ensure patients have obtained a suggested imaging study or referrals and that the result/comment has returned to the office/chart and has been reviewed by a medical personnel. Young women presenting with self-detected lesions must have appropriate evaluation although many will be found not to have any breast pathology. Practitioners must become familiar with risk assessment techniques and clinical options/alternative. Moreover, all practitioners are going to have a role in the delivery of genetic services and must be familiar with appropriate referral mechanisms.

As obstetrician gynecologists are becoming important members of the team caring for patients with breast cancer, we must become familiar with developing the concept of choosing a "captain" for the medical team Thus, when clinical concerns arise on physical examination, a referral system is already in place to ensure this information is relayed to a single practitioner who will analyze, evaluate, and initiate appropriate follow-up and care rather than assuming some other health care personnel is aware and will handle the episode of care.

Careful and thorough documentation is another important aspect of breast health care. Judgment calls that may result in an adverse outcome are more easily defensible with accurate and through documentation of examination and follow-up care. Be careful of descriptive terms that may mimic cancer when in actuality your examination does not support such diagnosis such as the use of lump, lesions, nodule, or irregular margins when describing an area of fibrocystic in nature. We do not have "microscopes" in our fingertips and thus such a level of discernment may be impossible and may require additional evaluation including imaging or observation. Be sure to have a plan of follow-up and document your reason and clinical thought process. Patients should always be a part of the decision-making process and thorough informed consent is necessary as well as documentation of reasons for refusal and noncompliance with care and your resolution of the matter. Documentation of refusal of care should include a thorough discussion of the consequences of noncompliance with care and the patient's understanding. Health literacy and cultural context must be included as an important part of meticulous and comprehensive education for the patient. Strict adherence to these principles will foster better physician/patient relationship and mitigate against increased damages if a claim is filed against you. Do not be lulled into a false sense of security in the face of lack of a family history (80% of patients have no risk factor for breast cancer other than being female and their age), lack of abnormal imaging, or lack of distinctive mass on initial evaluation. Be sure the patient is comfortable with your plan of management and refer as necessary.

TAKE HOME POINTS

- Delayed diagnosis of cancer and specifically breast cancer was the most frequent gynecologic allegation against obstetricians/gynecologists.
- Although breast cancer most commonly occurs in women over 50 years of age, the obstetrician gynecologist must realize that nearly 5% to 10% of breast cancer occurs in women under the age of 45 and 3% in women under the age of 35.
- The triad of a young patient with a self-detected breast mass and a negative mammogram is the most frequent scenario preceding the delayed diagnosis of breast cancer.
- Do not be lulled into a false sense of security in the face of lack of a family history.

SUGGESTED READINGS

American Cancer Society. *Cancer Facts and Figures 2008*. Atlanta, GA: American Cancer Society, Inc. 2008.

American Cancer Society. *Breast Cancer Facts and Figures 2007–2008*. Atlanta, GA: American Cancer Society, Inc. 2008.

American Cancer Society. *Cancer Facts and Figures for African Americans 2007–2008*. Atlanta, GA: American Cancer Society, Inc. 2008.

American College of Obstetrics and Gynecology. 2006. Accessed November 10, 2008. www.acog.org

American College of Obstetricians and Gynecologists. Breast cancer prevention and treatment: what's new, what's promising? *ACOG Today*. 2003;4(3):1.

Bland KI, Copeland EM III, eds. *The Breast: Comprehensive Management of Benign and Malignant Diseases*. 2nd ed. Philadelphia, PA: W.B. Saunders Company; 2004.

Burke W, Daly M, Garber J, et al. Recommendations for follow-up care of individuals with an inherited predisposition to cancer. II> BRCA1 and BRCA2. *JAMA*. 1997;277:120: 997–1003.

Green VL. *Liability in Obstetrics and Gynecology in Legal medicine*. 7th ed. American College of Legal Medicine. New York, NY: Elsevier, Inc.; 2007.

Green VL. Breast diseases: benign and malignant. In: Rock JA, Thompson J, eds. *Telinde's Operative Gynecology*. New York, NY: Elsevier Publications; 2006.

Kern KA. Causes of breast cancer malpractice litigation: a 20 year civil court review. *Arch Surg*. 1992;127:542.

Kern KA. Medicolegal analysis of the delayed diagnosis of cancer in 338 cases in the United States. *Arch Surg*. 1994;129:397–403.

Mandelson MT, Oestreicher N, Porter PL, et al. Breast density as a predictor of mammographic detection: comparison of interval- and screen-detected cancers journal. *Natl Can Inst*. 2000;92:1081.

Parents of Tay-Sachs infant win damage award in New Jersey "wrongful Birth" suit. East Brunswick Home News Tribune, Feb 9, 2001.

Physician Insurers Association of America. *Data Sharing Reports, Executive Summary* (1995, 2001). Washington, DC: PIAA; 1995, 2001.

Zoler ML. Take family cancer history in pregnancy or risk lawsuit. *OB/GYN news*, March 1, 2003.

49

BREAST CARE: MORE REASONS FOR DELAY IN DIAGNOSIS

FRANCIS KWARTENG, MD AND DIANA BROOMFIELD, MD, MBA, FACOG, FACS

A 36-year-old female, G2P2002, LMP 14 weeks ago, presents for her first prenatal case with complaints of swelling in the left lower quadrant of the left breast. She has diabetes mellitus type II for 8 years and is on glyburide 7.5 mg daily. Her maternal aunt and her younger sister both died of breast cancer at age 42 and 23 respectively. She smokes a pack of cigarettes daily. She has no history of illicit drug use. She appears worried on examination. She has normal vitals. The lower left quadrant of the left breast shows minor erythema with no appreciable mass. Mammogram results are negative. The patient is apprehended and states, "My younger sister's mammogram was normal and she had similar breast swelling, am I going to die?"

Diseases of the breast are manifold. Common benign conditions encountered are mastalgia, mastitis, cellulitis, and breast abscess. The most concerning problem to both health care providers and patients is the presence of breast mass which may prognosticate a diagnosis of breast cancer.

Breast cancer is the commonest female cancer in all age group and second to lung cancer in mortality, considering cancer-related deaths in the United States. Between 2004 and 2005, 216,000 new cases of breast cancer were reported and a little over 40,000 breast cancer–related deaths were documented. Indeed, to most families, the diagnosis of breast cancer presents great moments of anxiety and thought about possibilities of death. Furthermore, 1 in 8 females are at risk of developing breast cancer (12.5%) in a lifetime and 1 in 28 are at risk of dying from the disease.

This underscores why current preventive guidelines regarding breast care are all directed at early detection of breast masses and subsequent diagnosis of breast cancer.

The screening and diagnostic methods currently expounded by the U.S. Preventive Service Task Force (USPSTF), American Cancer Society (ACS), National Cancer Institute (NCI), and the American College of Obstetrics and Gynecology (ACOG) are summarized in *Table 49.1*. The most prevalent risk factors for developing the disease are illustrated in *Table 49.2*.

TABLE 49.1   SCREENING METHODS AVAILABLE AND THEIR POTENTIAL CLINICAL USEFULNESS

	BREAST SELF-EXAMINATION	CLINICAL BREAST EXAMINATIONS	MAMMOGRAPHY
Guidelines recommendations	ACS: Educate women about the benefit and limitations beginning at 20 y/o. ACOG: Recommend BSE despite no clear evidence for or against. USPSTF: Evidence is insufficient to recommend	ACS: 20–30 y; every 3 y after 40 y, annually. AGOG: All women should have clinical breast examination annually. ACP: To discuss with women risk and benefits. USPSTF: Does not recommend for or against.	ACS: 40–50 y; every 1–2 y 50 y and over, annually. As long as a woman is in reasonably good health and can undergo treatment, she should get mammography. ACOG: 40–49 y; every 1–2 y >50 y, annually. USPSTF: >40 y; every 1–2 y. NCI: >40 y; every 1–2 y.
Limitations	Higher number of biopsies and subsequent procedures done for benign lesions	Efficiency limited in obese individual, examine dependent, less specific compared to mammography.	1. Increase false + results in young women, increase breast density. HRT breast implants. 2. Less sensitive in faster growing tumors. 3. Less sensitive in radiation Ass. breast changes.
Efficacy in detecting breast cancer	Sensitivity in diagnosing breast cancer is 20%–30%.	Sensitivity ≥55%. Specificity ≥94%. Sensitivity and specificity increases if done in conjunction with mammography. May detect 5% of cancers not seen on mammograms.	1. Decrease breast cancer mortality by 15%–35%. 2. Sensitivity 75%–96%. 3. Specificity 89%–99%.
Clinical technique/ benefit	Required monthly preferably the first 7–10 d of cycle (follicular phase)	Needs to be done by trained health care provider. Axillary and supraclavicular nodes required. Effective if coupled risk factors.	1. Detect lesion otherwise not palpable on BSE/CBE. 2. May detect microcalcifications.

Above screening guidelines were derived from National Guidelines Clearinghouse, United States Preventive Service Task Force (USPSTF), American College of Obstetrics and Gynecology (ACOG), National Cancer Institute (NCI), and American Cancer Society (ACS). www.nationalguidelinesclearinghouse for in-depth information and patients at high risk such as BRCA mutations and use of adjunctive screening and diagnostic tools such as MRI and ultrasonography.

TABLE 49.2	RISK FACTORS FOR BREAST CANCER

- Old age
- Family history of breast cancer
- Older age at time of first birth
- Younger age of menarche
- History of breast biopsy
- Two or more first-degree relatives with breast cancer
- Two previous breast biopsies
- First-degree relative with breast cancer and one previous biopsy
- Previous diagnosis of breast cancer
- Ductal carcinoma in situ (DCIS)
- Atypical hyperplasia of the breast
- Previous chest irradiation

In spite of the available screening and diagnostic tools to aid early detection, breast cancer still remains the most expensive and common medicolegal claims against clinicians. This is attributed to delay in diagnosis of breast cancer.

IGNORANCE OF MOST PATIENTS TO RISK FACTORS AND COMPLICATIONS OF THE DISEASE

There is a lack of appropriate preventive health care education to patients in regard to risk factors whose avoidance would constitute primary prevention. In addition to the risk factors outlined in Figures I and II, smoking, ionizing radiation exposure, and alcoholic consumption have been implicated as risk factors whose exposure in adolescence would increase development of breast cancer in adulthood. Education and review of risk factors for breast cancer with patients during annual routine examination will help determine which patients require further evaluation.

LACK OF STRICT ADHERENCE TO SCREENING GUIDELINES

Studies show only 40% of females who meet the criteria for screening mammograms pursue it regularly. Health care providers may require more logistics to enhance health promotion and education to increase public awareness to the importance and need for mammography in early detection of breast cancer.

DENIAL ON THE PART OF PATIENTS TO FOLLOW-UP EVALUATION FOR SUSPECTED BREAST LESIONS

This relates to personal fears and misconceptions about treatment of breast cancer that borders on religion and cultural beliefs. Studies from 1996 conducted in Stony Brook, New York, on the reasons for delay in breast cancer diagnosis attributed 25% of such delays to the patients themselves, because they did not consider the diagnosis as important. Health care providers on suspicion of breast lesions should stress the importance of follow-up and at best explain the prognosis. This may occur in patient family setting to provide support and encouragement to the patient to follow up.

ACCESS TO TREATMENT

Difficulties associated with scheduling an office visit accounted for 45% of delays in treatment in the same study from Stony Brook. Often, it takes an average of 4 to 6 weeks for most patients to secure a visit in a busy practice. Appropriate health care must ensure frequent follow-up visits in an expeditious manner especially for patients with diagnosis that carry a grave prognosis such as breast cancer.

REPEAT BREAST EXAM

Several studies have attributed over 50% of delays in diagnosing breast cancers to an ambiguous initial examination by the physician and no follow-up breast exam to compare or confirm findings. Such patients may present later with advanced breast cancer. The onus lies with health care providers to refer such patients for diagnostic studies especially if there are serious risk factors.

FAILURE TO FOLLOW UP NEGATIVE MAMMOGRAM IN PATIENTS WITH HIGH INDEX OF SUSPICION ON THE BASIS OF CLINICAL OR FAMILY HISTORY

A screening mammogram has a 5% to 15% false-negative rate. A negative screening mammogram in the face of high risk factors should attract further investigation with magnetic resonance imaging (MRI). The ACS recommends MRI for patients with BRCA mutations, first-degree relatives of BRCA carriers who are untested, and for patients with 20% to 25% risk by the BRCAPRO model.

COMORBID CONDITIONS

Physician attention to other comorbid and compelling health conditions of the patient that present concurrently with breast lesions has been implicated as a cause of delay in diagnosing breast cancer. Although all disease conditions should be managed with equal attention, those with grave prognosis such as breast cancer require similar serious attention.

- All patients with ovarian cancer should be closely followed for development of breast cancer. This will help in early detection of heredity-related breast cancer that account for 5% to 10% of all breast cancer.

- The incidence of breast cancer in pregnancy is 1:3,000, though pregnancy does not seem to alter the natural history of breast cancer, delay in diagnosis occurs because of increased density of the breast. All breast lesions suspected during pregnancy should be aggressively worked up with clinical examination and appropriate clinical tools (mammography, fine needle aspiration, and biopsy) to avoid delays in diagnosis.

TAKE HOME POINTS

- Diagnosis of advanced breast cancer is almost invariably associated with death in <5 years.

- Early detection is key in improving long-term survival. Avoidance of delays in diagnosis should constitute the primary goal of providers who specialize in women's health.

SUGGESTED READINGS

American Cancer Society. Cancer facts and figures. http://www.cancer.org/docroots/STT/content/STT_1x_Cancer_Facts_Figures_2005.asp. Assessed 2006.

American Medical Association. *Current Procedural Terminology: CPT*. Chicago, IL: American Medical Association; 1998.

Anderson I, Aspengren K, Janzon L, et al. Mammographic screening and mortality from breast cancer: the Malmo Mammographic screening trial. *Br Med J*. 1988;297:943–948.

Caplan LS, Helzlsouer KJ, Shapiro S, et al. System delay in diagnosis of cancer in whites and blacks. *Am J Epideminol*. 1995;142:804–812.

Caplan LS, Helzlsouer KJ, Shapiro S, et al. Reasons for delay in breast cancer diagnosis. *Prev Med*. 1996;25:218–224.

Facione NC, Miaskowski C, Dodd MJ, et al. The self-reported likelihood of patient delay in cancer: new thoughts for early detection. *Prev Med*. 2002;34:397–407.

Freeman JL, Goodwin JS, Zhang D, et al. Measuring the performance screening mammography in community practice with Medicare claims data. Women Health. 2002;37(2):1–15.

Goodson WH III, Moore DH II. Causes of physician delay in the diagnosis of breast cancer. *Arch intern Med*. 2002;162:1343–1348.

Gregorio DI, Cummings KM, Michalek A. Delay, stage of disease, and survival among whites and black women with breast cancer. *Am J Public Health*.1983;73:590–593.

Gwyn K, Bondy ML, Cohen DS, et al. Racial differences in diagnosis, treatment, and clinical population-based study of patients with newly diagnosed breast carcinoma. *Cancer*. 2004;100:1.

Harlan LC, Abrams J, Warren JL, et al. Adjuvant therapy for cancer: practice patterns of community physicians. *J Clin Oncol*. 2002;20:1809–1817.

Harris DM, Miller JE, Davis DM. Racial differences in breast cancer screening, knowledge and compliance. *J Natl Med Assoc*. 2003;95:693–701.

Jenner DC, Middleton A, Webb WM, et al. In-hospital delay in the diagnosis of cancer. *Br J Surg*. 2000;87:914–919.

Kern KA. The delayed diagnosis of symptomatic breast cancer. In: Bland KI, Copeland EM III, eds. *The Breast: Comprehensive Management of Benign and Malignant Disease*. 2nd ed. Philadelphia, PA: WB Saunders Co.; 1998:1588–1631.

Lannin DR, Harris RP, Swanson FH, et al. Difficulties in diagnosis of carcinoma of the breast in patients less than fifty years of age. *Surg Gynecol Obstet*. 1993;177:457–462.

Mann BD, Giuliano AE, Bassett LW, et al. Delayed diagnosis of breast cancer as a result of normal mammograms. *Arch Surg*. 1983;118:23–24.

Meechan G, Collins J, Petrie KJ. The relationship of symptoms and psychological factors to delay in seeking medical care for breast symptoms. *Prev Med*. 2003;36:374–378.

Miller AB, Baines CJ, To T, et al. Canadian National Breast Screening Study: 2. Breast cancer detection and death rates among women aged 50 to 59 years. *Can Med Assoc J*. 1992;147:1477–1488.

Ries L, Eisner M, Kosary C, et al., eds. *SEER Cancer Statistics Review, 1975–2000*. Bethesda, MD: National Cancer Institute; 2003.

Swann CA, Kopans DB, McCarthy KA, et al. Mammographic density and physical assessment of the breast. *Am J Roentgenol*. 1987;148:525–526.

U.S. Preventive Services Task Force. Screening for breast Cancer Release Date: February 2002 available at: http://ahrq.gov/clinic/uspstf/uspsvbrca.htm. Last assessed December 10, 2004.

U.S. Preventive Services Task Force. *Guide to Clinical Preventive Services*. 2nd ed. Baltimore, MD: Williams & Wilkins; 1996:73–87.

50

PERTUSSIS, TDAP, AND WHOOPING COUGH: DO NOT FORGET TO VACCINATE

JESSICA ARLUCK, MD

Pertussis, also known as whooping cough, is caused by the coccobacilli, *Bordetella pertussis*, and is a highly contagious respiratory infection. The initial catarrhal stage includes symptoms similar to a "common cold" including sneezing, coughing, malaise, and a runny nose. The cough is a dry hacking one. After 1 to 2 weeks, the cough changes to the characteristic "whoop," which is due to an intake of air after coughing. This second stage called the paroxysmal stage can last from 2 to 6 weeks. The typical high-pitched "whoop" is usually heard in children and not adults. The coughing fits manifest as 15 rapid coughs in sequence. During this stage, coughing tends to occur at night and the coughing fits can cause vomiting. The energy expended during these coughing fits typically results in fatigue. Sometimes the coughing is severe enough to cause rib cage bruising or rib fractures. The final stage, known as the convalescent stage, can last up to 6 months. During this time, the coughing becomes less severe and finally subsides.

Pertussis is an airborne pathogen, which persists in mucus droplets for up to 3 days. Adolescents and adults are the primary source of transmission. People are most infectious during the catarrhal stage. For most patients, pertussis has a benign clinical course. Major complications in infants and young children include middle ear infections, pneumonia, syncope, dehydration, seizures, encephalopathy, and even death. The complication rate is higher for those <12 months of age.

The incidence of pertussis is increasing due to children who have not completed their immunization schedule (normal schedule for DTaP is 2, 4, 6, and 15 to 18 months of age) or with adolescents and adults whose immunity has waned. In 1976, there were only 1,000 reported cases of pertussis; however, by 2004, the number of reported cases increased to nearly 25,000. In 2005 and 2006, the CDC reported that 93% of pertussis-related deaths occurred in infants <12 months of age, with infants <6 months at the highest risk. Premature and low–birth-weight infants are at an increased risk of severe complication and death rates are higher when compared to term infants. Parents were identified as the source of the pertussis in >25% of these cases.

The best treatment of pertussis is prevention. Ideally, evaluation and vaccination should occur during a well-woman visit for those in the reproductive age range. In 2006, the Advisory Committee on Immunization

Practice (ACIP) recommended that all new mothers get vaccinated with the Tdap vaccine (tetanus, diphtheria and acellular pertussis) prior to discharge from the hospital. If not done during the immediate postpartum period, then vaccination should occur as soon as possible postdelivery. There is no isolated vaccine that contains only acellular pertussis antigens. ACIP recommends that the interval between the last Td vaccine and Tdap can be as short as 2 years when given to adults in close contact with infants in order to achieve immunity to pertussis. Breast-feeding is not a contraindication to vaccination with the Tdap vaccine.

ACIP recommends a single dose of Tdap vaccine be given to adults and adolescents who will be in contact with infants. Fathers should be encouraged by the obstetrician to seek vaccination from their primary care providers in anticipation of delivery of their newborn.

Contraindications to the vaccine include a history of allergic reaction to any of the components of the vaccine or latex. Patients who have a history of encephalopathy (coma, prolonged seizures) within 7 days should also not get the vaccine. Reasons to consider deferring the vaccine include a history of Guillain-Barre syndrome after the Td vaccine, progressive neurologic conditions, or a history of an arthus reaction (hypersensitivity reaction causing a local vasculitis). Arthus reactions are characterized by severe pain, swelling, induration, edema, hemorrhage, and occasionally by necrosis.

TAKE HOME POINTS

- The incidence of pertussis is increasing due to nonvaccinated children and adults who have lost immunity.
- The vaccination schedule is 2, 4, 6, and 15 to 18 months of age.
- Breast-feeding is not a contraindication to Tdap vaccination.
- Contraindications include allergic reaction to components of the vaccine and anaphylaxis to latex, progressive neurologic conditions and epilepsy, and history of hypersensitivity reactions following tetanus toxoid administration.

SUGGESTED READINGS

Bisgard KM, Pascual FB, Ehresmann KR, et al. Infant Pertussis: who was the source? *Pediatr Infect Dis J.* 2004;23(11);985–989.

Clark S, Adolphe S, Davis MM, et al. Attitudes of US obstetricians toward a combined Tetanus-Diptheria-Acellular Pertussis vaccine for adults. *Infect Dis Obstet Gynecol.* 2006;1–5.

Vitek CR, Pascual FB, Baughman AL, et al. Increase in deaths from pertussis among young infants in the United States in the 1990's. *Pediatr Infect Dis J.* 2003;22(7):628–634.

Vaccines and Preventable Diseases: Combined Tdap Vaccine. Combined Tetanus, Diphtheria and Pertussis (Tdap) Vaccines. Available at: http://www.cdc.gov/vaccines/vpd-vac/combo-vaccines/DTaP-Td-DT/tdap.htm, 2009.

Combined Tetanus, Diphtheria and Pertussis (Tdap) Vaccines. Available at: http://www.cdc.gov/vaccines/vpd-vac/combo-vaccines/DTaP-Td-DT/tdap.htm

51

FOCUSING ON PATIENT EDUCATION WITH DIABETES MANAGEMENT

JESSICA B. SPENCER, MD, MSc

You review your patient's most recent lab tests. Because of her obesity and family history, you had ordered a 2-hour glucose tolerance test. Her 2-hour glucose comes back at 221 and her HgA1c is 8.5. She has diabetes. So now you have to discuss her diagnosis and medical management, set her up with a dietician, arrange glucometer teaching with the nurse, and make a close follow-up appointment to review her sugars. Do not forget, however, that this is an important opportunity to educate your patient. Patient education in diabetes management has been proven to improve compliance and reduce long-term complications. You must consider her needs, fears, resources, and value systems.

Threatening the patient with statistics of diabetic complications often has the opposite effect of the practitioner's intension. The patient may withdraw into illness denial. Instead, start by determining what the patient knows about diabetes. Explore her fears and misconceptions. Do not overwhelm her with too much information at once, and ask her to explain back important concepts so that you can assess her understanding.

Next, discuss the treatment options available and develop a *shared* decision-making plan for her care. Adherence will likely be higher if she can assert her own opinion. Do not set the bar too high initially, especially when discussing weight loss. Set realistic smaller goals that she can meet and be sensitive to any financial burden she may experience. Be particularly sensitive to any cultural differences in her management. If applicable, a dietician familiar with her traditional cuisine may be more effective in suggesting realistic alternatives to high-carbohydrate or high-fat dishes that may be a staple in her diet.

Motivating the noncompliant patient is a particular challenge. Common contributing obstacles to motivation include overcomplicated plans, a sense of lost autonomy, lack of self-esteem or sense of inefficacy, and financial burden. Cognitive-behavioral therapy may help address the vicious cycle of binge eating with negative thoughts and guilt. Be on the look out for patients with depression, which is common among diabetic patients. If you suspect depression, have her evaluated and treated immediately.

Since many patient visits have to occur in <15 minutes, the use of questionnaires may assist identifying specific problem areas a particular patient may have (e.g., the 20-item PAID [Problem Areas in Diabetes] questionnaire). Keep in mind that 5 minutes of empathy can go a long way.

TAKE HOME POINTS

- Patient education has been proven to improve compliance and reduce long-term complications in diabetic patients.
- Be empathetic with your patient, go slow, and be sensitive to cultural and socioeconomic differences that may play a role in her care.
- Screen for depression and consider cognitive-behavioral therapy for patients with persistent negative thoughts.
- To provide the most comprehensive care possible in a short visit, utilize the team-based approach and tools such as patient questionnaires.

SUGGESTED READINGS

Dagogo-Jack S, Funnell MM, Davidson J. Barriers to achieving optimal glycemic control in a multi-ethnic society: a US focus. *Curr Diabet Rev.* 2006;2:285–293.

Golay A, Lagger G, Chambouleyron M, et al. Therapeutic education of diabetic patients. *Diabet/Metabol Res Rev.* 2008;24(3):192–196.

Peyrot M, Rubin RR. Behavioral and psychosocial interventions in diabetes: a conceptual review. *Diabetes Care.* 2007;30(10):2433–2440.

Welch GW, Jacobson AM, Polonsky WH. The problem areas in diabetes scale: an evaluation of its clinical utility. *Diabetes Care.* 1997;20:760–766.

52

THIS THYROID SEEMS BIGGER THAN USUAL...
NOW WHAT?

JESSICA B. SPENCER, MD, MSc AND SUMATHI SRIVATSA, MD

Do not forget to check the thyroid. Look at it, and palpate it from the front or the back as the patient swallows. Ask your patient about tenderness, voice changes, discomfort on swallowing, symptoms of thyroid dysfunction, and family history of autoimmune thyroid disorders. The thyroid exam is an essential part of every woman's annual or pregnancy intake exam since thyroid dysfunction, nodules, and cancer are more prevalent in women than in men. Once you find a mass or enlarged thyroid, further evaluation is necessary even in an asymptomatic patient. Remember that approximately 5% of nodules will be malignant. A patient is more likely to have a malignant nodule if she has a history of childhood radiation exposure, a family history of thyroid cancer (e.g., medullary thyroid cancer), hoarseness of voice, and cervical lymphadenopathy. Screening for hypothyroidism or hyperthyroidism is also very important since autoimmune thyroid disorders such as Hashimoto disease and Graves disease are very common in women. Pregnant women with hypothyroidism are at particular risk of adverse pregnancy outcomes such as preterm delivery and poor fetal brain development. Euthyroid women with antithyroid antibodies have higher miscarriage rates and are more likely to develop postpartum thyroiditis.

GOITERS AND ABNORMAL THYROID-STIMULATING HORMONE

Initial assessment should include a thorough exam (heart rate, hair pattern, reflexes) and blood tests for thyroid-stimulating hormone (TSH), free thyroxine, and antibodies: thyroid peroxidase (TPO-Ab), thyroglobulin (TG-Ab), and TSH receptor (TR-Ab). If the patient is or is trying to become pregnant, the TSH should be kept below 2.5 µU/mL (3.0 in the second or third trimester) with thyroxine replacement. Consider increasing a woman's thyroxine dose by 30% to 50% automatically when she becomes pregnant and then monitoring TSH in 4 to 6 weeks. Pregnant women preferably should take their thyroid pills separately from prenatal vitamins since the latter may interfere with thyroid hormone absorption. Likewise, they will need a lower dose automatically after delivering. Women who have TPO antibodies but are euthyroid should be monitored at least once per trimester since they are at risk of developing overt hypothyroidism in pregnancy.

A suppressed TSH is often seen in first trimester of pregnancy (the high levels of hCG cross-react with TSH) and this should improve after the first trimester. Alternatively, low TSH can also be a sign of hyperthyroidism especially in a pregnant woman. The presence of TR-Ab and a goiter is more consistent with Graves disease. A woman should be treated in pregnancy if her free T4 is above the normal range propylthiouracil ((PTU) is first line) but not for subclinical hyperthyroidism alone. Thyroid levels should be checked at least every 3 to 4 weeks to make dose adjustments. If her Graves' cannot be managed medically, a subtotal thyroidectomy in the second trimester may be indicated. Since the TR-Ab can cross the placenta, the fetus should be monitored carefully for signs of growth restriction, hydrops fetalis, and cardiac failure.

Women who are TPO-antibody positive and women with type 1 diabetes should be screened for postpartum thyroiditis at 3 and 6 months after delivery. Women with postpartum depression should be screened for hypothyroidism. Exacerbation of Graves disease is also seen commonly after delivery.

NODULES

Pregnancy does not seem to alter the course or prognosis of malignant thyroid nodules, but pregnancy may change your management depending on the patient's gestational age. Initial diagnostic management should include an ultrasound (US) of the thyroid. This can help you determine if it is a solitary nodule or diffuse goiter and differentiate from solid versus cystic nodule and give accurate measurements. Certain US characteristics of a nodule are associated with malignancy (microcalcifications, irregular borders, hypogenicity, or increased intranodular vascularity seen on Doppler exam), either way a Fine Needle Aspiration (FNA) should be performed for any nodule >1 cm. US-guided FNAs may reduce the likelihood of obtaining an unsatisfactory result. A benign result carries a <1% risk of developing thyroid cancer. A radioisotope uptake scan in nonpregnant women may aid in your suspicion of malignancy in intermediate cases. Benign nodules are more prevalent in the population (>90%). The most common kinds of thyroid cancers are papillary and follicular thyroid cancers (differentiated thyroid cancers).

If an FNA reveals features of papillary thyroid cancer, surgery (i.e., near total thyroidectomy) is the first line of treatment followed by remnant ^{131}I ablation in some high-risk patients. In pregnant women, the American College of Obstetrics and Gynecology guidelines recommend performing the thyroidectomy preferably in the second trimester and deferring radiation treatment until postpartum. Patients need thyroxine supplementation life long and in high-risk patients, suppressive doses of L-thyroxine may prevent the thyroid cancer recurrence. Mothers should be advised to discard breast milk for 120 days after radiation ^{131}I treatment and avoid getting pregnant again for 6 months to 1 year after treatment for thyroid cancer.

TAKE HOME POINTS

- All women need to have their thyroid palpated as part of their routine exam.
- Hypothyroid women trying to conceive or pregnant women should have their TSH kept below 2.5 μU/mL (3.0 in the second or third trimester).
- Consider increasing a newly pregnant woman's thyroxine dose by 30% to 50% and confirm normal TSH 4 to 6 weeks later, since subclinical hypothyroidism is associated with multiple adverse pregnancy outcomes.
- PTU is used to treat overt hyperthyroidism and aim for a high normal T4 level.
- Thyroid nodules that are >1 cm should be biopsied. An US-guided biopsy reduces nondiagnostic aspirations.
- Mothers should not breastfeed for 4 months after ^{131}I treatment.

SUGGESTED READINGS

Abalovich M, Amino N, Barbour LA, et al. Management of thyroid dysfunction during pregnancy and postpartum: an endocrine society clinical practice guideline. *J Clin Endocrinol Metab*. 2007;92:s1–s47.

American College of Obstetricians and Gynecologists. ACOG Practice Bulletin No. 37: thyroid disease in pregnancy. Clinical Management Guidelines for Obstetrician-Gynecologists. *Obstet Gynecol*. 2002;100(2):387–396.

American Thyroid Association. ATA guidelines in THYROID. Volume 16, Number 2, 2006.

Moosa M, Mazzaferri EL. Outcome of differentiated thyroid cancer diagnosed in pregnant women. *J Clin Endocrinol Metab*. 1997;82:2862–2866.

Roman SA. Endocrine tumors: evaluation of the thyroid nodule. *Curr Opin Oncol*. 2003;15(1):66–70.

53

DOMESTIC VIOLENCE AND SEXUAL ASSAULT

DAPHNE P. BAZILE, MD

Marie is a 32-year-old female, gravida 4 para 3, at 25 weeks' gestation who presents to your OB/GYN office for her routine prenatal visit. This is her third visit to the office. At each visit, Marie is accompanied by her husband Michael. This morning, she is being seen by you as your partner is on vacation. In reviewing her chart, you notice that Marie's previous three pregnancies were all preterm deliveries before 32 weeks; all were low–birth-weight infants. You have also noticed that Marie has failed to gain any weight with this current pregnancy. In evaluating Marie, she does not answer any questions, instead her husband answers all inquires. As you exam her, Marie flinches as you touch her wrist. When questioned, Marie states she fell on her hand running after her 2-year-old daughter. Her husband quickly states that he has to get back to work. You quickly finish your evaluation, instructions are given, and Marie and her husband leave the office.

Domestic violence or intimate partner violence is a worldwide health problem and continues to be underreported. As obstetricians and gynecologists, this is of special concern because the majority of the victims are women. The violence has no barriers. It affects women of all economic, educational, ethnic, religious, and racial backgrounds as well as all age groups. It is a sensitive issue, that many physicians, when faced with the signs, choose to ignore them or do not know the steps to help the patient.

WHAT IS DOMESTIC VIOLENCE?

Domestic violence is not just hitting, pushing, or any form of physical manifestation. It is a series of behaviors that controls the victim by calculated threats and intimidation. It encompasses sexual and emotional abuse. The violence occurs between two individuals in a close relationship, whether married or dating. Oftentimes, the abuse starts as emotional and progresses to physical and sexual abuse.

Approximately 30% of women who present to the emergency room are thought to be victims of abuse. Thirty percent of all murdered women are killed by their partners.

The victim is controlled by her abuser because in many cases her "freedoms" are taken away. She may have no access to money. She is isolated from her family and friends. She completely relies on her abuser for transportation and other means of communication. The patient may have attempted to confide to family and friends and was told to "deal with it" or simply ignored. Again, the victim presenting to her doctor may be looking for help, but in the physician's haste to see patients quickly, signs are overlooked.

As obstetricians and gynecologists, we evaluate patients with pathology related to the genitalia and reproductive system. These pathologies can be the nonspecific presentations of abuse. These include chronic pelvic pain, urinary complaints, sexual dysfunction, irritable bowel syndrome, vaginitis, and so many others.

With the above patient, there are signs for future evaluation of the patient. Marie is 25 weeks in gestation and yet had failed to gain any weight. Her previous pregnancies all resulted in preterm deliveries. Abuse during pregnancy places the mother and her fetus at risk. There is an increased risk of miscarriage, low birth weight, vaginal bleeding, and poor maternal weight gain.

Marie shows signs of injury when she flinches at the touch of her wrist. Oftentimes, to avoid injury to their abdomen, many victims use their limbs to block assaults. Their limbs, such as Marie's wrist, are often the site of abuse.

For many women, pregnancy is the time when the abuse decreases. Some will state that they feel safer during pregnancy and as a result have repeated pregnancies. The theory is that the abuser will not hit them as long as they are pregnant; however, it resumes once the baby is born.

WHAT DO WE DO?

As health care providers, we are required to screen EVERYONE. Every woman who walks through the door in your office gets asked about violence. Every woman should be questioned regarding safety. Laws regarding mandatory reporting vary from state to state. BEFORE inquiring about violence, it is important that you learn the details about your state's mandatory reporting.

When suspected, the following steps can help:

- Acknowledge the trauma
- Assess immediate safety of patient and children
- Help establish a safety plan
- Review options
- Offer educational materials and a list of community and local resources (including toll-free hotline)
- Provide referrals
- Document interactions
- Provide ongoing support at subsequent visits

- Questions to ask include the following:
  - Has anyone close to you ever threatened to hurt you?
  - Has anyone ever hit, kicked, choked, punched, or hurt you physically?
  - Has anyone ever forced you to have sex against your will?
  - Do you feel safe at home?
  - Since you became pregnant, have you been physically, emotionally, or sexually hurt by anyone?
  - Do you fear for the safety of you and/or your children and/or unborn child?

TAKE HOME POINTS

- Domestic abuse is any series of behaviors that controls a victim by calculated threats and intimidation.
- Approximately 30% of women who present to the emergency room are thought to be victims of abuse.
- Domestic abuse pathology can be the nonspecific including but not limited to chronic pelvic pain, urinary complaints, sexual dysfunction, irritable bowel syndrome, and vaginitis.
- It is important that you learn the details about your state's mandatory reporting for abuse cases.

SUGGESTED READINGS

American College of Obstetricians and Gynecologists. *Guidelines for Women's Health Care*. 2nd ed. Washington, DC: ACOG; 2002.

Centers for Disease Control and Prevention (CDC). Costs of intimate partner violence against women in the United States. Atlanta, GA: CDC, National Center for Injury Prevention and Control; 2003. [cited 2006 May 22]. Available at: URL: www.cdc.gov/ncipc/pub-res/ipv_cost/ipv.htm

Centers for Disease Control and Prevention National Center for Injury Prevention and Control 1-800-CDC-INFO. Available at: www.cdc.gov/injury; cdcinfo@cdc.gov

Heise L, Ellsberg M, Gottemoeller M. Ending violence against women. *Population Reports*; Series L, No. 11. Baltimore, MD: Johns Hopkins University; 1999. Available at: http://www.infoforhealth.org/pr/l11/violence.pdf

54

FEMALE SEXUAL DYSFUNCTION

DIANA BROOMFIELD, MD, FACOG, FACS

Connie has always been a "go-getter." She graduated in the top 10% of her medical school class and now serves as the Chair of a major metropolitan hospital. She has been married for the past 10 years to Tom, another physician who is the Chair of his department. This couple is considered one of "power couples" in the area. They have two children. Connie has been fortunate to have had the same nanny to help with the children since their birth several years ago. Like so many busy physicians, Connie really has not had much time to herself and even less time to spend intimate moments with her husband. In the earlier years of their marriage, Tom and Connie went on "dates" at least once per month and engaged in sexual or intimate activities at least once per week. However, since having the children and becoming Chair Connie has noted a reluctance to engage in any sexual activities. On a scale of 0 to 10 (0 being no desire for sexual activity and 10 being desirous of sexual activity at least three to four times per week), Connie rates her desire for sexual activity as 0 to 1. She states that if she engaged in sexual activity once per year that would be okay and really prefers that her husband just "leaves her alone."

Sexual health is a complex and multifactorial disorder. Sexual dysfunctions and disorders may be caused by endocrinopathies, vasculogenic, neurogenic, musculogenic, or psychogenic factors. Medications such as antidepressants may cause sexual dysfunctions as well as chronic disease such as diabetes, neurological diseases, hormonal imbalances, menopause, hypothyroidism, liver failure, hypertension, heart disease, and alcoholism.

Sexual health is impacted by a women's sense of well-being, her overall health status, her general perception of well-being, and her previous sexual and relationship experiences (bad, good, or indifferent). Interestingly, when couples are questioned about their relationship, if they are "happy" or contented with their relationship, they will attribute the sexual aspect as having very little to do with their happiness. However, couples who have poor communications and consider their relationship as "unhappy" will attribute sex as a significant part of that relationship. Sexual health can be divided into concerns, dysfunctions, or disorders. A sexual disorder is a sexual dysfunction that results in personal distress to the patient. Thus, a woman may have sexual concerns, discontent, or even dysfunctions without having a sexual disorder.

One of the most important aspects of sexual well-being is education. Many women believe that the "normal" sexual response is the traditional Masters and Johnson's desire-arousal-orgasm-resolution process. However, women must realize that normal sexual functioning is quite variable. Sexual activity, and/or desire, may also encompass the desire for intimacy and not only the desire for and the act of intercourse. This revelation is often enlightening to many women and brings a sense of normalcy to what was once deemed abnormal. Thus, having the desire for intimacy constitutes normal sexual functioning even if the woman is not interested in actual sexual activity.

Masters and Johnson defined the normal physiologic sexual response in 1957 as consisting of four phases:

- Excitement
- Plateau
- Orgasm
- Resolution

Clearly, discontent, dysfunctions, and disorders may occur in any or all four phases of the sexual response. Kaplan later modified this classification to include Desire as a fifth phase preceding the Excitement phase. The female sexual response phases are known to be mediated by the activity of the autonomic nervous system (ANS) via neurotransmitters. Increased activity of the ANS results in:

- Tachycardia
- Skin flushing

Positive effects on the ANS are mediated through the following neurotransmitters:

- NE
- Dopamine
- Oxytocin

Neurotransmitters having "negative" effects on the female sexual response include:

- Prolactin
- GABA

The neurotransmitter serotonin may have both negative and positive effects on the female sexual response.

Thus, during the postpartum period when prolactin secretion is increased, this neurotransmitter will have a negative effect on the female sexual response. This perhaps serves as a natural protective mechanism so that the women in the immediate postpartum period refrain from sexual activity.

ROLE OF THE PHYSICIAN

It is imperative that the physician is nonjudgmental and supportive when interviewing patients. Questions should be open ended. There are patient intake tools such as questionnaires and checklist tools used to facilitate ease of communication and comprehensiveness. The PLISSIT (Permission, Limited Information, Specific Suggestions, Intensive Therapy) or ALLOW (Ask, Legitimize, Limitations, Open up, Work together) method can be used to facilitate discussions about sexual concerns and initiation of treatment.

HYPOACTIVE SEXUAL DESIRE DISORDER

According to the *DSM IV*, 35% to 45% of all women (about 40 million) report some level of sexual dysfunction. Of the many sexual dysfunctions, certainly the most frequent dysfunction is decreased libido. This is also known as hypoactive sexual desire disorder or "low sexual desire." Hypo-active sexual desire disorder is the most common type of all female sexual dysfunction disorders. Hypoactive sexual desire disorder is frequently linked to a psychological or physiologic etiology. The psychological etiologies are usually treated with psychotherapy, behavioral modification, stress management, education, and lifestyle changes. Pharmacologic management has limited value. Transdermal application of 300 μg testosterone daily may have some benefit in postmenopausal women in combination of hormone replacement therapy (HRT). This indication is not FDA approved in women for hypoactive sexual desire disorder.

SEXUAL AROUSAL DISORDER

Sexual arousal disorder is the recurrent or persistent inability to achieve sexual arousal or excitement, which causes personal distress. This may be manifested as a subjective lack or reduction in sexual excitement or the inability to have vaginal lubrication with sexual, visual, tactile, emotional, or other sensory stimulus. In April 2000, the FDA approved a clitoral device, the Eros Therapy Clitoral Device for female sexual dysfunction. Eros Clitoral Therapy Device (FDA Approved Device for Female Sexual Dysfunction, *http://healiohealth.com/tek9.asp?pg=products&specific=jnnpjqfrk&gclid =CJqC5d6q9Z0CFZho5QodXQymKA*) is a small, handheld female sexual health medical device that is placed over the clitoris and external genitalia. It can be purchased over the internet for $395.00. The device causes a small suction or vacuum over the clitoris, which increases the blood flow to the clitoris and external genitalia leading to engorgement, increasing vaginal lubrication, thus increasing sexual stimulation and ability to achieve orgasm.

ORGASMIC DISORDER

Many women suffer from anorgasmia, the inability to achieve an orgasm. Anorgasmia is typically associated with sexual activity with a partner. Many women are misinformed and are led to believe that orgasm should be achieved with intercourse without any collateral or direct clitoral, breast, or other sensate organ stimulation. These women must be educated that orgasm for most women requires direct clitoral or other organ stimulation (e.g., the breasts) during intercourse, and rarely does isolated intercourse without any clitoral (or sensate organ) stimulation lead to orgasm. Most women are able to achieve an orgasm through masturbation. Thus, a treatment option of anorgasmia is directed masturbation, cognitive behavior therapy, and sensate focus. Cognitive behavior therapy focuses on decreasing anxiety and promoting changes in attitudes and sexual thoughts, which increase the ability to achieve orgasm and to gain satisfaction from orgasm. Sensate focus is a form of sexual therapy that guides a woman and her partner through a series of exercises, moving from nonsexual to sexual touching.

Anorgasmia or arousal disorders may also be caused by chronic diseases, medications, or a woman's sexual inhibition, lack of experience or knowledge, and psychological factors such as guilt, anxiety, depression, or a past sexual trauma or abuse.

SEXUAL PAIN DISORDERS

Dyspareunia is defined as genital pain caused during sexual intercourse. Dyspareunia has many potential etiologies, pelvic factors such as infection, endometriosis, or vestibulodynia (formerly called vulvar vestibulitis); Lichen sclerosis; chronic candidiasis vulvovaginitis; sexually transmitted infections (STI); and vaginal atrophy. It is imperative that a thorough pelvic examination is done to identify any contributing pathologies. Thus, treatment is dependent on the underlying disorder.

Vaginismus is the painful contractions of the musculature of the lower third of the vagina in response to vaginal penetration including tampons but typically sexual intercourse. It is important to rule out underlying pathologies such as vestibulitis or even a history of incest or rape.

Sexual pain disorders may improve with some pharmacologic agents such as tricyclics and other antidepressants, anticonvulsants, and topical estrogen cream. Many patients also may benefit from desensitization therapy through behavioral modification techniques, sensate therapy, hypnotherapy, or use of vaginal dilators.

The clinician must not be afraid to ask female patients about their sexual function and be prepared to rule out underlying pathologies, some of which have specific medical treatments (hypothyroidism, hyperprolactinemia, endometriosis, peripheral vascular disease, and the like). When pharmacologic agents fail to correct the disorder, a referral to an appropriate sex therapist, behavioral therapist, or psychologist may be most beneficial for those women who suffer from sexual disorders.

TAKE HOME POINTS

- Thirty-five to forty percent of all women (about 40 million) report some level of sexual dysfunction.
- The female sexual response phases are known to be mediated by the activity of the ANS via neurotransmitters.
- Sexual health is a complex and multifactorial disorder.
- A sexual disorder is a sexual dysfunction that results in personal distress to the patient.
- The most frequent dysfunction is decreased libido. This is also known as hypoactive sexual desire disorder or "low sexual desire."
- The physician's role is to provide education, search for underlying pathologies, and conduct interview that is nonjudgmental, and questions should be open ended.
- Many causes of sexual dysfunctions are treatable.

SUGGESTED READINGS

American Psychiatric Association. *Diagnostic and Statistical Manual of Mental Disorders.* 4th ed. Arlington, VA, American Psychiatric Association; 1994.

Feldman J, Striepe M. Women's sexual health. *Clin Fam Pract.* 2004;6(4):839–861.

Frank JA, Mistretta P, Will J. *Diagnosis and Treatment of Female Sexual Dysfunction.* American Academy of Family Physicians; Leawood, KS. 2008.

Laumann EO, Paik A, Rosen RC. Sexual dysfunction in the United States. *JAMA.* 1999;281(6):537–544.

Masters WH, Johnson VE. *Human Sexual Response.* Toronto, ON; New York, NY: Bantam Books; 1966. ISBN 0–553–20429–7.

Meston CM, Hull E, Levin RJ, et al. Disorders of orgasm in women. *J Sex Med.* 2004;1(1): 66–68.

Nicolosi A, Laumann EO, Glasser DB, et al. Sexual behavior and sexual dysfunctions after age 40: the global study of sexual attitudes and behaviors. *Urology.* 2004;64(5):991–997.

Ragucci KR, Culhane NS. Treatment of female sexual dysfunction. *Ann Pharmacother.* 2003;37(4):546–555.

55

ADNEXAL TORSION CAN STILL HAVE BLOOD FLOW

THINH H. DUONG, MD

Adnexal torsion is a common cause of acute pelvic pain, with a reported prevalence rate as high as 3%. It occurs when the ovary or tube rotates upon its axis resulting in either complete or partial occlusion of blood flow to the tube and ovary. It is the fifth most common gynecologic surgical emergency. Although women of all ages may be affected, it most commonly occurs in women aged 20 to 40 years.

Several preexisting conditions predispose a patient to adnexal torsion. The presence of an ovarian mass, pregnancy, pelvic trauma, pelvic adhesive disease, pelvic inflammatory disease, and ovarian hyperstimulation syndrome have all been associated with adnexal torsion. Of these, the presence of an ovarian mass is the most common. Regardless of etiology, the resulting torsing of the ovary and/or fallopian tube results in occlusion of vascular flow. If left untreated, the lack of perfusion may result in end-organ damage and eventual death of the tissue.

Although the diagnosis of adnexal torsion is made clinically, its varied presentation may make the diagnosis difficult. The classic presentation of intermittent waxing and waning pain in the pelvis may represent a torsing and untorsing adnexa. Other possible symptoms include fevers, chills, nausea, vomiting, and anorexia. The time frame from onset of symptoms to presentation may range from hours to months. Unfortunately, most patients may have few or none of these symptoms.

Aside from a detailed history of the patient's pain and associated symptoms, a careful physical examination may assist in making the diagnosis. Physical findings include abdominal pain (either direct or rebound), voluntary and involuntary guarding on abdominal palpation, pelvic pain, and cervical motion tenderness. Laboratory findings may include an elevated white blood cell count, abnormal markers of inflammation (C-reactive protein or erythrocyte sedimentation rate), and even abnormal electrolytes, if emesis is severe.

An ultrasound may be of assistance in making the diagnosis. A finding of an enlarged adnexal mass on pelvic ultrasound is often present. The absence of Doppler flow to an ovary may represent torsing of the adnexa. Despite of the usefulness of modern ultrasound, the diagnosis of adnexal torsion remains a clinical one. This is of particular importance given that the majority of patients presenting with a possible adnexal torsion are of childbearing age and wish to preserve their future fertility potential.

Prompt diagnosis and treatment are critical in young women desiring to preserve their fertility potential. Delayed diagnosis may lead to an ovary damaged beyond recovery requiring surgical removal. Given the grave nature of an untimely diagnosis, prompt diagnosis and treatment are critical. Given this, when a clinical diagnosis of adnexal torsion is made in a woman desiring to preserve her fertility, operative intervention is indicated. At the very least, a prompt diagnostic laparoscopy is indicated.

Once the definitive diagnosis of adnexal torsion is made at the time of surgery, the decision of removal of the tube and/or ovary versus detorsion and resection of any pathology is a clinical one. Traditionally, removal of the torsed tissue was advocated secondary to the concerns of persistent necrotic tissue, potential malignancy, or potential propagation of a blood clot. In postmenopausal women or women who have completed their childbearing, adnexal resection is perhaps faster surgically and potentially wrought with less complications. In women wishing to preserve their fertility options, the decision is more difficult. These concerns are beginning to be answered by science and not just opinion. Several case series have reported viable ovarian tissue of up to 92% of ovaries in women with adnexal torsion and presumed dead tissue. Furthermore, women with necrotic-appearing ovaries have been followed after detorsion with minimal to no subsequent complications (other than febrile morbidity that generally resolved after 2 days). Given this, however, the choice of radical removal versus conservative restoration remains a difficult one. Some have advocated untorsing the adnexa and assessing for reperfusion (i.e., restoration of blood flow and the red or pink appearance).

Unfortunately, even viable tissue may remain black or blue in appearance when perfusion is restored. The use of fluorescein may aid in the diagnosis of flow to the adnexa. In general, 5 mL of 10% fluorescein is injected intravenously and the affected adnexa are visualized under an ultraviolet light. If perfusion is absent, there will be an absence of fluorescent tissue under the light. Unfortunately, this tool is not foolproof and may lead to unnecessary removal of viable ovary.

The obvious downside to ovarian removal is decreased fertility and potential early hormonal cessation. The downsides to not removing a non-viable adnexa are the concerns for infection, malignancy, and possible propagation of a formed thrombus. Prospective research is lacking; however, several retrospective studies show minimal complications of not removing the affected adnexa. Given this, preservation of an ovary in reproductive age women should always be considered first.

TAKE HOME POINTS

- Adnexal torsion is a common cause of acute pelvic pain.
- Diagnosis is generally clinical although an ultrasound may be useful.
- Prompt surgical treatment is critical for the preservation of ovarian function and future fertility.
- Intravenous fluorescein may aid in the diagnosis of nonviable ovarian tissue.
- When in doubt, favor conservative detorsion in women wishing to preserve their fertility.

SUGGESTED READINGS

Ben-Ami M, Perlitz Y, Haddad S. The effectiveness of spectral and color Doppler in predicting ovarian torsion. A prospective study. *Eur J Obstet Gynecol Reprod Biol.* 2002;104:64–66.

Eitan R, Galoyan N, Zuckerman B, et al. The risk of malignancy in postmenopausal women presenting with adnexal torsion. *Gynecol Oncol.* 2007;106:211–214.

Houry D, Abbott J. Ovarian torsion: a fifteen year review. *Ann Emerg Med.* 2001;38:156–159.

McGovern PG, Ralph N, Koenigsberg R, et al. Adnexal torsion and pulmonary embolism: case report and review of the literature. *Obstet Gynecol Surv.* 1999;54:601–608.

Oelsner G, Cohen SB, Soriano D, et al. Minimal surgery for the twisted ischaemic adnexa can preserve ovarian function. *Hum Reprod.* 2003;18:2599–2602.

Oelsner G, Shashar D. Adnexal torsion. *Clin Obstet Gynecol.* 2006;49:459–463.

Pena J, Ufberg D, Cooney N, et al. Usefulness of Doppler sonography in the diagnosis of ovarian torsion. *Fertil Steril.* 2000;73:1047–1050.

Rody A, Jackisch C, Klockenbusch W, et al. The conservative management of adnexal torsion—a case report and review of the literature. *Eur J Obstet Gynecol Reprod Biol.* 2002;101:83–86.

Shalev E, Bustan M, Yaro I, et al. Recovery of ovarian function after laparoscopic detorsion. *Hum Reprod.* 1995;10:2965–2966.

Shalev E, Peleg D. Laparoscopic treatment of adnexal torsion. *Surg Gynecol Obstet.* 1993;176:448–450.

56

You cannot diagnose everything with a speculum: Appendicitis

Thinh H. Duong, MD

Appendicitis remains a common problem affecting approximately 7% of the U.S. population. The overall mortality rate is 0.2% to 0.8% but rises above 20% in individuals over 70 years old. Luminal perforation is higher among patients under 18 and over 50 years of age, likely secondary to the delay in diagnosis and treatment. Overall, the incidence of appendicitis is slightly lower in women than men (1.4 times less) while the incidence of primary appendectomy is about the same.

Appendicitis occurs as a result of obstruction of the appendiceal lumen. The most common causes of obstruction are fecaliths and lymphoid follicle hyperplasia. Other possible causes of obstruction include parasites, foreign ingested materials, tuberculosis, and cancer. The resulting obstruction results in accumulation of intestinal fluids and subsequent distension. Bacteria invade the walls of the appendix secondary to poor lymphatic and venous drainage resulting in infection of the organ. In advanced cases, perforation and development of peritonitis may occur.

While the classic presentation of anorexia, periumbilical pain followed by nausea, right lower quadrant (RLQ) pain, and vomiting may occur in 50% of patients, the initial presentation of appendicitis is generally inconsistent. Fevers, chills, diarrhea, constipation, and irritative voiding symptoms may also be presents. The different presentations are secondary to the varied positions of the appendix, age of the patient, and the extent of inflammation present. Given this, migration of pain from the periumbilical region to the RLQ is the most discerning feature, with sensitivities and specificities approaching 80%. Nausea may be present in 90% of patients while anorexia is present 75% of the time. The duration of these symptoms are generally <48 hours but may be longer in elderly patients and those with a perforated lumen. Pain lasting longer than 2 weeks is rare; however, it may occur in a minority of patients.

A detailed history and physical exam are of paramount importance in making the diagnosis of an appendicitis. A patient may present with the aforementioned symptoms. On abdominal exam, RLQ pain is often elicited. In addition, rebound tenderness, boardlike rigidity, and involuntary guarding may be present.

Although they may be absent, severe signs are associated with an appendicitis:

1. Rovsing sign—RLQ pain with palpation of left lower quadrant (LLQ)
2. Obturator sign—RLQ pain with internal rotation of the flexed right hip
3. Psoas sign—RLQ pain with hyperextension of the right hip
4. Dunphy sign—increased abdominal pain with coughing
5. Markle sign—abdominal pain when a standing person drops from her toes to her heals

Laboratory tests may reveal evidence of infection. A complete blood cell count may reveal an elevated white blood cell count. A left shift with an increased neutrophil count of >75% is also commonly present. These findings may be inconsistent in the elderly and immunocompromised patient, however. Although a C-reactive protein may be nonspecific, a normal value in a patient with >24 hours of symptoms virtually rules out an appendicitis. A urinalysis may be useful to diagnosing a urinary tract infection; however, studies show that pyuria may be present in one in seven patients.

A computed tomography (CT) scan has become the imaging study of choice for the diagnosis of appendicitis. Although abnormal findings are present in normal patients, correlation with clinical examination often will reveal the diagnosis, preventing avoidable morbidities and mortalities. The addition of contrast improves the sensitivity and specificity of the CT scan. Findings suggestive of appendicitis include lack of contrast filling, thickened diameter, and enhancement.

Other imaging modalities have been used for the diagnosis of appendicitis. They are compression ultrasound, radionuclide tagged cell scan, and MRI. While noninvasive and potentially accurate in the diagnosis of appendicitis, the operator-dependent nature of ultrasound has limited their use. A tagged cell scan has the benefit of very high sensitivities as the cells will accumulate in the infected appendix. The slow acquisition time (upwards of 5 hours) and relative lack of immediate availability also limit its use. MRI shows promise as it is relatively accurate in diagnosing appendicitis, although its cost is significantly higher than a CT scan.

Despite these diagnostic modalities, appendicitis is misdiagnosed 25% of the time. In addition, a normal appendix is present in upwards of 40% of patients undergoing emergent appendectomy. Thus, other diagnoses must also be considered. Other differential diagnoses include ectopic pregnancy, adnexal torsion, mittelschmerz, pelvic inflammatory disease, cholecystitis, gastroenteritis, diverticulitis, pancreatitis, perforated duodenal ulcer, renal colic, urinary tract infection, small bowel obstruction, and other inflammatory bowel disease (e.g., Crohn disease).

Once the diagnosis of an appendicitis is made, it is not a matter of if, but when surgical intervention will take place. With prompt diagnosis and swift surgical treatment, mortality from an appendicitis is very rare. However, in rare circumstances, sepsis may occur and warrant antibiotic therapy prior to surgical intervention.

The decision for laparoscopic versus open laparotomy depends on various parameters, the most import of which is the stability of the patient and the comfort level of the surgeon performing the surgery. Currently, however, laparoscopic appendectomy is a relatively standard procedure and exhibits decreased morbidity compared to a laparotomy.

TAKE HOME POINTS

- Appendicitis is a common problem in the United States with an incidence of 7%.
- Diagnosis is generally clinical although a CT can help considerably.
- Prompt surgical treatment considerably reduces morbidity and mortality.
- Despite modern diagnostic modalities, upwards of 40% of appendix emergently removed are normal.

SUGGESTED READINGS

Bickell NA, Aufses AH, Rojas M. How time affects the risk of rupture in appendicitis. *J Am Coll Surg*. 2006;202(3):401–406.

Eriksson S, Granstrom L. Randomized controlled trial of appendicectomy versus antibiotic therapy for acute appendicitis. *Br J Surg*. 1995;82(2):166–169.

Fuchs JR, Schlamberg JS, Shortsleeve MJ, et al. Impact of abdominal CT imaging on the management of appendicitis: an update. *J Surg Res*. 2002;106(1):131–136.

LeBlond RF, DeGowin RL, Brown DD. *DeGowin's Diagnostic Examination*. 8th ed. New York, NY: McGraw-Hill; 2004.

Lin HF, Wu JM, Tseng LM, et al. Laparoscopic versus open appendectomy for perforated appendicitis. *J Gastrointest Surg*. 2006;10(6):906–910.

57

A BLACK CAT ON A DARK NIGHT: ECTOPIC PREGNANCY

VICTOR M. FELDBAUM, MD
AND THINH H. DUONG, MD

Pregnancy in the fallopian tube is like a black cat on a dark night. It may make its presence felt in subtle ways and leap at you or it may slip past unobserved. Although it is difficult to distinguish from cats of other colors in darkness, illumination clearly identifies it. Mc Fadyen (1981)

Ectopic pregnancy comes from Greek word "Ektopos," which means out of place and was first described by Abulcasis in 936 A.D. It is one of the leading causes of maternal mortality and morbidity, accounting for 9% of all maternal deaths. Ectopic pregnancy is a complication of pregnancy where an early identification and proper management can significantly impact morbidity and mortality. The most common site of ectopic implantation is the ampullary segment of the fallopian tube (80%), followed by the isthmic segment of the fallopian tube (12%), fimbrial segment of the fallopian tube (5%), cornual/interstitial segment of the fallopian tube (2%), abdominal (1.4%), ovarian (0.2%), and cervical (0.2%). The etiology of an ectopic pregnancy has been associated with any process that injures or scars the tube:

- Acquired—PID, septic abortion, puerperal sepsis, tuberculosis, previous ectopic
- Surgical—tubal reconstructive surgery or recanalization of tubes
- Neoplastic—broad ligament myoma, ovarian tumor
- Congenital—tubal hypoplasia, congenital diverticuli, accessory ostia, partial stenosis
- Miscellaneous—endometriosis, cigarette smoking

Ectopic pregnancy most commonly presents with complaints of abdominal pain (80%–90%), amenorrhea (75%–90%), and/or vaginal bleeding (50%–80%). It is important to administer RhoGAM (50 μg if <12 weeks of gestational age) if the patient is Rh negative to prevent Rh alloimmunization in a future pregnancy. Pelvic ultrasound can detect an intrauterine pregnancy with serum β-hCG levels as low as 1,500 to 2,000 mIU/mL. If the patient is stable and has low β-hCG level, she can be closely followed, rechecking a β-hCG in 48 hours. Be aware that an abnormal increase in serum β-hCG of <53% over 48 hours has a 99% sensitivity for an abnormal pregnancy. A gestational sac on ultrasound by itself does not confirm intrauterine pregnancy as one could be looking at a pseudosac (present in 10% of ectopic pregnancies). One should look for the presence of a yolk sac or fetal pole to confirm an intrauterine pregnancy. A common error in the diagnosis of ectopic pregnancy is not considering multiple gestation pregnancy with implantations in one tube, both tubes, or the tube and the uterine cavity (heterotopic pregnancy).

If the patient is hemodynamically stable and an ectopic pregnancy is suspected, she may be offered expectant management, methotrexate therapy, or surgical management. Expectant management is effective in a stable patient presenting with β-hCG level of <200 mIU/mL, as spontaneous resolution is seen in approximately 80% of cases. β-hCG levels >200 mIU/mL will spontaneously regress in <25% of cases. In expectant management, β-hCG levels should be monitored biweekly.

Methotrexate has been FDA approved since 1996 and affects the synthesis of purine nucleotides and thymidylate, thus interfering with DNA synthesis, repair, and cellular replication. It can be offered to hemodynamically stable patients with an unruptured mass and works best in people with β-hCG levels under 10,000 mIU/mL. It is contraindicated in women who are breastfeeding or have immunodeficiency, blood dyscrasias, renal, hepatic, or active pulmonary disease. It is relatively contraindicated in women with a gestational sac >3.5 cm or positive fetal heart tones. Prior to administration, dilation and curettage or manual vacuum aspiration should be performed to ensure that the patient with a spontaneous abortion is not treated unnecessarily. Patients who receive methotrexate should avoid pregnancy for at least 3 months. Methotrexate should be given 50 mg/m^2 IM as a single dose. After administration of methotrexate on day 1, β-hCG levels should be assessed on days 4 and 7. Another error in the management of an ectopic pregnancy is not recognizing methotrexate treatment failure:

- β-hCG levels that do not decline by at least 15% between day 4 and day 7 after administration
- Significantly worsening abdominal pain, regardless of change in β-hCG levels
- Hemodynamic instability

If the patient is stable and β-hCG levels did not decline appropriately, a second dose of methotrexate may be offered.

Surgical management is needed in all patients who are unstable or who do not meet the above criteria for conservative or methotrexate management. Surgery offers a firm diagnosis, offers less prolonged and less demanding follow-up, and allows patients to attempt to conceive as soon as they recover from the operation. The disadvantages include fallopian tube scar formation, pelvic adhesions, and general surgical and anesthesia risks. When choosing between laparoscopy and laparotomy, one should consider the patient's surgical history, the surgeon's experience, and the location of the ectopic. Pelvic adhesions, hematoperitoneum, mass >4 cm, and hemodynamic instability are contraindications to laparoscopic management. There is no difference in the rate of subsequent intrauterine and ectopic pregnancies between the two surgical methods.

Finally, as with any pregnancy, order a type and screen to check the patient's Rh status. Do not forget to follow up on result and give RhoGAM if the patient is Rh negative.

TAKE HOME POINTS

- Give RhoGAM if the patient is Rh negative.
- Methotrexate works best in patients with β-hCG levels under 10,000 mIU/mL.
- An abnormal increase in serum β-hCG of <53% over 48 hours has a 99% sensitivity for an abnormal pregnancy.
- There is no difference in the rate of subsequent intrauterine and ectopic pregnancies between laparoscopic and laparotomy treatments.

SUGGESTED READINGS

ACOG Practice Bulletin No. 94. *Ectopic pregnancy.* 2008;111(6):1479–1485.

Barnhart KT, Gosman G, Ashby R, et al. The medical management of ectopic pregnancy: a meta-analysis comparing "single dose" and "multidose" regimens. *Obstet Gynecol.* 2003;101: 778–784.

Fernandez H, Vincent SCY, Pauthier S, et al. Randomized trial of conservative laparoscopic treatment and methotrexate administration in ectopic pregnancy and subsequent fertility. *Hum Reprod.* 1998;13:3239–3243.

Hajenius PJ, Mol F, Mol BW, et al. Interventions for tubal ectopic pregnancy. *Cochrane Database Syst. Rev.* 2007 (1): CD000324.

Laure S. The history of the diagnosis and treatment of ectopic pregnancy: a medical adventure. *EJOGRB.* 1992;43:1–7.

McFadyen IR. Gynaecological pain in the lower abdomen. *Clin Obstet Gynaecol.* 1981(1): 33-47.

Mol BW, Matthijsse HC, Tinga DJ, et al. Fertility after conservative and radical surgery for tubal pregnancy. *Hum. Reprod.* 1998;13:1804–1809.

Rock JA, Jones HW. *Te Linde's Operative Gynecology.* 9th ed. Philadelphia, PA: Lippincott Williams & Wilkins; 2003.

Ying TL. Tubal disease and fertility outcome. *Reprod Biomed.* 2007;15(4):396–402.

58

ACUTE PELVIC PAIN

NAA SACKEY, MD AND DIANA BROOMFIELD, MD, MBA, FACOG, FACS

A 25-year-old G1P0010 female with a last menstrual period of 3 weeks ago presents to the ER with acute pelvic pain that started 72 hours prior to admission. The patient states her pain is localized to the right lower quadrant and describes the pain as a constant, dull pain. She also experienced one episode of nausea. Medical history is significant for gonorrheal infection 2 years ago. On physical exam, the vitals are stable, and the abdomen is nontender with normoactive bowel sounds. A pelvic exam shows normal external genitalia, closed cervix, no discharge, no cervical motion tenderness; however, right adnexal tenderness is noted. Pregnancy test is negative. A transvaginal sonogram reveals an empty uterus and adnexal fluid. The patient is sexually active and uses condoms occasionally.

Acute abdominal and pelvic pain is one of the most common gynecologic emergency complaints. Pain can be described as visceral or somatic pain. Visceral pain is caused by irritation of the visceral peritoneum, and the pain is transmitted by the afferent fibers of the autonomic nervous system. On the contrary, somatic pain originates from the parietal peritoneum, and it is transmitted through the afferent fibers of the somatic nervous system.

The first step in diagnosis of acute pelvic pain is the history and physical exam. The history provides pertinent information that can help lead to diagnosis. There is certain useful information that should be obtained while gathering the history such as the characterization of the pain. Somatic pain is usually described as sharp pain that is worse with movements while visceral pain is characterized as a generalized dull, aching pain. The onset of pelvic pain can be sudden or gradual. Sudden pain is indicative or suggestive of an acute event, a rupture of viscera or mass, and the like. The duration of the pain can be described as constant, intermittent, or colicky. Location of the pain can also help guide the diagnosis; visceral pain is often referred and somatic pain is localized to the site of the affected muscle or organ. Frequency, severity, and relationship to the menstrual cycle are other important factors to consider in the diagnosis of pelvic pain. Other constitutional symptoms associated with pelvic pain are fever, chills, nausea, vomiting, vaginal discharge, and vaginal bleeding.

A focused physical exam should be performed promptly during the management of acute pelvic pain. It is important to be aware of signs that can differentiate the diagnosis and to determine the severity of the condition. General appearance such as diaphoresis, pallor, a grimacing facial expression, and agitation might be a clue to the severity of the pain. Vital signs that are consistent with fever may suggest an infection. Tachycardia and hypotension are other alarming signs in acute pain. On exam, the abdomen should be inspected for surgical scars, which might suggest a diagnosis of obstruction or adhesions. The abdomen should be auscultated for high-pitched bowel sounds, which are suggestive of intestinal obstruction. Palpation of all four quadrants should be performed and should begin away from the site of pain; rebound tenderness, psoas sign, and other signs of peritoneal inflammation are clues to the diagnosis. Pelvic exam should include a careful examination of vaginal or cervical discharge. Purulent discharge may be suggestive of vaginitis and inflammatory disease; bloody discharge may suggest pregnancy. Microscopic inspection of vaginal or cervical discharge should be performed. Uterine size, shape, consistency, tenderness, and cervical motion tenderness are also important signs to aid in the differential diagnosis.

Laboratory results and radiological imaging are the next steps in the management. Laboratory findings such as an elevated white blood count and erythrocyte sedimentation rate suggest an infection. A serum pregnancy test and a urinalysis should also be performed in the management of pelvic pain. Radiological imaging such as computed tomography, MRI, or sonography with or without Doppler is essential in the diagnosis of pelvic pain.

A ruptured ovarian cyst is a common diagnosis for acute pelvic pain. The pain is usually described as midcycle pelvic pain that is noticed near or during ovulation. Pain is caused by peritoneal irritation by the ovarian follicular cyst fluid; therefore, the pain is characterized as somatic pain. The pain is described as sudden onset of a unilateral pelvic pain that may be associated with initial nausea, diaphoresis, and vaginal bleeding. The pain usually lasts for hours to days. On physical exam, adnexal tenderness without a mass is present. The diagnosis is frequently a diagnosis of exclusion and is usually made by ultrasonography, which shows free fluid in the cul-de-sac. A common error in the management of ruptured ovarian cyst is missing the signs of hemorrhage. It is crucial to consider performing exploratory laparoscopy or laparotomy if there are signs of hemorrhage or hemodynamic instability. The treatment should include an analgesic if conservative management is warranted.

Ectopic pregnancy is the development of a fertilized ovum outside of the uterus usually in the fallopian tube, ovaries, or the abdominal cavity. Risk factors for ectopic pregnancy include tubular anomalies, pelvic inflammatory disease, tubal adhesions, history of previous tubal surgery (ligation, anastomosis), intrauterine devices, and previous ectopic pregnancy. The classic triad for ectopic pregnancy includes lower quadrant or pelvic pain that is associated with one or two missed periods and palpable mass; other associated features are cervical motion tenderness, vaginal bleeding, uterine enlargement, and shoulder pain. The definitive diagnosis is made by ultra-sonography, which shows an empty uterus with a high serum beta human chorionic gonadotropin (beyond the discriminatory zone, usually >2,000 U/mIU) with or without a pelvic mass. A culdocentesis, aspiration of blood from the cul-de-sac (looking for nonclotting blood), might be performed if sonography is not possible. Management includes blood work for blood typing and screening and Rh sensitivity should be performed, as all Rh-negative mothers are given RhoGAM. Treatments for ectopic pregnancy include surgical removal or medical treatment with methotrexate (a folate antagonist). A common error is to forget to have the patient discontinue prenatal vitamins, which contain folate.

Ovarian torsion is another common differential diagnosis for pelvic pain. Pain is described as sudden, colicky, lower quadrant pain that is asso-ciated with a history of intermittent cramping or history of ovarian cyst, nausea and vomiting, dyspareunia, and painful defecation. Ovarian torsion is also common in pregnancy especially during first trimester. Transvagi-nal ultrasound or CT scan is important for diagnosis of ovarian torsion. A common error is to exclude the diagnosis of ovarian torsion due to positive Doppler studies showing the presence of blood flow to the ovaries; remem-ber it is the absence of blood flow that suggests torsion; however, the pres-ence of blood flow does not exclude torsion. Ovarian torsion is a medical emergency and requires immediate operative laparoscopy or laparotomy to prevent necrosis of the ovary. During surgery, the torsed ovary is untwisted and may be tacked to prevent recurrence of torsion.

TAKE HOME POINTS

- History and physical exam are crucial in pelvic pain.
- Vital signs should be taken in all patients to determine the acuity of their medical condition.
- Any sign of hemodynamic instability requires exploratory laparoscopy or laparotomy; it is imperative to stop the bleeding and ensure hemody-namic stability.
- It is important to administer antibiotics when there are signs of infection.
- In ectopic pregnancy, administer RhoGAM to all Rh-negative mothers.
- Ovarian torsion is a medical emergency and should be treated promptly.

SUGGESTED READINGS

DeCherney AH, Nathan L. *Current Diagnosis and Treatment: Obstetrics and Gynecology.* 10th ed. New York, NY: McGraw Hill companies; 2007.

Gibbs RS, Karlan BY, Haney EF, et al. *Danforth's Obstetrics and Gynecology.* 10th ed. Philadelphia, PA: Lippincott Williams & Wilkins; 2008.

Katz VL, Lentz GM, et al, *Katz: Comprehensive Gynecology.* 5th ed. Philadelphia, PA: Mosby Elsevier; 2007.

Mcintyre-Seltman K, Ectopic pregnancy. In: Evans AT, ed. *Manual of Obstetrics.* 7th ed. Philadelphia, PA: Lippincott Williams & Wilkins; 2007.

Schorge JO, Schaffer JI, Halvorson LM, et al. *Williams Gynecology.* New York, NY: McGraw Hill Companies; 2008.

59

ACUTE PELVIC INFLAMMATORY DISEASE: MANAGEMENT ISSUES

MICHAEL OWOLABI, MD AND DIANA BROOMFIELD, MD, MBA, FACOG, FACS

A 27-year-old homemaker presents with fever, abdominal tenderness, and malaise for 2 days. Her temperature is 101.8°F. Her abdomen is moderately tender. She exhibits guarding and rebound tenderness and an ultrasonographic evaluation was consistent with a thin endometrial stripe and a right adnexal mass. The pregnancy test was negative. She is taken to the operating room with a presumptive diagnosis of acute appendicitis and undergoes a laparoscopic procedure. Laparoscopic findings are consistent with an enlarged tubo-ovarian complex that is surrounded by filmy adhesions. The appendix was normal, and the gynecologic surgeon is called. The tubo-ovarian abscess (TOA) was drained and she was admitted and continued on an antibiotic regimen.

The diagnosis of pelvic inflammatory disease (PID) must be considered when abdominal pain and pelvic tenderness are present in a sexually active female especially if associated with fever or an elevated white count. Since patients infected with *Neisseria gonorrhoeae* (GC) often are coinfected with *Chlamydia trachomatis*, dual therapy should be considered as a routine approach as soon as the clinical diagnosis is made. Antibiotics should be started and continued for 24 hours after the patient improves clinically. Oral antibiotics then should be given for a total of 14 days of treatment.

CLINICAL CRITERIA FOR THE DIAGNOSIS OF PELVIC INFLAMMATORY DISEASE

Pelvic organ tenderness, leukorrhea with or without mucopurulent endocervicitis

Additional Criteria:

Elevated C–reactive protein or erythrocyte sedimentation rate
Temperature >38°C (100.4°F)
Leukocytosis
Positive test for gonococcal or chlamydial infection
Ultrasonography documenting TOA
Laparoscopic visually confirming salpingitis

Treatment goals are to prevent tubal damage that leads to infertility and ectopic pregnancy and to prevent chronic infection. Treatment options include both outpatient and inpatient management. Ceftriaxone 250 mg IM single plus doxycycline 100 mg PO twice a day for 14 days is adequate for the outpatient regimen.

Criteria for Hospitalization include

Surgical emergency not excluded
Pregnancy
No clinical response to oral antimicrobial therapy
Inability to follow or tolerate outpatient oral regimen
Severe illness, nausea, vomiting, or high fever
Tubo–ovarian abscess
Nulliparous young patient

For hospitalized patients, Cefotetan 2 g IV every 12 hours plus Doxycycline 100 mg orally or IV every 12 hours is an adequate combination. In the presence of a TOA, add Cleocin or Metronidazole for more effective anaerobic coverage. When patients are unresponsive to intravenous antibiotics, CT-directed drainage may be considered. In rare cases, despite intravenous antibiotics and CT drainage, symptoms may worsen and lead to sepsis or significant peritonitis requiring operative intervention.

TAKE HOME POINTS

- High index of suspicion for diagnosis should be maintained.
- Coinfection with GC and *Chlamydia* is common.
- Early commencement of antibiotics is central to reduction in morbidity.
- Liberal admission for candidates who meet the criteria.
- Choice of antibiotics should follow recommendation.

SUGGESTED READINGS

American College of Obstetricians and Gynecologists. ACOG Educational Bulletin No. 236: HN prevention through early detection and treatment: Sexually transmitted diseases-United States. Recommendation Committee for HIV and STD Prevention. 1998;47 (RR-12):1–24.

Disease Control and Prevention. Sexually transmitted diseases treatment guidelines. *MMWR Recomm Rep.* 2002;(RR-6):1–78.

Soper DE. Genitourinary infections and sexually transmitted disease. In: Berek JS, Adashi EY, Hillard PA, eds. *Novak's Gynecology*. Baltimore, MD: Williams & Wilkins; 1996:211.

Soper DE. Genitourinary infections and sexually transmitted diseases. In: Berek JS, Adashi EY, Hillard PA, eds. *Novak's Gynecology*. 12th ed. Baltimore, MD: Williams & Wilkins; 1996:437.

60

CHLAMYDIA TRACHOMATIS: TEST OF CURE VERSES RESCREENING IN A NONPREGNANT PATIENT

MICHAEL OWOLABI, MD AND DIANA BROOMFIELD, MD, MBA, FACOG, FACS

An 18-year-old nulligravid, who takes oral contraceptives, tests positive for cervical Chlamydia *on a nucleic amplification test. She is treated with azithromycin, 1 g orally. She is instructed to ask her boyfriend to seek treatment and told to refrain from sexual intercourse for the next week. She is scheduled for test of cure in 2 weeks posttreatment.*

This infection is the most commonly reported notifiable disease. About 72% of reported cases occurred among teenagers and young adults aged 15 to 24 years. Most females (75%) are asymptomatic. Up to 40% of females with untreated Chlamydia or gonorrhea will develop pelvic inflammatory disease (PID). Of these women, 20% will become infertile, 18% of these women will experience debilitating chronic pelvic pain, and 19% will have a tubal ectopic pregnancy. Because the cervix of young girls and young women is not fully matured, they are at particularly high risk for infection if sexually active and exposed to *Chlamydia.*

Treatment with azithromycin, 1 g single oral dose, or doxycycline, 100 mg orally twice a day for 7 days, is equally effective. The single dose of azithromycin is a better treatment option if the physician is concerned about the patient's compliance. Patients should be counseled about the importance of referring their sexual partners for evaluation, testing, and treatment. *Chlamydia*-infected individuals should abstain from sexual intercourse until they and their partners have completed treatment; otherwise, reinfection is possible. A common error to avoid is doing a test of cue too early. *Chlamydia* testing at <3 weeks after completion of therapy with a nucleic acid amplification test (NAAT) can result in a false–positive result and so is not recommended. The improved sensitivity of NAATs is due to their ability to produce a positive signal from a single copy of the target DNA or RNA. A greater occurrence of *Chlamydia* is found in women who have had a previous *Chlamydia* infection in the preceding several months. Having multiple infections increases a woman's risk of serious reproductive health problems, including infertility.

An immediate test of cure is recommended only in pregnancy or questionable therapeutic compliance. However, the CDC recommends that repeat screening is always offered to women, especially adolescents, 3 to 4 months after treatment is completed to rule out reinfection. This is especially true if a woman does not know if her sex partner received treatment. STD treatment guidelines issued by CDC indicated that sexually active adolescent women should be screened for *Chlamydia* at least annually even if symptoms are not present.

TAKE HOME POINTS

- Chlamydia is the most commonly reported notifiable disease.
- Most infected females are asymptomatic.
- Up to 40% of females with untreated Chlamydia will develop PID.
- One fifth of infected women will become infertile.
- Adolescent and young women are particularly at risk.
- A single dose of azithromycin is preferred.
- Test of cure is recommended only in pregnancy/questionable therapeutic compliance.
- Repeat screening is recommended in nonpregnant adolescents and young women, 3 to 4 months after treatment is completed to rule out reinfection.
- Sexually active adolescent women should have annual chlamydial screening.

SUGGESTED READINGS

American College of Obstetricians and Gynecologists. *Sexually Transmitted Disease in Adolescents*. ACOG Committee Opinion No. 301. Washington, DC: ACOG; 2004.

Centers for Disease Control and Prevention. Sexually transmitted disease surveillance, 2003. Atlanta, GA: U.S. Department of Health and Human Services, Centers for Disease Control and Prevention, September 2003.

Hopkins RS, Jajosky RA, Hall PA, et al. Summary of notifiable diseases—United States, 2003. Centers for Disease Control and Prevention. *Morb Mortal Wkly Rep.* 2005;52:1–85.

Johnson RE, Newhall WJ, Papp JR, et al. Screening tests to detect Chlamydia trachomatis and Neisseria gonorrhea infections—2002. Centers for Disease Control and Prevention. *MMWR Recomm Rep.* 2002;51(RR-15):1–38; quiz CE 1–4.

Centers for Disease Control and Prevention. Sexually transmitted disease treatment guideline, 2006. *MMWR Recomm Rep.* 2006;55(RR-11):1–94.

Weinstock H, Berman S, Cates W Jr. Sexually transmitted diseases among American youths: incidence and prevalence estimates, 2000. *Perspect Sex Reprod Health.* 2004;36:6–10.

61

GONORRHEA: INEFFECTIVE COUNSELING

MICHAEL OWOLABI, MD AND DIANA BROOMFIELD, MD, MBA, FACOG, FACS

A 21-year-old college student presents for annual gynecologic exam. She is sexually active and takes oral contraceptives. She states that she has been treated for sexually transmitted diseases (STDs) three times in the past 12 months. She tests negative for Chlamydia but positive for cervical gonorrhea on a gene probe screening. She is treated with single-dose ceftriaxone, 125 mg intramuscularly. She is counseled to use condom as a backup contraception and instructed to ask her sex partners to seek treatment. She was also told to refrain from sexual intercourse for the next week. She is scheduled for test of cure in 2 weeks posttreatment.

Gonorrhea is an STD that is caused by *Neisseria gonorrhoeae*, a Gram-negative diplococcus bacterium that infects the columnar or pseudostratified epithelium affecting the urogenital tract. *N. gonorrhoeae* can grow and multiply easily in the warm, moist areas of the reproductive tract, including the cervix, uterus, fallopian tubes, and urethra. *N. gonorrhoeae* can also grow in the mouth, throat, eyes, and anus. Patients are often asymptomatic but may present with vaginal discharge, dysuria, or abnormal uterine bleeding. Culture with selective medium such as Thayer-Martin is the gold standard. DNA probes offer a rapid, low-cost alternative.

Treatment with single-dose ceftriaxone should be complemented with treatment of Chlamydia (because coinfection is common) unless the DNA amplification test is negative. Sexual partners should be referred for treatment.

TAKE HOME POINTS

- *N. gonorrhoeae* is the offending agent.
- The most common site of infection is the endocervix.
- Women are often asymptomatic.
- Symptomatic patients may present with vaginal discharge, dysuria, or abnormal uterine bleeding.
- Single-dose ceftriaxone is sufficient treatment.
- Coinfection with *Chlamydia* is common and should be sought and treated appropriately.
- Counseling on the use of condom as a backup contraception and referral of sex partners for treatment are essential parts of standard care.

SUGGESTED READINGS

Koumans EH, Johnson RE, Knapp JS, et al. Laboratory testing for *Neisseria gonorrhoea* by recently introduced nonculture tests: a performance review with clinical and public health consideration. *Clin Infect Dis*. 1998;27:1171–1180.

Centers for Disease Control and Prevention. Sexually transmitted diseases treatment guideline, 2006. *MMWR Recomm Rep*. 2006;55(RR-11):1–94 .

Van Dyck E, Ieven M, Pattyn S, et al. Detection of *Chlamydia trachomatis* and *Neisseria gonorrhoea* by enzyme immunoassay, culture, and three nucleic acid amplification tests. *J Clin Microbiol*. 2001;39(5):1751–1756.

62

FORGOTTEN MANAGEMENT OF ENDOMETRIOSIS

AIMEE S. BROWNE, MD, MSC AND ROBERT N. TAYLOR, MD, PHD

A 23-year-old woman presents for an urgent visit with a chief complaint of painful menses. The patient has had three other visits for similar complaints in the past year. She underwent a diagnostic laparoscopy at the age of 18 for an acute pain episode to rule out appendicitis. At that time, she was diagnosed with endometriosis and treated conservatively with surgical ablation of endometriotic implants, followed by depot leuprolide acetate, a gonadotropin-releasing hormone analogue (GnRH-a) that induces a hypoestrogenic state, for 6 months. She experienced 2 years of symptom relief but her pain recurred about 1 year ago. She was prescribed continuous oral contraceptive pills but reported that secondary to her busy school schedule she did not remember to take them consistently. Currently, she complains of severe pain not relieved with Motrin 800 mg TID. She presents today for management of her acute pain episode and also requests long-term therapy for her progressively worsening symptoms.

Her past medical history is significant for asthma, requiring frequent glucocorticosteroid administration and osteopenia diagnosed when bone densitometry was performed at the end of her leuprolide treatment 4 years ago. Her past surgical history is significant for a laparoscopy as noted above. The patient has been a social smoker in the past but currently denies any tobacco, alcohol, or drug use.

The most likely cause of the patient's pain is persistent or recurrent endometriosis. This was diagnosed 4 years ago based on direct laparoscopic visualization, the gold standard. Undergoing a repeat laparoscopy to confirm the diagnosis is not warranted; however, this clinical vignette illustrates some of the potential difficulties with hormonal management of endometriosis. Your discussion of possible treatment options includes continuous oral contraceptives, depot leuprolide acetate, depo-medroxyprogesterone acetate (DMPA), nonsteroidal anti-inflammatories, and the levonorgestrel-releasing intrauterine device.

Based on her bone loss findings, likely a result of long-term glucocorticosteroids and possibly exacerbated by her past treatment with leuprolide acetate, she should not be offered a GnRH-a or DMPA. While both of these agents have been shown to be highly effective in relieving dysmenorrhea, dyspareunia, and nonmenstrual pain in women with endometriosis, they have a negative impact on bone mineral density (BMD). The side effect profile of GnRH-a is due to hypoestrogenism. Although DMPA might be a convenient and effective way to manage the patient's dysmenorhea for the long term, evidence shows that its use significantly decreases BMD; however, this effect may be reversed after discontinuation. Although the effects may be reversed, a medication that decreases BMD in a patient at risk for osteoporosis who has not reached peak bone mass is not the best option.

Many clinicians use oral contraceptive pills (OCPs) as first-line therapy for endometriosis. The progestin-dominant hormones found in modern OCPs induce a state of pseudopregnancy, resulting in decidualization and atrophy of endometriotic lesions, inhibition of pituitary gonadotropins, and decreased estradiol synthesis and secretion. In the endometrium, another salutary effect of progestins is inhibition of estrogen receptor expression and their growth promoting effects. However, as she reports a history of difficulty remembering daily medications, this may be a poor option for this patient.

Our patient may be an ideal candidate for the levonorgestrel intrauterine system (LNG-IUS). Although hormonal IUSs are the most popular contraceptive worldwide, <2% of women in the United States use an IUS for birth control. Additionally, there are many other benefits and treatment options offered by the IUS that are often overlooked. Their application in the treatment of endometriosis is underutilized.

The medicated IUS slowly releases levonorgestrel into the uterine cavity. While endometrial concentrations of the contraceptive steroid are quite high, systemic levels remain low, allowing normal follicular function and endogenous estradiol production. Levonorgestrel is a 19-nortestosterone causing decidualization and acyclicity of the endometrium and endometriotic tissue. A Cochrane review of LNG-IUS treatment of endometriosis-associated pain postoperatively revealed one randomized controlled trial showing a significant reduction in the recurrence of painful periods when compared to GnRH-a. After pelvic organ–sparing laparoscopy, an open-label pilot study found a 10% recurrence in the group treated with LNG-IUS compared to 45% recurrence in the control group. The LNG-IUS appears to be an excellent long-term option for treatment. In a cross-sectional study comparing LNG-IUS users to controls using nonhormonal IUDs, BMD was unaffected after 7 years of use.

TAKE HOME POINTS

- Effective endometriosis therapy must take into account the patient's symptoms, desires, and full clinical history.
- Although OCPs are often used as the first-line treatment for pain, they are not always the best option.

- The LNG-IUS has many noncontraceptive benefits that are often overlooked and provide a unique treatment option for endometriosis pain symptoms.
- LNG-IUS has been shown to effectively treat endometriosis-related pain.
- GnRH-a and DMPA have possible negative effects on BMD and should be used with caution in patients with or at high risk for osteoporosis.

SUGGESTED READINGS

Abou-Setta A, Al-Inany H, Farquhar C. Levonorgestrel-releasing intrauterine device for symptomatic endometriosis following surgery. *Cochrane Database System Rev.* (Online) 2006.

Bahamondes L, Espejo-Arce X, Hidalgo M, et al. A cross sectional study of the forearm bone density of long-term users of levonorgestrel-releasing intrauterine system. *Hum Reprod.* 2006;21:1316–1319.

Scholes D, Lacroix A, Ichikawa L, et al. Change in bone mineral density among adolescent women using and discontinuing Depot medroxyprogesterone acetate contraception. *Arch Pediatr Adolesc Med.* 2005;159:139–144.

Vercellini P, Frontino G, De Giorgi O, et al. Comparison of a levonorgesterel-releasing intra-uterine device versus expectant management after conservative surgery for symptomatic endometriosis: a pilot study. *Fertil Steril.* 2003;80:305–309.

Winkel C. Evaluation and management of women with endometriosis. *Am J Obstet Gynecol.* 2003;102:397–408.

Winkel C, Scialli A. Medical and surgical therapies for pain associated with endometriosis. *J Women's Health Gender-Based Med.* 2001;10:137–162.

63

ENDOMETRIOSIS-RELATED PAIN

AIMEE S. BROWNE, MD, MSC AND ROBERT N. TAYLOR, MD, PhD

A 21-year-old nulliparous woman with a history of endometriosis presents to your office complaining of 2 days of worsening lower abdominal pain. Her period started 3 days ago. The patient reports some nausea at home but is mostly concerned with nonrelenting central pelvic pain. Past medical history is negative except for a laparoscopy for pelvic pain at the age of 18 when she was diagnosed with endometriosis. Her current medications include cyclic oral contraceptive pills since the time of her surgery. In the office, the patient is noted to have a temperature of 101°F. Her exam is significant for lower abdominal pain without rebound and right adnexal tenderness. You order all appropriate tests and admit the patient for further evaluation and management.

While you assess the patient, should she be empirically treated with any medications?

Endometriosis is defined as the presence of endometrial glands and stroma outside of the endometrial cavity. Ten to fifteen percent of all reproductive-age women have endometriosis and the most common symptom of this disease is pain. Endometriosis is associated with several forms of pelvic pain including painful periods (dysmenorrhea), painful intercourse (dyspareunia), pain with bowel movements (dyschezia), and chronic pelvic pain. Although these symptoms are associated with endometriosis, their relatively nonspecific nature requires that gynecologists acknowledge that the findings of endometriosis overlap with a variety of different gynecological, genitourinary, and gastrointestinal diseases.

The heterogeneity of symptoms associated with endometriosis commonly results in delayed diagnosis and frank misdiagnosis of the disease. Similarly, there may be a misdiagnosis of endometriosis when women with related symptoms actually suffer from another process.

In the above example, our patient previously had laparoscopically confirmed endometriosis. Her symptoms of lower abdominal pain around the time of menses may lead the practitioner to believe that she is having a flare of her endometriosis. Unfortunately, while endometriosis is often associated with dysmenorrhea and pelvic pain, there are other gynecologic conditions that present with these signs and symptoms. Adenomyosis, ovarian cysts, pelvic adhesive disease, leiomyoma, hydrosalpinx, and pelvic infection are just a few of the gynecologic disorders that may present with pain. It is important to evaluate patients for other causes of pelvic pain and treat accordingly. Based on her clinical findings, this patient is likely suffering from an episode of pelvic inflammatory disease (PID). Delayed treatment for PID can have a deleterious impact on future reproductive outcomes.

Endometriosis symptoms often overlap with the urinary tract system. Chronic calculi, urethral syndrome, and interstitial cystitis (IC) are just a few disease processes that can mimic endometriosis. IC is commonly overlooked by gynecologists treating women with pelvic pain. Pain impulses emitted from the urinary bladder travel to the spinal cord and may be perceived as pain in many locations throughout the pelvis. In addition, IC may also be associated with dyspareunia and may be cyclically exacerbated during the menstrual cycle. Similar to other organ systems, gastrointestinal diseases such as diverticulitis, inflammatory bowel disease, and irritable bowel syndrome (IBS) commonly present with pelvic pain. An evaluation of endometriosis patients reveals the prevalence of IBS symptoms in approximately 32% of women with endometriosis without bowel lesions and in 100% of endometriosis cases in which endometriosis infiltrates through the serosal layer of the bowel. Based on these findings, one should always consider endometriosis as a cause of pelvic pain and GI symptoms in women of reproductive age.

Musculoskeletal, psychiatric, and neurologic causes of pelvic pain also have been identified. The differential diagnosis of endometriosis and pelvic pain includes nearly every organ system. An awareness of different possible disease processes is required to adequately treat patients with pelvic pain and to avoid a misdiagnosis or a delay in diagnosis.

TAKE HOME POINTS

- Endometriosis is a common cause of pelvic pain and may present with dysmenorrhea, dyspareunia, dyschezia, and chronic pelvic pain.
- Disorders of many other organ systems can generate overlapping symptomatology that may delay diagnosis of endometriosis or result in its misdiagnosis.
- PID may present with pelvic pain and should be treated immediately to prevent future sequelae. (For up-to-date recommendations, refer to the CDC STD/PID treatment guidelines).
- The bladder may be a source of pain in up to 85% of women with pelvic pain.
- Gastrointestinal diseases often present with abdominal/pelvic pain and should be considered and evaluated in these patients.

SUGGESTED READINGS

Centers for Disease Control. *Sexually Transmitted Diseases Treatment Guidelines.* 2006. Available at: http://www.cdc.gov/std/treatment/2006/pid.htm

Ferrero S, Abbamonte L, Remorgida V, et al. Irritable bowel syndrome and endometriosis. *Eur J Gastroenterol Hepatol.* 2005;17:687.

Hadfield R, Mardon H, Barlow D, et al. Delay in diagnosis of endometriosis: a survery of women from the USA and the UK. *Hum Reprod.* 1996;11;878–880.

Hillis S, Joesoef R, Marchbanks P, et al. Delayed care of pelvic inflammatory disease as a risk factor for impaired fertility. *Am J Obstet Gynecol.* 1993;168:1503–1509.

Parsons CL, Dell J, Standford EJ, et al. Increased prevalence of interstitial cystitis: previously unrecognized urologic and gynecologic cases identified using a new symptom questionnaire and intravesical potassium sensitivity. *Urology.* 2002;60:573–578.

Standford E, Dell J, Parsons L. The emerging presence of intersitial cystitis in gynecologic patients with chronic pelvic pain. *Urology.* 2007;69:41–47.

Winkel C. Evaluation and management of women with endometriosis. *Am J Obstet Gynecol.* 2003;102:397–408.

64

BARTHOLIN DUCT CYST

STEPHEN H. WEISS, MD, MPH

A 26-year-old comes in with a chief complaint of a 3-day history of a tender mass at the back of the vaginal opening. An exam reveals a 4-cm cystic tender mass under the posterior third of the labial minus on the patient's right side. How do you acutely resolve the cyst and try to prevent recurrence?

The Bartholin duct may enlarge with or without infection due to blockage of the duct opening in the lower third of the vestibule of the vagina. Scarring of the duct opening from infection, surgery, and a stone are common causes of cyst formation. The duct opening also can be congenitally small. When infected, there may be heat and erythema over the duct. Simple drainage can resolve the current symptoms and infection but usually will not prevent recurrence. If there is coincident cellulitis or suspicion of a sexually transmitted disease, antibiotics should be given.

The gland itself is pea sized and very deep below the vestibular bulb. It is very difficult to locate, and massive hematomas are possible. Removal requires a trip to the operating room. The only indication for removal is to rule out the very rare cancer of this gland, which occurs primarily in postmenopausal women who have a mass, not just a duct cyst.

The office surgeries include the following procedures as treatment options:

1. Marsupialization involves removing an ellipse of epithelial tissue in the vestibule of the vagina over the cyst and then incising the cyst and suturing the edge of the cyst wall over the epithelium (eversion), to induce a new permanent duct opening once healed. There is no improvement in cure compared to the Word catheter and the procedure is technically challenging and time consuming.

2. The Word catheter is a 4-cm-long latex inflatable balloon-tip catheter. After cleansing and local anesthesia, the cyst is stabbed with a 15 scalpel blade. This blade makes the perfect-size opening for the Word catheter

and will not go very deep due to its shape. Once fluid begins to escape, quickly insert the Word catheter to prevent loss of the location of the cyst cavity that will occur after total collapse of the cyst. Now inflate the balloon with 3 to 5 mL of water and teach the patient how to tuck the loose end up into the vagina. One problem with the Word catheter design is that the balloon inflation port is made for an old style Luer slip syringe. The average office only stocks Luer lock syringes, so either buy some Luer slip syringes or use a knife to cut the female threads off existing syringes. Using a needle to fill the balloon will increase the chance of a slow leak and premature dislodgement of the catheter. Leave the catheter in for 2 to 3 weeks to allow a new opening to form into the duct. Prescribe sitz bathes for a few days and have the patient return to the office in 3 to 4 weeks for removal of the catheter.

3. Incision and drainage (I&D) may be done but is best avoided due to a high recurrence rate, even with packing.

TAKE HOME POINTS

- The Bartholin gland is pea sized and very deep below the vestibular bulb.
- Office procedures for a cyst include placement of a Word catheter, marsupialization, and I&D (not recommended).

SUGGESTED READING

Omole F, Simmons BJ, Hacker Y. Management of Bartholyn's duct cyst and gland abscess. *Am Fam Physician*. 2003;68(1):135–140.

65

DO NOT PERFORM A SIMPLE "I&D" FOR A RECURRENT BARTHOLIN CYST

COURTNEY ROWLAND, MD

The Bartholin glands are located at 4 and 8 o'clock portions of the introitus providing moisture to the area through secretion of mucus. Normally, the gland is 0.5 cm in size and drains into a duct approximately 2.5 cm long. Occasionally, the mucus can "build up" causing cyst formation due to vulvovaginal trauma or inflammation leading to distal obstruction. Typically, this leads to a painless dilation of the duct called a Bartholin "cyst." This does not need to be drained unless it is causing the patient pain or discomfort as it can spontaneously resolve. However, if the material inside the gland becomes infected, intervention is a necessity.

Treatment of a Bartholin cyst or gland involves either placement of a Word catheter or marsupialization. Simple incision and drainage (I&D) is inadequate as the lesion will frequently recur. Typically, Word catheter placement takes precedence over marsupialization in the initial therapy of choice as marsupialization must be performed in an operating setting.

Treatment of a Bartholin cyst or abscess first begins with informed consent. The patient must be aware of risks (bleeding, infection, scarring, dyspareunia, recurrence), benefits (decreased pain, resolution of the lesion), and alternatives (do nothing or marsupialization). Clean and anesthetize the area using Betadine and inject 1 to 3 mL of 1% lidocaine behind the hymenal ring at site of future incision. For Word catheter placement, make a stab incision with scalpel approximately 5 mm in length and 1.5 cm deep. Use hemostats to clear the duct of all mucus and remove loculations. Then culture duct material and fully insert Word catheter. Inject 2 to 3 mL of sterile water into Word catheter and inflate. Place distal end of catheter in the vagina to minimize discomfort as epithelialization occurs (2 to 4 weeks). Recommended antibiotic coverage for abscesses includes ceftriaxone 125 mg IM and clindamycin 300 mg PO every 6 hours for 7 days. This antibiotic regimen can be adjusted based on results of culture sensitivities.

If Word catheter placement fails, marsupialization is indicated. This is an operative procedure and involves larger stab incision (1 to 3 cm) over the lesion with eversion of incision edges that are approximated to normal vulvar tissue using interrupted sutures.

TAKE HOME POINTS

- Do not I&D Bartholin cysts.
- Culture Bartholin abscesses.
- Place Word catheter for Bartholin abscess.
- Use marsupialization technique for recurrent Bartholin abscesses.
- Cover the patient with ceftriaxone 125 mg IM and clindamycin 300 mg PO every 6 hours for 7 days; tailor coverage to culture sensitivities.

SUGGESTED READING

Eckert LO, Lentz GM. Infections of the lower genital tract: vulva, vagina, cervix, toxic shock syndrome, HIV infections. In: Katz VL, Lentz GM, Lobo RA, et al., eds. *Comprehensive Gynecology*. 5th ed. Philadelphia, PA: Mosby Elsevier; 2007:chapter 22.

66

ALWAYS BIOPSY A VULVAR LESION

COURTNEY ROWLAND, MD

The vulvar lesion often proves to be a diagnostic challenge to the gynecologic practitioner. Benign, premalignant, and malignant lesions often present similarly and can fool even the experienced eye. Initial evaluation of the patient with a vulvar lesion involves a detailed history and physical. Key points to the history include

1. Duration of lesion
2. Treatments (including home remedies) attempted
3. Associated symptoms (itching; pain; changes in color, size, or appearance, etc.)
4. Hygiene habits (including douching, shaving, waxing, etc.)
5. History of similar lesions or presence of similar lesions on other parts of the body

On physical exam, one must characterize lesion. Symmetry, borders, color, size, and dermatologic description of lesion may help elucidate a diagnosis. With an assistant in the room and good lighting, the vulva and surrounding areas should be systematically examined. Oftentimes, it helps to have the patient point out the area of concern. A complete pelvic exam including speculum and bimanual exam should be performed as the lesion may not be in isolation or may be associated with other occult findings. Separating the blades of the speculum many assist in visualizing lesions of the anterior and posterior vaginal vault. Finally, colposcopic evaluation of the lesion is useful in delineating benign from malignant and premalignant conditions. Acetic acid (5%) should be applied to the vulva and cervix followed by saturation of the area with Lugol solution. Affected areas will turn white and red, respectively, due to the increased nuclear-to-cytoplasmic ratio of cells with increased mitotic activity.

The differential diagnosis of vulvar lesions is broad. *Table 66.1* lists many types of common vulvar lesions along with their morphologic appearance.

As shown in *Table 66.1*, presentation may be misleading in diagnosing a benign versus malignant lesion. Vulvar cancer is rare, comprising approximately 5% of female genital malignancies. However, vulvar cancer can be terminal, unlike other common lesions of the vulva, and should not

TABLE 66.1	TYPES OF COMMON VULVAR LESIONS AND THEIR MORPHOLOGIC APPEARANCE
VULVAR LESION	**APPEARANCE**
Atrophic vaginitis	Erythematous, dry mucosa with possible abrasions due to hypoestrogenic state
Bartholin cyst	Inflamed, raised, pustular lesion with extreme tenderness to palpation
Candida	Beefy red, moist, pruritic lesions
Chancroid ulcer	Gray purulent lesion with draining buboes from lymph nodes
Condyloma accuminata	Flesh colored, polypoid, raised lesions
Dermatitis	Erythematous lesions associated with irritation, pruritus, and possible excoriation
Folliculitis	Small, raised pustular lesions surrounding the hair follicle
Herpes simplex virus	Small, ulcerated lesions that may be vesicular or denuded, associated with extreme tenderness
Hidradenitis suppurativa	Pustular draining lesions or tracts that may become chronic sinuses, associated with moderate tenderness
Hyperkeratosis	Thickened, raised white plaques associated with chronic pruritus
Lichen sclerosis	White, fine, paperlike lesions
Lymphogranuloma venereum	Shallow ulcers that may be associated with draining sinus tracts and fluctuant lymph nodes; nontender
Melanoma	Asymmetric, irregular border, black or colored lesion that may be elevated
Pilonidal cyst	Small white to yellow sharply demarcated, raised lesions
Skin tags	Small fleshy pedunculated lesions with uniform stalk
Syphilitic chancre	Painless, ulcerated, indurated lesion with associated lymphadenopathy
Vulvar cancer	Ulcer, scale, plaque or fleshy, polypoid mass; may be associated with bleeding and/or pruritus
Vulvar intraepithelial lesion	Typically on non–hair-bearing areas; may be white or colored, raised, verrucous, or ulcerative

be missed. Routine punch biopsy of vulvar lesions is a prudent measure and should be performed to exclude malignancy. The area should be anesthetized with 1% lidocaine. As the vulva is highly vascularized, aspirate before injecting lidocaine to avoid intravascular injection. With a standard punch biopsy, the metallic, round head is inserted into the lesion by carefully twisting and pushing the punch biopsy until the head can no longer be advanced. It may be necessary to use your nondominant hand or a forceps to stabilize the labia as the skin in the area has redundancy. Also, a portion of the normal dermis should be captured with the biopsy of the lesion for pathologic comparison. The forceps may then be used to remove the specimen from the punch biopsy and placed in formalin for pathologic examination. Pressure from a large cotton-tipped swab or 4 × 4 should be used to achieve hemostasis. If the site continues to bleed, Monsel solution, silver nitrate, or an interrupted delayed absorbable suture may be used.

TAKE HOME POINTS

- Benign and malignant lesions of the vulva may present similarly.
- Detailed history and physical may assist in diagnosing vulvar lesions.
- Punch biopsy should be used to confirm diagnosis of vulvar lesions.
- Vulvar biopsy should include a portion of normal tissue.

SUGGESTED READING

Eckert LO, Lentz GM. Infections of the lower genital tract: vulva, vagina, cervix, toxic shock syndrome, HIV infections. In: Katz VL, Lentz GM, Lobo RA, et al., eds. *Comprehensive Gynecology.* 5th ed. Philadelphia, PA: Mosby Elsevier; 2007:chapter 22.

67

VULVA DISEASES

JOHN-CHARLES AKODA, MD, AND
DIANA BROOMFIELD, MD, MBA, FACOG, FACS

A 52-year-old G3P3 postmenopausal female presents to your office with a chief complaint of a group of small, red brown to dark blue color lesions on vulva that bleeds easily during strenuous exercise. She is worried that it is cancer. What is your differential diagnosis?

BACKGROUND

For the clinician, the differences between benign and malignant disorders of the vulva are not always clear. When the diagnosis from the history, physical exam, and lab tests is clear, management is usually self-evident. Thus, the clinical approach to many of these problems must be broad and not so focused as to prematurely exclude dangerous pathologies within the differential diagnosis, though they may be less common. This presentation (*Tables 67.1 and 67.2*) is not encyclopedic; rather, lesions are selected based on their clinical importance and prevalence.

TAKE HOME POINTS

- Vulvar cancer accounts for approximately 5% of malignancies of the lower genital tract ranking it fourth in frequency after
  - Endometrial
  - Ovarian
  - Cervical
- Paget disease appears as grossly diffused erythematous eczematoid lesions that are usually chronic.
- Squamous cell carcinoma represents 90% of primary vulvar cancers.
- Melanoma is the most common nonsquamous cell of the vulva.

TABLE 67.1	BENIGN DISEASES OF THE VULVA	
DISORDER	**CHARACTERISTICS**	**DIAGNOSIS/TREATMENT**

Urethral caruncle	Small, fleshy, friable outgrowth of the distal edge of the urethra
	Usually single and sessile
	Maybe pedunculated and grows to be 1–2 cm
	Most common in postmenopausal women
	Arises from ectropion of the posterior urethral wall
	Associated with retraction and atrophy of the postmenopausal vagina
	Growth is secondary to chronic irritation by infection
	Histologically composed of transitional and stratified squamous epithelium
	Usually subdivided by histological types
	  1. Papillomatous
	  2. Granulomatous
	  3. Angiomatous
	Often secondarily infected producing ulceration and bleeding
	Not precursors for urethral cancer though confused for urethral cancers
	~1:40 women with a diagnosis of urethral caruncles have urethral cancers
		Diagnosis: Biopsy under local anesthesia
		Treatment: Warm sitz bath and antibiotics
		Oral or topical Estrogen
		If no regression, or is symptomatic, it may be destroyed by cryosurgery, laser therapy, fulguration, or operative excision.
		Postoperatively, a Foley catheter should be left in place for 48–72 h to prevent urethral stenosis.
		May mimic urethral prolapse, which is a predominant disease of premenarcheal female, not as bright red and well circumscribed as the caruncle.

Cysts (a) Bartholin's (b) Skene's (c) Epidermal or sebaceous (d) Rare cysts (i.e., wolffian duct or mesonephric duct)	(a) Commonest is cystic dilation of the obstructed duct. (b) Rare; may present with symptoms of discomfort or found on routine exam; arise secondary to infection and scarring of the small ducts; compression of the duct unlike in urethral diverticula should not produce fluid from the urethral meatus. (c) Most common on anterior of the labia majora; usually multiple, freely movable, round, slow growing, and nontender; grossly white or yellow in color—contents are caseous like a thick cheese. (d) Occur near the clitoris or lateral to the hymenal ring. They contain clear serous fluid.	(a) Treatment not necessary in women <40 y old unless the cyst becomes infected or enlarged enough to cause symptoms. (b) If asymptomatic: conservative management in premenopausal women; excision with careful dissection to avoid urethral injury. (c) Most require no treatment. If it becomes infected, local heat application with incision and drainage is to be done.

(Continued)

TABLE 67.1   BENIGN DISEASES OF THE VULVA (*CONTINUED*)

DISORDER	CHARACTERISTICS	DIAGNOSIS/TREATMENT
Nevus	Arise from embryonic neural crest and are present from birth. Commonly called a "mole" and may become pigmented at puberty. Vulvar nevi are one of the most common benign neoplasms in females. Have a wide range of colors from blue to dark brown to black. Some are even amelanotic. Diameter ranges from a few millimeters to 2 cm. Generally asymptomatic. Nevi that are raised or contain hair seldom undergo malignant changes. Recent changes in growth or color, ulceration, pain, bleeding, or depth of satellite lesions mandate biopsy. Think ABCD for clinical features of malignant melanoma: asymmetry, border irregularity, color variegated, and diameter >6 mm. Lifetime risk of melanoma forming in women with dysplastic nevi is 15× that of the general population. Dysplastic nevus characterized by being >5 mm in diameter, irregular borders, and patchy variegated pigment.	*Treatment:* Excisional biopsy including 5–10 mm of normal surrounding skin.
Hemangiomas (a) Strawberry (b) Cavernous (c) Senile or Cherry (d) Angiokeratomas (e) Pyogenic granulomas	Rare malformations of blood vessels, rather than true neoplasms. Discovered initially during childhood. Usually single, 1–2 cm in diameter, flat and soft. Color ranges from brown to red or purple. Mostly asymptomatic but may become ulcerated and bleed. 60% of vulvar hemangiomas discovered during the 1st y of life spontaneously regress by school age. (a) Congenital and mainly in children; bright red to dark red in color; rarely increases in size after the age of 2 y. (b) Usually purple, appears in the first few months of life; spontaneously regresses by the age of 6. (c) More common in postmenopausal women; most often <3 mm in diameter, multiple, red brown to dark blue color.	(e) *Diagnosis:* Usually by gross inspection. *Treatment:* Asymptomatic in children—usually requires no treatment; in adults and if bleeding or infected, may require subtotal resection; if in doubt, do excisional biopsy.

(d) Purple or dark red color; occurs in women between 30 and 50 y old; rapid growth, bleeds easily during strenuous exercise; DDx—Kaposi sarcoma, angiosarcoma

(e) ~1 cm diameter; deep excision to prevent recurrence

Fibromas

Slow growing (few centimeters to gigantic, weighing 250 lb)
Majority are 1–10 cm
Often firm but may be cystic after myxomatous degeneration → pain
Most common benign solid tumors of the vulva
More common than lipomas
Most common in all age group
Arise from deep connective tissues, hence classified by some as dermatofibromas

Treatment: Operative removal if symptomatic

Lipomas

Benign, slow growing circumscribed tumors of fat cells
Arise from the subcutaneous tissue of the vulva
Similar to lipomas of other parts of the body
Present usually softer and larger than fibromas
Usually <3 cm (largest recorded is 44 lb)
Second most frequent benign vulva mesenchymal tumors
Cut section appears soft, yellow, and lobulated
Usually asymptomatic (unless large)

Diagnosis: Excisional bx

Hidradenoma

Rare, small, benign vulvar tumor of apocrine sweat glands of the inner surface of the labia majora and nearby perineum
Occasionally, may originate from eccrine sweat glands
Exclusively seen in white females aged 30–70 (most commonly in the fourth decade of life)
Occasionally seen at puberty
55% of them are cystic
38% arise from labia majora, 26% from labia minora
50% are <1 cm in diameter
Well-defined, sessile, pinkish gray nodule
Generally asymptomatic, may cause pruritus or bleeding if undergoes necrosis

Diagnosis: Excisional bx

(Continued)

TABLE 67.1	BENIGN DISEASES OF THE VULVA (CONTINUED)	
DISORDER	**CHARACTERISTICS**	**DIAGNOSIS/TREATMENT**
Syringoma	Very rare, cystic asymptomatic tumor. Adenoma of the eccrine sweat glands. <5 mm in diameter, may coalesce to form cords of firm tissues. Usually skin colored or yellow. Usually located in the labia majora. DDx: Fox-Fordyce disease, a condition of multiple retention cysts of apocrine glands accompanied by inflammation of the skin, usually produces intense pruritus while syringoma is asymptomatic.	*Treatment:* Excisional bx or cryosurgery. Topical or oral estrogens and topical retinoic acid.
Endometriosis	Rare, only 1 in 500 women c/ endometriosis presents c/ vulvar lesions. May be solid or cystic. May be blue, red, or purple depending on their size, activity, or closeness to the surface of the skin. Usually found at site of old, healed obstetric laceration, episiotomy site, area of removal of Bartholin cyst, or along canal of Nuck. May be 2° to metaplasia, retrograde lymphatic spread or implantation of endometrial tissues during surgery. Sx: Pain, dyspareunia, cyclic discomfort, and enlargement of mass c/ menses.	*Treatment:* Wide excision or laser vaporization.
Granular cell myoblastoma	Originates from neural sheath (Schwann cells). Sometimes called schwannoma. Usually in the labia majora (may be on the clitoris). Usually subacute nodules 1–5 cm in diameter. Benign but infiltrate the local surrounding tissue. Slow growing, skin may ulcerate. Cut surface is yellow, not encapsulated. Tumor nodules are painless.	*Treatment:* Wide excision (otherwise high recurrence rate).
von Recklinghausen Disease	Gen. neurofibromatosis and café au lait spots. Vulvar lesions are fleshy, brownish red, and polypoid. ~18% of female c/ von Recklinghausen disease have vulvar involvement.	*Treatment:* Excision.

Hematomas	Usually 2° to blunt trauma, that is, straddle injury from a fall, automobile accident, physical assault, or recreational activities Spontaneous hematomas are rare and usually occur from rupture of a varicose vein during pregnancy or postpartum period.	*Treatment:* Mgt of nonobstetric vulvar hematoma is usually conservative unless >10 cm or is rapidly expanding. Bleeding is usually venous in origin and can therefore be controlled by direct pressure compression or application of ice pack to the area. If continues to expand, then surgery to ligate the bleeder is indicated. Careful inspection during surgery to r/o associated urinary bladder or rectosigmoid injury
Dermatologic Diseases (a) Contact dermatitis (b) Neurodermatitis (c) Psoriasis (d) Seborrheic dermatitis (e) Cutaneous candidiasis (f) Lichen planus	The skin of the vulva is similar to the skin of any surface of the body and is therefore susceptible to any generalized skin disease or involvement by systemic disease. Majority are red, scalelike rashes, and the 1° complaints are pruritus. Combination of moisture and heat of the intertriginous areas may produce irritation, maceration, and a wet weeping surface. The patient will commonly apply ointments and lotions c/ may → 2° irritation therefore important to examine the skin of the entire body.	
Vulvar pain syndrome/ vulvar vestibulitis/ vulvodynia	One of the most common gynecological problems. 15% of women have had chronic severe vulvar pain in their lifetimes. Wide range of causes, including neurologic diseases (esp. of the nerve roots), herpes simplex, vulvar vestibulitis, vulvar dysesthetia; contact dermatitis; and psychogenic causes Chronic pain may be designated as vulvodynia, once the diagnosis of infection, invasive disease, or inflammation has been excluded.	*Treatment:* Medical—TCA, Gabapentin, biofeedback, topical lidocaine gel Surgical—removal of the vulvar and vestibule and reapproximation of tissue
Vulvar edema	May be a symptom of either local or generalized disease Most common are inflammation or lymphatic blockage. The loose connective tissue of the vulva and its dependent position predispose to development of edema. Systemic causes are circulatory and renal failure, ascites, and liver cirrhosis.	

TABLE 67.2	MALIGNANT DISEASES OF THE VULVA (CONTINUED)	
DISEASE	CHARACTERISTICS	DIAGNOSIS/TREATMENT
Granular cell myoblastoma	Extremely rare Invariably benign	Local excision is the treatment of choice.
Vulvar cancer	Accounts for ~5% of malignancies of the lower genital tract ranking it fourth in frequency after 　1. Endometrial 　2. Ovarian 　3. Cervical Well-defined predisposing factors have not been identified. Associated c/ 　1. HPV in young patients 　2. Granulomatous disease of the vulva 　3. Diabetes mellitus 　4. HTN 　5. Obesity 　6. Smoking Current data do not provide consistent evidence regarding their association. Occurs w/ increasing frequency in those who have been treated for squamous cell carcinoma of the cervix or vagina, presumably as a result of the increased risk of carcinogenesis in the squamous epithelium of the lower genital tract in these patients. Incident increases c/ age: >50% of pts are older than 60 y. Those with carcinoma in situ are 40–55 y old.	Possible treatments are (a) CO_2 laser to a depth of 1–3 mm resulting in healing without scarring. (b) 5-FU cream. This leads to severe burning hence not generally used. (c) 5% imiquimod cream may also be used. (d) Excisional biopsy but this leads to scar formation.

Vulvar atypias (a) **Intraepithelial neoplasia** (b) **Lichen sclerosis**	Vulvar atypias present c/ variety of symptoms and signs. Irritation and itching are common. Whitish change due to thickened keratin layer Lichen Sclerosis: Whitish change in the vulvar skin; microscopically, epithelium becomes think with a loss or blunting of the rete ridges. In some cases, may be thickening or hyperkeratosis of the surface layers. Inflammation is usually present 5% risk of becoming malignant Atypias are classified as: VIN I—mild VIN II—moderate VIN III—severe (carcinoma in situ)	Diagnosis is by biopsy; may use colposcopy as means of f/u After biopsy and diagnosis, topical testosterone can be used for atrophic conditions. Like lichen sclerosis, side effects may be clitoral hypertrophy and increased hair growth. If positive response to testosterone, continue indefinitely. Another option is topical steroids 0.05% clobetasol. In addition to topical steroids, local skin irritation can be diminished with cotton underclothes, avoidance of strong soaps and detergents, and avoidance of synthetic undergarments. In some pts with lichen sclerosis with severe contracture, surgery may be indicated.
Advanced vulvar tumors		Large tumors of the vulva especially those encroaching on the anorectal area or the urethra may require extensive surgery than radical vulvectomy (i.e., removal of the anus or urethra as part of the primary surgery in which case a diversion procedure is required). It is also prudent to debulk with external radiation and perform the radical vulvectomy about 5 wk later in such large tumors. Other approach to stage III and IV disease is chemoradiation with cisplatin or 5-FU. Radiation therapy and recurrences: In a few instances, the medical condition of the patient precludes and radiation therapy may be employed as the sole treatment. However, the vulvar skin is prone to radiation dermatitis, fibrosis, and ulceration, making this a less desirable treatment option.

(Continued)

TABLE 67.2	MALIGNANT DISEASES OF THE VULVA (CONTINUED)	
DISEASE	**CHARACTERISTICS**	**DIAGNOSIS/TREATMENT**
		To manage recurrences, reoperation is often done. The most common recurrence is local. Chemoradiation may also be used. No effective agent for disseminated disease. Quality of Life: No published data. But, body image disturbance is significant and may account for decreased or absent sexual activities in women who have undergone vulvectomy. The extent of surgery or type of vulvectomy did not correlate with the degree of sexual dysfunction.
Vulvar intraepithelial neoplasia	Although diagnosed more commonly in younger women, the risk of progression to invasive cancer is higher for those who are older and for those who are immunocompromised. Associated with HPV 16, 18, 31, 33, and 35, especially 16.	Mgt of HPV is complicated because it is prevalent and the risk of progression from HPV infection to VIN is small. The best approach is to restrict therapy to individuals with clinically bothersome symptoms such as warts or to eradicate lesions with VIN, particularly 11 and 111. Cytologic or histologic evidence of asymptomatic HPV is not an indication for therapy.
Paget disease	Occurs generally in postmenopausal women. Appears as grossly diffused erythematous eczematoid lesions that are usually chronic. Itching is a problem. More common in whites (average age is 65 y). Once a diagnosis of Paget disease is made, it is important to r/o other. Malignancies since they are usually associated with other invasive cancers	*Treatment:* Wide excision, if no local or distinct primary malig-nancy is uncovered

| Squamous cell carcinoma | 90% of primary vulvar cancers. Grossly usually appears as raised, flat, ulcerated, plaquelike or polypoid masses on the vulva. Two classifications: TNM and FIGO Natural History: The vulvar area is rich in lymphatics with numerous cross connections. Tumors located in the middle of either labium drain initially to the ipsilateral femoral-inguinal nodes. Tumors in the clitoral, urethral, or perineal areas can spread to either side. From the femoral-inguinal nodes, the lymphatic spread of tumor is cephalad to the deep pelvic iliac and obturator nodes. Prognosis: Related to the stage of disease, lesion size, and regional node involvement. 5-y survival: Stage I = 76.9% Stage II = 54.8% Stage III = 30% Stage IV = 8.3% The status of the regional lymph nodes is the most important prognostic and therapeutic factor. Others are stage, thickness, location on the vulva, microscopic differentiation, vascular space involvement, and age of the patient. | Management: IA: Wide excision with 1-2-cm margin IB, II, Early III: Wide radical excision with femoral-inguinal node dissection Lesions located >2 cm from the midline typically need only an ipsilateral femoral-inguinal lymphadenectomy, whereas midline lesions require bilateral nodal dissection. Because the deep pelvic nodes are virtually never involved, only the femoral-inguinal nodes are removed at the time of primary surgery. The deep pelvic nodes are subsequently treated with external radiation. If the nodes above the cribriform fascia are negative, the deep nodes are spared and so are the saphenous veins, thus reducing lower extremity edema. If the nodes particularly in the upper femoral ring are involved, the pelvic nodes need be treated. |

(Continued)

TABLE 67.2	MALIGNANT DISEASES OF THE VULVA (CONTINUED)	
DISEASE	CHARACTERISTICS	DIAGNOSIS/TREATMENT
Melanoma	Most common nonsquamous cell of the vulva 5% of vulvar cancers 5-y survival = 50% Average age is 50 y. Clinically appear as brown, black, or blue-black masses on the vulva. Can be flat or ulcerated Most occur on the labia minora or clitoris. Depth of invasion is the most useful prognostic factor. *Types:* 1. *Superficial spreading* is a more common type with better prognosis. 2. *Nodular melanoma* is less common but more invasive. Breslow reported that overall prognosis is excellent and spread to regional lymph node less likely if thickness is <0.76 mm.	*Treatment:* Wide excision with 1- to 3-cm margin
Bartholin gland carcinoma	Usually adenocarcinoma 1%–2% of vulvar cancers More common in postmenopausal women	*Treatment:* Radical vulvectomy with bilateral femoral–inguinal lymphadenectomy
Verrucous carcinoma	Rare Special variant of squamous cell ca. Appear as large condylomatous mass on the vulva	*Treatment:* Wide local excision Radiation is contraindicated as it can cause anaplastic changes in the tumor.
Sarcoma	Extremely rare (<3%) Leiomyosarcomas are the most common followed by liposarcomas.	*Treatment:* Surgical removal

SUGGESTED READINGS

Aghajanian A, Bernstein L. Bartholin's duct abscess and cyst. *South Med J*. 1994;87:26–29.

American College of Obstetricians and Gynecologists. ACOG Committee No. 345: Opinion: Vulvodynia. October 2006.

Beutner KR. External genital warts. *West J Med*. 1998;169(4):227–228.

Chamorro T. Cancer of the vulva and vagina. *Semin Oncol Nurs*. 1990;6(3):198–205.

Curtin JP, Rubin SC, Jones WB, et al. Paget's disease of the vulva. *Gynecol Oncol*. 1990;39:374–377.

Katz, Lentz, Lobo, Gershenson. *Comprehensive Gynecology*. 5th ed.

68

THE INCOMPLETE ABORTION

CARRIE CWIAK, MD, MPH

A 17-year-old white woman G1P0 presented to her physician for an elective abortion at 11 weeks estimated gestational age per her last menstrual period. She underwent a vacuum aspiration. She was given a prescription for ibuprofen to take as needed for cramping. She had moderate vaginal bleeding for 7 days, requiring five to six sanitary pads per day. On the 7th day, she also noted a subjective fever and suprapubic abdominal cramping that did not respond to ibuprofen. She presented to the emergency room with a temperature of 37°C. Her urine hCG was positive, and serum quantitative hCG was 1,200 mIU/mL. Her pelvic exam noted blood clots in the vagina and an enlarged and tender uterus. Vaginal ultrasound noted an endometrial stripe thickness of 3 cm.

She underwent a repeat vacuum aspiration for retained products. Examination of the aspirated tissue revealed retained placental tissue. She was also treated with oral doxycycline for endometritis.

In the United States, 49% of pregnancies that occur annually are unintended. Forty percent of these pregnancies end in abortion. Therefore, in an American woman's lifetime, she has a one in two likelihood of having an unintended pregnancy and a one in three likelihood of having an abortion. Not surprisingly, induced abortion is one of the most common minor surgeries in the United States. Complications of induced abortion are rare, with only 0.3% of cases having complications that require hospitalization. Yet, although complications are rare, the fact that abortion is such a common procedure means that patients presenting to the emergency room or gynecology clinic with a complication is not that uncommon. In addition, the surgical management for early pregnancy failure (EPF) is the same as surgical management for early induced abortion, namely, vacuum aspiration (also referred to as dilation and curettage [D&C]). Therefore, even if a clinician does not perform induced abortions, the ability to manage the complications is important.

PREVENTING COMPLICATIONS OF INDUCED ABORTION

Abortion-related complication rates and mortality rates are much lower when the pregnancy is early in gestation; the risk of death is 1 per 1,000,000 at ≤8 weeks of gestation. In comparison, this is approximately 1/100th of the risk of death when carrying a pregnancy to term. Appropriate preoperative evaluation for abortion should include a careful patient history, pelvic examination to determine flexion and size of the uterus, and screening for pelvic infection. Many clinicians routinely use ultrasound preoperatively to determine gestational age. At the very least, ultrasound should be utilized if there is a discrepancy between menstrual dating and uterine size. The use of local anesthesia and/or sedation is safer than general anesthesia. During vacuum aspiration, care must be taken to completely empty the uterus of all products of conception. The aspirated products should be examined immediately afterward to assure that the evacuation was in fact complete.

POSTOPERATIVE INFECTION

Prophylactic antibiotics reduce the incidence of postabortal infection. A meta-analysis by Sawaya et al. concluded that providing antibiotics reduces the risk of postabortion infection by 42%, even among low-risk populations. Though the most common etiology of postabortion infection is chlamydial cervicitis and/or pelvic inflammatory disease, most commonly treated with doxycycline, effective regimens against bacterial vaginosis have also proven to reduce infection risk.

RETAINED INTRAUTERINE PRODUCTS

The most common cause of heavy bleeding after abortion is retained products in the uterus, which can occur in as many as 2% of abortions. Diagnosis is made by pelvic exam and can be facilitated by the use of ultrasound. Qualitative and quantitative HCG tests are not useful for diagnosis as HCG levels, though declining, can still be present for up to 8 weeks after an uncomplicated abortion. Although minimal amounts of tissue or blood clot can typically be present after induced or spontaneous abortion, the presence of a thickened endometrial stripe on ultrasound in a woman symptomatic for bleeding and infection is an indication for reaspiration. As with the original surgery, pain control with local anesthesia and/or sedation will decrease the risks associated with reaspiration.

Occasionally, only blood clot rather than tissue is obtained on reaspiration, indicative of postabortal hematometra. This is also known as "postabortal syndrome" and can occur in 1 in 200 abortions, most commonly at or after 11 weeks of gestation. Patients similarly present with cramping and an enlarged and tender uterus, but bleeding is minimal in contrast. Ultrasound will not be able to differentiate between retained tissue and hematometra, but aspiration is nonetheless indicated per the patient's symptoms of pain and tenderness. Studies investigating reproductive health after abortion indicate that sexually transmitted infections (STIs) and pelvic inflammatory disease are factors that increase risk of later infertility. Since hematometra can be a nidus for intrauterine infection, antibiotics should be initiated following reaspiration, whether retained tissue or clot is obtained. Most patients with postabortion infection can be treated as an outpatient; if fever or peritoneal signs are present, admission for intravenous antibiotics is warranted.

POSTABORTION CONTRACEPTION

Over half of women who have abortions were not using a contraceptive method in the month they conceived. This may be the result of lack of access to and education about contraception or perceived low risk for pregnancy. The mean day of ovulation after a first-trimester abortion is 22 days, though it can occur as early as day 10. By day 36, almost all women will have resumed ovulation, and so contraceptive counseling and provision at the time of abortion is paramount in preventing further unintended pregnancy. All forms of hormonal contraceptives, including estrogen-containing methods, can be initiated immediately after first- or second-trimester abortion. Intrauterine contraceptives (IUCs) can be safely inserted immediately after first-trimester aspiration without an appreciable increase in complications. And certainly, barrier methods for pregnancy prevention and/or infection protection may be resumed without delay.

TAKE HOME POINTS

- Vacuum aspiration for induced abortion is a common procedure and management is primarily the same as with aspiration for EPF.
- Prevention of complications from abortion begins with correct determination of gestational age and assurance that the uterus has been completely evacuated at the time of surgery.
- Providing antibiotics at the time of surgery decreases the risk of postoperative infection.
- Retained intrauterine products are the most common cause of heavy bleeding postabortion and require reaspiration.
- Contraceptive counseling and/or provision should occur at the time of induced abortion in order to prevent further unintended pregnancies.

SUGGESTED READINGS

Boyd EF Jr, Holmstrom EG. Ovulation following therapeutic abortion. *Am J Obstet Gynecol.* 1972;113:469–473.

Guttmacher Institute. *Facts on Induced Abortion in the United States.* Available at: www. guttmacher.org/pubs/fb_induced_abortion.pdf, 2008.

Hatcher RA, Trussell J, Stewart F, et al. *Contraceptive Technology.* 18th rev. ed. New York, NY: Ardent Media; 2004.

Paul M, Lichtenberg ES, Borgatta L, et al. *A Clinician's Guide to Surgical and Medical Abortion.* Philadelphia, PA: Churchill Livingstone; 1999.

Sawaya GF, Grady D, Kerlikowske K, et al. Antibiotics at the time of induced abortion: the case for universal prophylaxis based on a meta-analysis. *Obstet Gynecol.* 1996;87:884–890.

Speroff L, Darney PD. *A Clinical Guide for Contraception.* 4th ed. Philadelphia, PA: Lippincott Williams & Wilkins; 2005.

World Health Organization (WHO). *Selected Practice Recommendations for Family Planning.* Geneva, Switzerland: WHO; 2004.

69

CREATING UNNECESSARY BARRIERS TO EFFECTIVE CONTRACEPTIVE USE

CARRIE CWIAK, MD, MPH

A 36-year-old African American married woman G2P1011 had been using Depo-Provera for 5 years, since her last pregnancy, which had been an ectopic pregnancy. She and her family had recently relocated to start a new position in a new city. She was due for her next Depo-Provera injection but the soonest she could get an appointment with a new physician for an annual examination and Pap smear was in 1 month. She arrived at the appointment, now late for her next injection. The physician told her he could not prescribe any contraception for her because she was over 35 years old, had already used Depo-Provera for several years, and had had an ectopic pregnancy. He suggested she use male condoms. She used condoms for the next 6 months, until she missed her menses for the month. A home pregnancy test was positive.

Although we cannot control the economic and social changes our patients experience, we can utilize the principles of evidence-based medicine to decrease barriers in the health care we provide, including safe and effective contraception. Male condoms are associated with a 15% failure rate with the 1st year of typical use, compared to 3% for Depo-Provera (DMPA). Therefore, while there are many benefits of male condoms, including protection from sexually transmitted infections (STIs) and human immunodeficiency virus (HIV), they are not the most effective method for women who are primarily looking to avoid pregnancy.

SCREENING PRIOR TO CONTRACEPTIVE USE

Although annual screenings, including Pap smears, may provide other preventative benefits for our female patients, they are not a prerequisite to providing contraceptive methods. In fact, if a patient's principal need is immediate, effective contraception, then with few exceptions, very little workup is required other than a careful history. Before initiating any hormonal contraceptive, a blood pressure (BP) measurement is suggested. Before inserting an intrauterine contraceptive (IUC), a pelvic exam and assessment for STIs or high-risk practices are essential. In addition, a hemoglobin (Hgb) level can significantly improve contraceptive counseling in regard to the type of IUC best suited for the patient (Copper T vs. levonorgestrel releasing). Finally, preoperative evaluation for surgical sterilization should include all these elements (BP, Hgb, and pelvic exam).

MEDICAL RESTRICTIONS TO CONTRACEPTIVE USE

The vast majority of combined oral contraceptives (OCs) currently available in the United States contain <50 μg of ethinyl estradiol. These low-dose formulations are associated with a three- to fourfold increased risk of venous thromboembolism (VTE) in current users. For healthy, nonsmoking women, this translates to a VTE incidence of 12 to 20 per 100,000 women. Risks are increased by additional cardiac risks such as smoking or hypertension. The risks of stroke and myocardial infarction (MI) are also increased in OC users who have cardiac risk factors but not in those without risk factors. In the absence of smoking or other cardiac risk factors, women over 35 years of age need not be restricted from using estrogen-containing contraceptives. And although estrogen-containing contraceptives modestly increase a woman's baseline risk of thromboembolic complications, progestin-only contraceptives do not confer the same risk. Large, international, multicenter trials have shown that, in the absence of hypertension, progestin-only contraceptives are not associated with an increased risk of VTE, stroke, or MI.

LONG-TERM USE OF DEPO-PROVERA

DMPA is associated with a decrease in bone mineral density (BMD) during its use. The main mechanism of action of DMPA is to block the luteinizing hormone (LH) surge in order to inhibit ovulation. A simultaneous effect is that estrogen levels in the serum are decreased, and therefore, estrogen-dependent bone growth is suppressed. The BMD loss is progressive for the first 18 to 24 months of DMPA use before it begins to plateau. After discontinuation of DMPA, normal estradiol and BMD levels are regained within 2 years. This temporal effect on estrogen and BMD mirrors the effect that occurs during lactation.

RISK OF ECTOPIC PREGNANCY

A woman's baseline risk of ectopic pregnancy is nearly 2%. However, after one ectopic pregnancy, the risk of recurrence is substantially increased. Use of combined OCs and DMPA is associated with decreased risk of ectopic pregnancy, because pregnancy overall is effectively prevented. Therefore, history of ectopic pregnancy is not a contraindication to contraceptive use. With the use of an IUC, the risk that a failure will result in an ectopic pregnancy is increased as much as 1 in 16. However, because IUCs are the most effective reversible contraceptive methods, with typical-use failure rates of <1%, a woman's overall risk is decreased 70% to 80% relative to nonuse of contraception.

- Pelvic exams and Pap smears are not necessary prior to initiating most contraceptive methods.
- Estrogen-containing contraceptives are associated with few risks when used by healthy, nonsmoking women.
- Progestin-only contraceptives are safe alternatives for women who are concerned about additional cardiovascular risks.
- BMD loss associated with Depo-Provera use is reversible upon discontinuation and does not appear to result in increased osteoporosis or fracture risk.
- Use of effective contraception decreases a woman's risk of ectopic pregnancy compared to nonuse.

SUGGESTED READINGS

Curtis KM, Martins SL. Progestogen-only contraception and bone mineral density: a systematic review. *Contraception.* 2006;73:470–487.

Hatcher RA, Trussell J, Stewart F, et al. *Contraceptive Technology.* 18th rev. ed. New York, NY: Ardent Media; 2004.

Heinemann LAJ, Assmann A, DoMinh T, et al. Oral progestogen-only contraceptives and cardiovascular risk: Results from the Transnational Study on Oral Contraceptives and the Health of Young Women. *Eur J Contracept Reprod Health Care.* 1999;4:67–73.

Speroff L, Darney PD. *A Clinical Guide for Contraception.* 4th ed. Philadelphia, PA: Lippincott Williams & Wilkins; 2005.

World Health Organization Collaborative Study of Cardiovascular Disease and Steroid Hormone Contraception. Cardiovascular disease and use of oral and injectable progestogen-only contraceptives and combined injectable contraceptives. *Contraception.* 1998;57:315–324.

World Health Organization (WHO). *Medical Eligibility Criteria for Contraceptive Use.* 3rd ed. Geneva, Switzerland: WHO; 2004.

World Health Organization (WHO). *Selected Practice Recommendations for Family Planning.* Geneva, Switzerland: WHO; 2004.

Zieman M, Hatcher RA, Cwiak C, et al. *Managing Contraception. 2007–2009 ed.* Tiger, GA: Bridging the Gap; 2007.

70

PERMANENT STERILIZATION: INCOMPLETE PREOPERATIVE COUNSELING

CARRIE CWIAK, MD, MPH

A 24-year-old Latina woman G3P3003 requests permanent sterilization. She is currently using combined oral contraceptives (OCs) but often forgets to take them. She explains that she and her husband do not want anymore children. Her physician explains the risks and benefits of surgery. She consents to and receives a laparoscopic tubal ligation 4 weeks later.

Five years later, she returns with her husband and requests a reversal of her tubal ligation. They explain that their financial situation has substantially improved, and they now want a larger family. They ask what options are available to them.

Permanent sterilization is one of the most frequently used contraceptive methods in the United States, with 28% of contracepting reproductive-aged females and 9% of contracepting reproductive-aged males relying on sterilization. Sterilization provides highly effective protection from pregnancy; tubal ligation is associated with a failure rate of 0.5% in the 1st year and a cumulative failure rate of 1.85% at 10 years.

ELEMENTS OF PRESTERILIZATION COUNSELING

Counseling a woman who requests permanent sterilization should include a review of the benefits, risks, and available options for permanent sterilization. The obvious benefit is highly effective long-term contraception that requires no coital or daily administration. Risks of female sterilization include risks of surgery and/or anesthesia, risk of failure with the possibility of ectopic pregnancy, and risk of regret. Surgical complications are rare but can include minor complications (infection, wound dehiscence) as well as major complications (hemorrhage, bowel injury, anesthesia reactions). Postpartum sterilization is performed via partial salpingectomy at the time of cesarean section or immediately after vaginal delivery. Options for interval sterilization (i.e., not immediately postpartum) include laparoscopic tubal ligation (via Filshie clip, Falope ring, or bipolar cautery), hysteroscopic tubal occlusion (via Essure coils), and male sterilization. In addition, all available options for reversible contraception and their failure rates should be reviewed.

INCIDENCE OF REGRET AFTER STERILIZATION

Frank discussion emphasizing that sterilization is a permanent procedure is important. The clinician should confirm that the patient does not desire any more children, regardless of potential changes in her relationship, family size, or financial situation. A U.S. multicenter study followed women for up to 14 years after sterilization and found a cumulative risk of regret of nearly 13%. The probability of regret was higher among women who at the time of sterilization were 30 years of age or younger, nonwhite, unmarried, or immediately postpartum, postabortion, or within 1 year of the birth of their youngest child. Other risk factors for regret include marriage and starting a family at a young age and remarriage with desire for more children.

MALE STERILIZATION

Benefits of vasectomy in relation to tubal sterilization include lower failure rate, lower complication rate, less cost, and less need for anesthesia. The failure rate in the 1st year is 0.15%. The most common procedure is no-scalpel vasectomy, typically performed in an office setting under local anesthesia. Hence, complications are rare and primarily consist of minor events such as hematoma and infection. Vasectomy is one of the three most cost-effective methods of contraception at 5 years of use, with costs that typically range from 60% to 70% less than costs of female sterilization.

LONG-ACTING REVERSIBLE CONTRACEPTION

Like sterilization, the levonorgestrel-releasing intrauterine contraceptive (IUC), the Copper T IUC, and the progestin implant are methods that provide highly effective long-term contraception for up to 5, 10, and 3 years, respectively, without the need for coital or daily administration. Failure rates for the three methods are each less than 1% in the 1st year of use, prompting the World Health Organization (WHO) to categorize them in the top tier of contraceptive efficacy along with female and male sterilization. Current IUCs are not associated with increased risk of pelvic inflammatory disease. Therefore, similar to the progestin implant, IUCs are associated with rapid return to baseline fertility upon removal. Despite the fact that long-acting reversible contraceptives provide equivalent efficacy to sterilization without the risk of regret, patient counseling is often lacking in this respect. In one survey, 37% of women who had chosen postpartum tubal ligation for contraception had not discussed long-acting methods with their providers.

TAKE HOME POINTS

- Female and male sterilizations are highly effective, albeit permanent, methods of contraception.

- Presterilization counseling should include a review of all available options for reversible contraception.
- Risk of regret after sterilization is high. Regret is more likely among young, minority, or unmarried women.
- The option of male sterilization should also be presented as a method that is associated with fewer complications and less need for anesthesia.
- Long-term reversible contraception provides equivalent efficacy in pregnancy protection, without a decrease in future fertility.

SUGGESTED READINGS

Cwiak C, Gellasch T, Zieman M. Peripartum contraceptive attitudes and practices. *Contraception*. 2004;70:383–386.

Hatcher RA, Trussell J, Stewart F, et al. *Contraceptive Technology*. 18th rev. ed. New York, NY: Ardent Media; 2004.

Hillis SD, Marchbanks PA, Tylor LR, et al. Poststerilization regret: findings from the United States Collaborative Review of Sterilization. *Obstet Gynecol*. 1999;93:889–895.

Leader A, Galan N, George R, et al. A comparison of definable traits in women requesting reversal of sterilization and women satisfied with sterilization. *Am J Obstet Gynecol*. 1983;145:198–202.

Peterson HB, Xia Z, Hughes JM, et al. The risk of pregnancy after tubal sterilization: findings from the U.S. Collaborative Review of Sterilization. *Am J Obstet Gynecol*. 1996;174:1161–1170.

Sivin I, Stern J. Health during prolonged use of levonorgestrel 20 mcg/day and the Copper T380Ag intrauterine contraceptive devices: a multicenter study. *Fertil Steril*. 1994;60:70–77.

Speroff L, Darney PD. *A Clinical Guide for Contraception*. 4th ed. Philadelphia, PA: Lippincott Williams & Wilkins; 2005.

Zieman M, Hatcher RA, Cwiak C, et al. *Managing Contraception. 2007–2009 ed*. Tiger, GA: Bridging the Gap; 2007.

71

WHEN DOES BREAST-FEEDING FAIL FOR POSTPARTUM CONTRACEPTION?

TARA P. CLEARY, MD

Your pregnant patient informs you that she plans on breast-feeding after she delivers. You commend her for her plans, telling her that breast-feeding can be easier to do than bottle feeding, especially in the middle of the night or while out at the supermarket. You educate her that studies have shown that infants who are breast-fed have decreased infections early in life and may have increased IQ levels.

You then ask her what she plans to use for contraception following delivery. She says she plans on breast-feeding and she thought that that was sufficient as long as she does not get her period. Right?

In order to practice the lactational amenorrhea method (LAM), three basic criteria must be achieved. As long as menses have not returned, as long as the patient is not supplementing regularly or allowing for long intervals between breast-feeding, and as long as the infant is no more than 6 months old, she has only a 1% to 2% chance of pregnancy.

Should your patient meet these criteria, she must be further educated as to what these criteria really mean. Return to menses is defined as 2 contiguous days of bleeding considered equal or heavier than menstrual flow, 2 contiguous days of spotting and 1 day of menstrual-like bleeding, OR 3 contiguous days of spotting. To meet definition of fully or nearly fully breast-feeding, all of the following must be met: (a) breast-feeding frequency must be a pattern comparable to at least ten short or six long breast-feeding episodes within 24 hours, an episode being feeding that continues at least 4 minutes post letdown; (b) supplemental feeding of no more than 1 oz (30 mL) per week in 1st month, no more than 2 oz (60 mL) in 2nd month, 3 oz (90mL) in 3rd month, etc.; (c) no replacement of breast-feeds with other feeds and no more than 10% of feeds or food can be other than direct breast-feeding; and (d) breast-feeding must be maintained with both day and night feeding and no long intervals between feeds, that is, no more than 10 hours or frequent interval greater than two times per week of 6 hours between feeds.

Expressed milk either by manual or electric methods is considered supplemental feeding by strict LAM definitions. A recent study was performed that included 71 working mothers who returned to work at average day 92 postpartum to determine the efficacy of LAM with mothers separated from their infants at long intervals. These women worked an average of 7.2 hours per day and while at work manually expressed milk every 4 hours. They continued normal breast-feeding practices for the remainder of the day and at night. For these women, their risk of pregnancy at 6 months was found to be 5.2% with only 50% of these women being amenorrheic at 6 months and only 18.8% using LAM at 6 months. Thus, working mothers may also use LAM but must understand the increased risk of pregnancy and the increased likelihood that they will not meet criteria at 6 months.

Therefore, there are several questions you must ask your patient to select her as a candidate for LAM. Does she plan on being separated from her infant, which would require she express her milk? Is she willing to accept the increased risk of pregnancy with manual expression? If she will not be separated from her infant, will she be able to breast-feed every 4 hours?

When a woman decides LAM will be her contraceptive method of choice, she must still be counseled in complimentary contraception. In women who are following LAM, approximately 75% remain amenorrheic at 6 months and if continued, 42% are still amenorrheic at 12 months. It is impossible to predict at what time point your patient will no longer meet criteria for LAM and she should be prepared to start another method as soon as LAM is no longer effective for her. Should she continue breast-feeding while using another method of contraception, you should inform her that methods containing estrogen are likely to decrease the quantity of breast milk that she produces.

TAKE HOME POINTS

- LAM is highly effective with a 2% pregnancy rate as long as menses has not yet returned, the infant is <6 months old, and the woman is exclusively breast-feeding every 4 hours.
- LAM can also be effective for working mothers who manually express milk while separated from the infants but there is an increased pregnancy rate.
- Women should be prepared to start a complimentary contraceptive method once they no longer meet criteria for LAM.
- Estrogen-containing contraceptive methods may decrease milk production.

SUGGESTED READINGS

Hatcher R, Trussell J, Nelson AL, et al. *Contraceptive Technology*. New York, NY: Ardent Media; 2004.

Labbok M, Hight-Laukaran V, Peterson AE, et al. Multicenter Study of the Lactational Amenorrhea Method (LAM): I. Efficacy, duration, and implications for clinical application. *Contraception*. 1997;55:327–336.

Valdés V, Labbok MH, Pugin E, et al. The efficacy of the lactational amenorrhea method (LAM) among working women. *Contraception*. 2000;62:217–219.

72

CAN TEENAGERS AND NULLIPAROUS WOMEN GET INTRAUTERINE CONTRACEPTIVE DIVICES?

FRANCIS KWARTENG, MD AND DIANA BROOMFIELD, MD, MBA, FACOG, FACS

A 17-year-old obese nulligravid female presented to her physician's office for contraceptive counseling. She denies any significant medical history and states that she has no desire of becoming pregnant. She vehemently rejects intrauterine contraceptive device (IUD) because she feels that she would have infertility issues upon removal. The physician agrees and prescribes the Ortho-Evra patch.

Intrauterine contraceptive is effective and is a long-term device that is currently used by 3% of reproductive age women seeking contraception in the United States. Currently, two commonly available IUDs are the Levonorgestrel and Paragard T380A variants. Failure rates are 0.1 and 0.1% for the Levonorgestrel type and 0.6 and 0.8% for Cu T380, when used as prescribed. Contrary to earlier notion, many health care providers are beginning to appreciate and accept their use in teenagers and especially nulliparous women with no contraindications.

In 1998, the World Health Organization's (WHO's) annual report on contraception recommended the use of IUD in teenagers and nulliparous women especially if they are in stable relationships. The decision of WHO is based on the benefits of IUD in teenagers and nulliparous women, which clearly outweigh the risk and promote increased compliance especially in teenagers who account for a huge proportion of unintended pregnancies around the world. This recommendation is also supported by ACOG's Committee on adolescence health. Currently, the food and drug administration (FDA) label for Mirena does not list nulliparity and nulligravidity as contraindications. Despite these recommendations, a number of physicians are still reluctant in using these devices in nulliparous and especially teenagers for fear of future infertility.

The July 2008 report from Bayer Healthcare Pharmaceuticals (manufacturer of Mirena), on indications to the use of Mirena, unequivocally states that the device is recommended for females who have at least one child. This proscribes nulliparous women from using the device. Ostensibly, this recommendation is to mitigate liability. Numerous misconceptions and myths surround IUD use, partly explaining why some clinicians and the manufacturers avoid its use. Infertility, infections, and ectopic pregnancy have long been associated with IUD use, but none of these have been confirmed in a large randomized prospective study. Indeed, fecundity returns immediately after IUD removal. The misconception about IUD and infection originated from the class action lawsuit that surrounded the use of the Dalkon shield IUD in the 1970s. Pelvic infection is believed to be increased slightly in the first 20 to 25 days postinsertion. Generally, IUD does not cause increased rates of ectopic gestation. Ectopic pregnancies are lower in IUD patients compared to the general population considering the fact that only 0.1% to 0.6% of IUD users fail, resulting in pregnancy.

TAKE HOME POINTS

- Research is underway looking at use of long-term reversible birth control options, IUD and implanon (subdermal implants), compared to short-term options with low compliance, resulting in unintended pregnancy in adolescence.
- Paragard is recommended for nulliparous female from 16 to 51 years provided they are monogamous in stable relationships.
- Available evidence, therefore, supports the use of IUD in these groups.

SUGGESTED READINGS

Chi IC, Balogh S. Interval insertion of intrauterine device in women with previous cesarean section. *Contraception.* 1984;30:209.

Chi IC, Farr G. Postpartum IUD contraception—a review of an international experience. *Contraception.* 1989;5:127.

Emans SJ, Grace E, Woods ER, et al. Adolescents compliance with the use of oral contraceptives. *JAMA.* 1987;257:3377.

Hayes JL, Cwiak C, Goedken P, et al. A pilot clinical trial of ultrasound-guided post placental insertion of a levonorgestrel intrauterine device. *Contraception.* 2007;76:292.

Hubacher D, Reyes V, Lillo S, et al. Pain from copper intrauterine device insertion: randomized trail of prophylactic ibuprofen. *Am J Obstet Gynecol.* 2006;195:1272.

Neinstein LS, Nelson AL. Contraception. In: Neinstein LA, ed. *Adolescent Health Care: A Practical Guide.* 4th ed. Philadelphia, PA: Lippincott Williams & Wilkins; 2000:834.

Toivonen J, Luukkainen T, Allomen H. Protective effect of intrauterine release of levonorgestrel on pelvic infection: three year's comparative experience of levonorgestrel-and cooper-releasing intrauterine devices. *Obstet Gynecol.* 1991;77:261.

Varila E, Wahlstrom T, Rauramo I. A 5-year follow-up study on the use of a levonorgestrel intrauterine system in women receiving hormone replacement therapy. *Fertil Steril.* 2001;76:969.

World Health Organization (WHO). Improving access to quality care in family planning. In: *Medical Eligibility Criteria for Contraceptive Use.* 3rd ed. Geneva, Switzerland: WHO; 2003.

73

APPROPRIATE CONTRACEPTION FOR SPECIAL MEDICAL AND SURGICAL PATIENTS

FRANCIS KWARTENG, MD AND DIANA BROOMFIELD, MD, MBA, FACOG, FACS

A 30-year-old G0 female with a history of mixed connective tissues disease, hypertension, and controlled diabetes mellitus type I presents for contraceptive counseling. She inquires if she could have combined contraceptive pills.

The contraceptive method appropriate for various medical conditions is usually determined by the underlying pathophysiology of the disease process and whether or not the active contraceptive hormone will deleteriously alter the pathophysiology of the disease. It may not be possible or appropriate to review all medical conditions and their most efficacious contraceptive method in each case. However, a common error is seen when health care providers fail to determine whether the disease process in their patients will reduce the efficacy of the agent to be prescribed or whether the agent will worsen the underlying disease process.

CHRONIC ESSENTIAL HYPERTENSION
The oral combined contraceptive pill is not recommended in patients with poorly controlled hypertension. However, patients with well-controlled hypertension may use oral contraceptive pills (OCP). Nevertheless, it is important to counsel such patients regarding the potential worsening of their hypertension. Such patients should be followed closely especially in first few months after onset of the OCP. All other contraceptive methods are appropriate alternatives.

PULMONARY HYPERTENSION
Another error to avoid is the use of OCPs in patients with primary or secondary pulmonary hypertension. This is contraindicated. These patients should be prescribed progestational agents or barrier contraceptives. Patients who have completed childbearing may consider permanent sterilization.

CARDIAC DISEASES
Combined oral contraceptive pills are not recommended in patients with congested heart failure (CHF) and valvular heart diseases. It is important that patient individualization and the degree of cardiac disease be considered when selecting a contraceptive method. Generally, all nonhormonal

agents are appropriate. Permanent sterilization is an option if childbearing is completed.

OBESITY

Another common error is not taking the woman's weight into consideration when recommending hormonal contraceptives. Women with a BMI of >29.5 may still consider OCPs or the Nuva ring after appropriate counseling. However, the Ortho Evra patch has reduced efficacy in women with weight >198 lb. Progesterone-only methods, intrauterine devices (IUDs), and permanent sterilization are also appropriate and alternate options for obese patients.

DIABETES

Low-dose OCPs can be used in patients with recent onset disease and well-controlled cases. Combined oral contraceptive agents are not advised in patients with poorly controlled diabetes and those with vasculopathic complications. Nonhormonal agents and permanent sterilization are appropriate options for these patients.

SUPERFICIAL VENOUS THROMBOSIS

OCP and progestational agents are recommended because their benefits outweigh the risk. The World Health Organization (WHO) categorizes progesterone-only pills and oral combined contraceptive pills as category 1 and 2 respectively; thus progesterone-only pills and OCPs may be prescribed when the benefits outweigh the risks.

SYSTEMIC SCLEROSIS

IUD is not advised because of increased tendency of adhesion formation around the device. OCP is not advised because of vascular complications associated with the disease process. The most appropriate contraception is permanent sterilization if patients are surgical candidates.

INFLAMMATORY BOWEL DISEASE

Several authorities recommend such patients to be offered the same contraception as the general population.

SURGICAL PATIENTS

Patients on progesterone-only pills (POPs) may continue taking their medication even when immobilization is anticipated postoperatively. Patients on OCPs should be counseled to discontinue 4 weeks prior to the procedure, especially where immobilization is anticipated. Candidates for elective minor surgical procedures can continue all hormonal contraception prior to surgery and postoperatively.

TAKE HOME POINTS

- Avoid not taking a thorough medical history.
- OCPs are contraindicated in patients with CHF and pulmonary hypertension.
- Weight affects efficacy of some hormonal contraceptives.

SUGGESTED READINGS

Cunningham FG, Leveno KL, Bloom SL, et al. *William Obstetrics.* 22nd ed. Available at: www. who.int/topics/contraception/en (Accessed February 6, 2008).

Dugdale M, Masi AT. Hormonal contraception. *J Chronic Dis.* 1971;23(10):775–790.

Martinez F, Avecilla A. Combined hormonal contraception and venous thromboembolism. *Eur J Contracept Reprod Health Care.* 2007;12:97.

Mohllajee AP, Cutis KM, Martins SL, et al. Does use of hormonal contraceptives among women with thrombogenic mutations increase their risk of venous thromboembolism? A systematic contraception. *Contraception.* 1998;57:315.

Vasilakiis C, Jick H. Rick of idiopathic venous thromboembolism in users of progestagrens alone. *Lancet.* 1999;354:1610.

GYNECOLOGIC ONCOLOGY AND PATHOLOGY

74

ULTRASOUND FINDING OF UNILOCULAR 5-CM OR LESS OVARIAN CYST IN PERIMENOPAUSAL WOMAN CAN USUALLY BE FOLLOWED WITHOUT SURGERY

PIERRE GORDON, MD AND DIANA P. BROOMFIELD, MD

A 49-year-old G2P2 perimenopausal woman presents complaining of lower abdominal pain for 2 days. The pain is a dull pressure, on the right. She also reports that her periods have been irregular over the past 6 months, and her last menstrual period was 2 weeks ago. On bimanual exam, the patient exhibits tenderness to palpation. A "fullness" is noted in the right adnexa. An ultrasound is performed and a single, thin-walled, unilocular cyst measuring 4.5 cm × 3.0 cm × 3.0 cm is found. Within 10 days, she is taken to the operating room for an ovarian cystectomy and possible oophorectomy. What is the error of management in this case? What is the most likely diagnosis?

This patient should not have undergone surgery for a case that is characteristic of a functional ovarian cyst. Being that this clinical presentation is not indicative of a malignancy and that such cysts often resolve on their own, surgery is not required at the time of diagnosis. This patient should be managed with a repeat ultrasound in 4 to 6 weeks expecting spontaneous resolution of the cyst if it is indeed functional. Additionally, one may consider prescribing oral contraceptives to promote regression of the cyst. If the cyst does not resolve or if it develops characteristics suggestive of malignancy on repeat ultrasound, then surgery may be indicated.

FUNCTIONAL CYST

At the top of the differential diagnosis of a unilocular cyst in a perimenopausal woman are functional ovarian cysts that include follicular cysts, the most common type, as well as lutein cysts, such as corpus luteum cyst and theca lutein cyst. A follicular cyst, filled with fluid and lined by granulosa cells, is derived from an ovarian follicle that is not fully resorbed after it ruptures or one that does not rupture at all. This cyst is more likely to be asymptomatic but may present with irregular menstrual cycle, which is oligomenorrhea or polymenorrhea, unilateral lower abdominal pain, or pelvic pain acutely if the cyst ruptures. A corpus luteum cyst, which arises from a persistent corpus luteum and produces progesterone, presents with unilateral abdominal tenderness and amenorrhea. Note that the lack of menstruation differentiates this cyst from the follicular cyst. A theca lutein cyst is derived from overstimulation of a follicle by high levels of human chorionic gonadotropin, especially that seen in gestational trophoblastic disease. This cyst may be multiple or bilateral.

ENDOMETRIOMAS AND NEOPLASIA

Low on the differential are endometrioma and neoplasia due to lack of multiple or thick septations, vegetations, and solid components within the cyst. One study of premenopausal and postmenopausal women showed only a 0.3% risk of malignancy in a unilocular cyst. It has also been shown that the highest probabilities of cancerous adnexal masses are in girls before the age of puberty and postmenopausal women. It must be noted that 80% of ovarian masses are benign. Even when large, 5 to 10 cm in diameter, most unilocular cysts are not malignant. If this patient was postmenopausal or ultrasound findings were suggestive of cancer, then a malignant process would be higher on the differential and more aggressive management would be warranted.

OVARIAN TORSION

Lastly, ovarian torsion, although not present in this case, would warrant emergent surgical intervention. Ovarian torsion is a twisting of the ovary with or without the fallopian tube as it cuts off its blood supply leading to ischemia and if prolonged, necrosis. Ovarian torsion may present as acute unilateral lower abdominal pain with, tenderness to palpation, rebound, nausea, vomiting, or leukocytosis. Risk factors include ovarian maneuverability and enlargement, as seen in a cystic ovary, but typically >6 to 8 cm. When the patient is stable, her pain controlled, and torsion is not diagnosed by Doppler ultrasound, repeat ultrasound without surgery is a justified plan.

TAKE HOME POINTS

- Simple, small unilocular cysts in reproductive-aged and perimenopausal women do not require aggressive initial management and can therefore be followed by ultrasound in 4 to 6 weeks.

- An ovarian cyst in a postmenopausal woman or one with multiple or thick septations, vegetations, or solid components should raise the suspicion for malignancy.
- Ovarian torsion is a surgical emergency.

SUGGESTED READINGS

Callahan TL, Caughey AB, Heffner LJ (eds). Ovarian and fallopian tube tumors. In: *Blueprints in Obstetrics and Gynecology*. Malden, MA: Blackwell Science; 1998:187.

Feig RL, Johnson NC. Benign ovarian masses. In: Stead L, Stead S, eds. *First Aid for the Obstetrics and Gynecology Clerkship*. New York, NY: McGraw-Hill; 2002:182–183.

Hoffman M. Overview of the evaluation and management of adnexal masses. UpToDate. [document on the internet]; updated [Oct 1, 2008]. Available from http://www.utdol.com/online/content/search.do

Mutch DG, Bleckman CR. Obg management: how to manage an adnexal mass. [serial on the Internet]. 2007 [cited Mar 24, 2009]:50–58. Available at: http://www.obgmanagement.com/

Sakala EP. Pelvic masses and pelvic pain. In: *Board Review Aeries: Obstetrics and Gynecology*. 2nd ed. Philadelphia, PA: Lippincott Williams & Wilkins; 2000:337.

Schraga ED, Blanda M. Ovarian torsion. Emedicine [document on the internet]; updated [Aug 4, 2008] [cited Mar 24, 2009]. Available at: http://emedicine.medscape.com

75

KNOW WHAT YOU ARE LOOKING FOR: BE CAREFUL WHEN ORDERING TUMOR MARKERS

PIERRE GORDON, MD AND DIANA BROOMFIELD, MD

A 33-year-old G3P3 African American female presents for her annual exam. Her past medical history is significant for multiple uterine fibroid and recurrent ovarian cysts. Her last menstrual period was 3 weeks ago. She reports that her cousin was diagnosed with ovarian cancer 2 years ago at the age of 40. She denies any significant history in her first-degree relatives. In an attempt to be proactive, her physician orders Carbohydrate Antigen 125 (CA 125) levels, which come back moderately elevated. He diagnoses ovarian cancer and recommends a prophylactic total abdominal hysterectomy with bilateral salpingo-oophorectomy. Distraught, the patient obtains a second opinion that refutes the initial physician's diagnosis and recommendation. Was the original physician wrong?

DISCUSSION

The initial physician should not have ordered CA 125 for two reasons. First, there are other factors besides ovarian cancer that could explain the elevation in CA 125. Three of these factors, the fibroid uterus, ovarian cysts, and menstrual cycle, are present in this patient. Second, the cousin's diagnosis is not significant because she is not a first-degree relative.

Tumor markers are biochemical products that are elevated in the presence of a neoplastic process. The substance measured by a tumor marker assay may be elevated because it is made by the tumor itself or is made by the body because of the tumor's presence. When ordering tumor markers, it should be clear how the information gained would be used. That is to say, will the levels be used to help screen or diagnose disease in an individual at increased risk or monitor disease response to treatment or disease recurrence?

Although tumor markers are used to help diagnose disease, at the moment, no marker is recommended for diagnostic purposes by itself. This is because the majority of tumor markers do not have high enough sensitivity to be good screening tests. Additionally, as seen in the case above, these assays are not very specific.

CA 125

Carbohydrate Antigen 125 is a marker sought out in ovarian epithelial tumors. It is increased in approximately 80% of nonmucinous ovarian carcinomas. It should be ordered preoperatively if there is a high index of suspicion that an ovarian malignancy is present. Values >35 U/mL are considered to be elevated. Factors that support getting CA 125 levels include personal or significant family history of cancer; a physical exam finding of an irregular, fixed, solid adnexal mass; the presence of ascites; septations >3 mm in thickness; and nonhyperechoic, solid components on ultrasound. Due to the low prevalence of disease (50/100,000) and low specificity, this marker is not currently recommended for use as a screening tool in the general population. The lack of specificity is exemplified by increased CA 125 levels seen in other gynecologic processes such as uterine fibromas, endometrial cancer, pelvic inflammatory disease, and endometriosis as well as kidney, liver, and cardiac diseases. Lastly, if levels are drawn in a premenopausal woman, one should keep in mind that CA 125 levels are not stable during the menstrual cycle and can be as high as 200 U/mL.

GERM CELL TUMOR MARKERS

While CA 125 is used for ovarian epithelial tumors, markers also exist for germ cell tumors. Human chorionic gonadotropin (hCG), for example, is physiologically elevated in pregnancy as it is produced by the syncytiotrophoblast of the placenta. Pathologically, hCG levels may be elevated in gestational trophoblastic disease in the adult or ovarian germ cell tumors in younger patients. HCG levels are important in management because they correlate well with tumor burden. Other tumor germ cell tumor markers include alpha-fetoprotein (AFP), which is elevated in endodermal sinus tumors, and lactate dehydrogenase (LDH), which is increased in dysgerminomas. Embryonal carcinomas and mixed germ cell tumors may show elevations in different combinations of these markers.

FAMILIAL CANCER SYNDROMES

A setting where one may think of ordering tumor markers would be in familial cancer syndromes. The BRCA mutations and Lynch syndrome are two examples. When BRCA1 and BRCA2 mutations are present, the lifetime risks for breast and ovarian cancers are increased significantly higher than that of the general population. Although no recommendation yet exists, a practical approach to management of a patient with these mutations should include annual transvaginal ultrasounds and CA 125 levels. While a history of breast cancer is a risk factor for endometrial cancer, nulliparity and obesity are shared risk factors, so currently, there is no consensus as to the association of BRCA mutations and endometrial cancer.

In Lynch syndrome, colon cancer develops in association with other malignancies such as endometrial and ovarian cancers. In this setting, approximately 40% of female patients develop ovarian or endometrial cancer by the age of 70. In approximately 50% of cases, the gynecologic malignancy precedes the appearance of colon cancer by 5.5 years for ovarian and 11 years for endometrial cancer.

TAKE HOME POINTS

- Ordering tumor markers hoping to pick up anything that is elevated can be deleterious as many markers can be nonspecifically elevated.
- Know the appropriate tumor markers for any condition.
- Know what physiologic and pathologic factors will cause tumor marker elevations.
- Tumor markers are not recommended as screening tools but as a preoperative tool to assess a patient's postoperative course.

SUGGESTED READINGS

Carlson KJ. Screening for ovarian cancer. UpToDate. [updated Oct 6, 2008; cited Mar 24, 2009]. Available at: http://www.utdol.com/online/content/search.do

Chen L. Endometrial cancer: clinical features, diagnosis, and screening. UpToDate. [updated Aug 18, 2008; cited Mar 24, 2009]. Available at: http://www.utdol.com/online/content/search.do

Chen L-M. Epithelial ovarian cancer: clinical manifestations diagnositic evaluation, staging, and hisopathology. UpToDate. [updated Sep 16, 2008; cited Mar 24, 2009]. Available at: http://www.utdol.com/online/content/search.do

Ferrini R. Screening asymptomatic women for ovarian cancer: American College of Preventive Medicine Practice Policy Statement. American College of Preventive Medicine 1996 [cited Mar 24, 2009]. Available at: http://www.acpm.org/ovary.htm

Hoffman M. Overview of the evaluation and management of adnexal masses. UpToDate. [updated Oct 1, 2008; cited Mar 24, 2009]. Available at: http://www.utdol.com/online/content/search.do

Holschneider C. Staging of cervical cancer. UpToDate. [updated Jun 6, 2008; cited Mar 24, 2009]. Available at: http://www.utdol.com/online/content/search.do

National cancer institute. National cancer institute fact sheet: Tumor markers: questions and answers. Feb 3, 2006 [cited Mar 24, 2009]. Available at: http://www.cancer.gov/cancertopics/factsheet/Detection/tumor-markers

Tc-cancer.com. Tumor markers; AFP, HCG, CA-125. 2006 [cited Mar 24, 2009]. Available at: http://www.tc-cancer.com/tumormarkers.html

76

ENDOMETRIAL ADENOCARCINOMA WITH CLEAR CELL CHANGE OR CLEAR CELL CARCINOMA OF THE ENDOMETRIUM

SANJAY LOGANI, MD

A 42-year-old female patient was seen in the clinic complaining of heavy vaginal bleeding of 3 months' duration. An office endometrial biopsy was performed. The pathologist reportedly diagnosed endometrial adenocarcinoma with clear cell differentiation. A hysterectomy with pelvic lymph node sampling was performed. On the hysterectomy specimen, the tumor was noted to be confined to the endometrium and predominantly a FIGO grade 1 endometrioid adenocarcinoma. No clear cell carcinoma was identified in the hysterectomy specimen.

Clinicopathologic studies suggest that endometrial adenocarcinoma can be divided into two types. Type 1 endometrial carcinoma is typically seen in reproductive age group patients and appears to be an estrogen-driven tumor. Risk factors include obesity, exogenous hormone administration, or any other cause of increased estrogen in the patient. On the other hand, type 2 endometrial carcinoma is seen in the sixth and seventh decade and does not appear to be estrogen driven. Endometrioid, mucinous, villoglandular, and secretory subtypes are considered to be type 1 tumors, while serous and clear cell carcinomas exemplify type 2 tumors. Prognostically, both serous and clear cell carcinomas are aggressive tumors and thus considered to be grade 3 in the FIGO grading system. Endometrioid adenocarcinoma is often associated with squamous or morular metaplasia, which when extensively glycogenated can show clearing of the cytoplasm and thus mimic clear cell carcinoma and in the authors experience is one of the most common causes of diagnostic confusion on a biopsy or a curettage (*Fig 76.1*). Another cause of clear cell change in endometrioid carcinoma is the rare secretory variant of endometrial carcinoma in which the clear cell change occurs in the tumor cell itself (*Fig 76.2*). The Arias-Stella reaction can show morphologic mimicry with the glands of a clear cell carcinoma, but the clinical history of recent pregnancy and lack of mitotic activity are helpful in distinguishing this nonneoplastic histologic finding from a clear cell carcinoma. Although mixed clear cell and endometrioid carcinomas exist, they are rare.

Distinguishing clear cell change in the squamous component of an endometrioid carcinoma from a true clear cell carcinoma on an endometrial

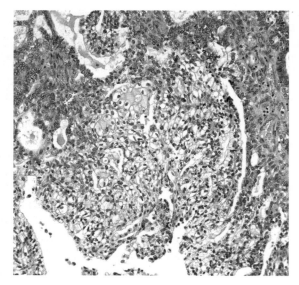

FIGURE 76.1. Endometrioid adenocarcinoma can mimic clear cell carcinoma.

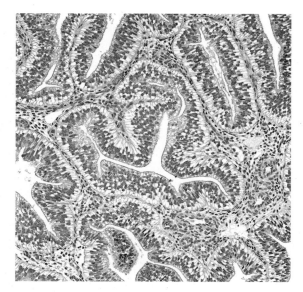

FIGURE 76.2. Rare secretory variant of endometrial carcinoma.

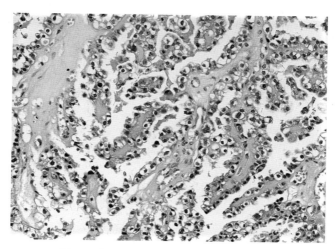

FIGURE 76.3. Clear cell carcinoma with hobnailed nuclei.

curettage is possible if careful attention is given to the cytologic characteristics of the tumor cells in the clear cell foci. Clear cell change in an endometrioid carcinoma often occurs on the surface or in-between the endometrioid glands within foci of morular metaplasia. Most often, the cells in the clear cell foci are arranged in sheets and the nuclei do not show the high-grade cytology or increased mitotic activity of a typical clear cell carcinoma. A true clear cell carcinoma tends to have an admixture of tubulocystic and papillary growth patterns along with sheetlike growth and the constituent cells show high-grade nuclei with prominent nucleoli. Hobnailed nuclei are characteristic of this tumor subtype (*Fig 76.3*). It is extremely important to distinguish an endometrioid carcinoma with clear cell change from a clear cell carcinoma from a therapeutic and prognostic standpoint. In order to avoid confusion, foci of clear cell change in an otherwise typical endometrioid adenocarcinoma should not be mentioned in the diagnostic line to avoid the potential of misinterpretation as a clear cell carcinoma by the treating physician. It is better explained in a comment or microscopic description. This is a common and avoidable error in the interpretation of endometrial adenocarcinoma on curettage or a biopsy specimen.

TAKE HOME POINTS

- Clear cell change in an endometrioid adenocarcinoma of the endometrium can potentially be confused for a clear cell carcinoma component in an otherwise low-risk tumor.

- If correctly identified, clear cell change in an endometrioid carcinoma should not be part of the diagnosis to avoid potentially being misinterpreted as a clear cell carcinoma.
- Therapy for clear cell carcinoma is different than that for an endometrioid adenocarcinoma with clear cell change.

SUGGESTED READINGS

Abeler VM, Vergote IB, Kjørstad KE, et al. Clear cell carcinoma of the endometrium: prognosis and metastatic pattern. *Cancer.* 1996;78:1740–1747.

Clement PB, Young RH. Endometrioid carcinoma of the uterine corpus: a review of its pathology with emphasis on recent advances and problematic aspects. *Adv Anat Pathol.* 2002;9(3):145–184.

Cirisano FD Jr, Robboy SJ, Dodge RK, et al. Epidemiologic and surgicopathologic findings of papillary serous and clear cell endometrial cancers when compared to endometrioid carcinoma. *Gynecol Oncol.* 1999;74:385–394.

Sherman ME. Theories of endometrial carcinogenesis: a multidisciplinary approach. *Mod Pathol.* 2000;13:295–308.

77

CLINICAL HISTORY AND SPECIMEN ADEQUACY: CLINICIANS ARE FROM MARS AND PATHOLOGISTS ARE FROM VENUS

GABRIELA M. OPREA-ILIES, MD AND BHAGIRATH MAJMUDAR, MD

A 45-year-old woman presents with heavy bleeding. An endometrial biopsy performed is sent to the pathologist with the clinical history of "vaginal bleeding". Histopathology examination shows small detached fragments of endocervix, lower uterine segment, and predominantly blood. No endometrial glands were present for evaluation. These findings were detailed in the pathology report. A laparoscopic hysterectomy with morcellation performed shortly after this biopsy revealed endometrial carcinoma, endometrioid type, FIGO grade II. Due to fragmentation, the depth of myometrial invasion could not be evaluated. In addition, dissemination of the carcinoma into the peritoneal cavity occurred.

At the time of the biopsy, there was no pertinent clinical history available: no ultrasound results of the uterine cavity and no communicating intent to perform hysterectomy. The fact that endometrial tissue was not present for evaluation raising the question of specimen adequacy did not induce the clinician to postpone or rethink the procedure.

The communications and close cooperation between the obstetrician-gynecologist and the pathologist are essential for the functioning of the health care team. The everyday management of the patient depends on the mutual understanding and communication between the pathologist and the clinician. Failure of this communication is the most frequent source of mistake in our practice and its consequences range from being the source of misunderstandings, mistrust, and ill feelings to serious consequences for the patient.

Pertinent clinical history is essential for an effective teamwork between clinicians and pathologists. We, as pathologists, cannot imagine a gynecologist/obstetrician performing any kind of procedure on a patient without talking first to the patient and obtaining the clinical history. Reciprocally, no clinician should expect a pathologic diagnostic without providing a pertinent clinical, imaging, and serologic history. The fear of biasing the pathologist is completely unjustified although it represents an international trend! Interpretation of complex morphologic pattern in a clinical context is akin to making a clinical diagnosis by interpreting imaging and laboratory findings in the context of the clinical presentation of the patient by the clinician. This constitutes adequate practice of medicine and not bias. It is frequently believed that the pathologist is doing an entirely objective work and can come up with the diagnosis in a vacuum. With more wide spread introduction of electronic medical record, pathologists may, in the future, have more access to clinical history. Despite this, the task of entering clinical history is frequently delegated to residents or nurses who have little understanding of the terms, as evidenced by frequent misspellings that may themselves give raise to additional misunderstanding. Even when the medical record is available, it still requires considerable time and effort form the pathologist who may be and frequently is overworked. It is, therefore, important to give a focused clinical history, where pertinent findings are included. The phone was the most important research tool for a pathologist for a long time. However, with advent of voice mail and Cerberus-like secretaries, it is less and less likely for the pathologist to reach a clinical colleague and still maintain the required turnaround time for the clinical specimen report.

The importance of the clinical history is widely recognized and led to a requirement to provide a clinical history accompanying the pathology specimen in the Clinical Laboratory Improvement Act (CLIA). Medicare-Medicaid audits, which will become more frequent in the future, will deny reimbursement and require restitution for so-called "illegitimate charges" when the specimen is read without appropriate clinical history available. Medicare-Medicaid audits, thus far limited only to some states, have recovered millions of dollars from such "illegitimate charges" with great damage to the provider. The "Joint Commission" also requires availability of a clinical history for the interpretation by the pathologist of all pathology specimens, including gynecologic specimen.

When referring a patient to a consultant, the referring practitioner is responsible to provide a summary of history, physical, and laboratory findings that may facilitate the evaluation of the patient. If this is true when sending a patient who can provide the same information herself, it is that much more important to provide such information with the biopsy specimen as this cannot be interrogated by the pathologist in charge of making a diagnosis.

The clinical history alerts the pathologist to the problem faced by the clinician and the question posed to the pathologist. The clinical history helps in the evaluation of specimen adequacy in relation to the clinical question. When pathologists notice discrepancies between clinical history and histopathology findings, they often resort to submitting additional material, getting additional sections from the paraffin block, and performing special stains. It may lead to a directed meaningful answer to the clinician's problem on the diagnosis line versus a long description of the histopathologic findings.

The largest volume of interaction between the clinician and the pathologist is the cervical, endocervical, and vulvar biopsies and endometrial biopsies or curetting. While they are performed for a variety of different reasons, they share the most frequent lack of communication/mistake in clinical/pathologic practice, due to a lack of pertinent and adequate clinical history.

Cervical biopsies are primarily performed to confirm squamous intraepithelial lesions that were diagnosed during a screening Pap test. As such, the date of the Pap test; its interpretation, including the high-risk HPV status, when available; and a brief statement on the colposcopic evaluation should be conveyed to the pathologist.

Information about recent cytology results provide for a quality control correlating the cytology and biopsy. Inadequate sampling may become obvious when the nature of the biopsy does not allow a clear answer to the question of interest. The history also should include information about recent procedures, cytology or biopsy. For example, information on a recent cervical cone biopsy may help in the interpretation of gynecologic specimen and avoids erroneous conclusions.

One cannot emphasize more the need for clinical information in the interpretation of endometrial biopsies or curettings. This includes information on the great variety of hormonal and related drugs used in medical practice. A clear statement of the question asked will avoid answers leading to long, descriptive diagnoses, for example, in the case of progestative drugs. Clinical history of breast cancer and tamoxifen treatments or other hormone action modifiers will alert the pathologist for possible endometrial polyps/malignancies.

In clinical pathology, bleeding disorders represent a frequent source of diagnostic and therapeutic mistakes. Menorrhagias and metrorrhagias are a relatively frequent symptom and may point to an underlying hemostatic defect, either congenital or acquired. When pregnancy, which is the most frequent cause of uterine bleeding in certain age groups, can be excluded, depending on the clinical history a coagulation or hemostasis workup may help to avoid unnecessary interventions and their potential complications.

Inadequate sampling is a frequent occurrence encountered by the pathologist. In the case of endocervical and endometrial biopsies, although the clinician may think that there was plenty of material submitted, sometimes a great part of it may be consisting of just mucus and blood.

Endocervical curettings are notorious in pathologic practice for their scarcity, and it is important for the pathologist to state the limitations of the material available to alert the clinician that additional material may be needed to answer the question to be examined.

Evaluation of adequacy of endometrial sampling will greatly depend upon the clinical presentation and the question asked. An unremarkable specimen that is adequate for one condition may not necessarily be sufficient for another. In case of atrophy, GnRH agonists, oral contraceptives, danazol, prolonged bleeding, or Asherman syndrome, the amount of endometrium is expectedly small and should be differentiated from an inadequate sampling of lower uterine segment.

Endometrial sampling before a scheduled hysterectomy may determine the nature and extent of the surgical procedure. An inadequate sampling may miss an endometrial carcinoma. Further mishaps may occur with a hysterectomy through morcellation as it spreads the carcinoma in the peritoneal cavity. Correlation with the clinical presentation, ultrasound endometrial evaluation and endometrial biopsy will lead to appropriate patient management.

Cervical biopsy specimens that do not include the transformation zone may be inadequate, again depending on the question asked. It is up to the pathologist to describe this potential inadequacy and for the clinician to read the pathology report from this viewpoint and evaluate the need for additional material.

The communications and close cooperation between the obstetrician-gynecologist and the pathologist are essential for the functioning of the health care team. The everyday management of the patient depends on the mutual understanding and communication between the pathologist and the clinician. Failure of this communication is the most frequent source of mistake in our practice, and its consequences range from being the source of misunderstandings, mistrust, and ill feelings to serious consequences for the patient. There are no well–established criteria for endocervical, endometrial, and cervical biopsy specimens' adequacy and many pathologists are reluctant to use the wording of inadequate or unsatisfactory in a diagnostic line. However, words such as minute, scant, and sliver of tissue are good indicators for questionable adequacy of the specimen. The use of modifiers such as suggestive of and consistent with have a different meaning to different people but reflect a degree of uncertainty from the part of the pathologist. Therefore, any discrepancy with the clinical picture should alert the clinician and lead to a phone conversation between the two practitioners. Keep in mind that the length of a diagnostic comment is inversely proportional to the pathologist's confidence in that diagnosis.

An important step forward in improving the communication between the clinician and the pathologist is a well–formatted pathology report. It is recommended to use diagnostic headlines to emphasize key points, maintain the layout of the report with continuity over time, optimize information density, and reduce "clutter". Pathologists are currently using the College of American Pathologists (CAP) guidelines in reporting malignancies, to uniformly and exhaustively address the Tumor, Node, Metastasis (TNM) staging elements used in patient management. For example, rather than descriptively reporting a "microinvasive carcinoma" of the uterine cervix, the horizontal spread and maximal depth of stromal invasions are reported to distinguish FIGO stage IA1 from IA2 with different risks of regional lymph node metastasis and relevance for patient outcome. The multidisciplinary institutional tumor boards represent a great setting for open and continuous communication within the care team for optimal patient management.

Proper communication and cooperation before, during, and after intraoperative consultation are key for the successful patient management. The surgeon has to know the detailed history of the patient and be aware of previous cytology and biopsy results (read the report). A previous inadequate endometrial biopsy may leave the team unprepared for a malignant endometrial tumor.

TAKE HOME POINTS

- Pertinent clinical history made available to the pathologist is essential for the interpretation of pathologic specimens.
- Adequate material has to be provided to the pathologist in conjuncture with the clinical setting.
- Quality of tissue preparations and, implicitly, of the diagnosis may be improved by good tissue fixation and avoidance of artifacts.
- No hysterectomy without preoperatively adequate cervical and endometrial sampling.
- Complete, well-formatted pathology reports should be understood by clinicians.
- Patients with and after hysterectomy for CIN should be followed for VaIN and VIN.
- Clinicians should review the slides with the pathologists in all doubtful cases.
- Pathologists should communicate by telephone any unexpected findings and document them:
  - No fallopian tube lumens in a tubal ligation procedure
  - No products of conception in curettage
  - Adipose tissue in a uterine curettage
  - Endometrial malignancy or atypia on curettage

SUGGESTED READINGS

American College of Obstetricians and Gynecologists. ACOG Committee Opinion. Seeking and giving consultation. *Obstet Gynecol.* 2007;109(5):1255–1259.

Ducatman BS. Pathologic diagnosis of the abnormally bleeding patient. *Clin Obstet Gynecol.* 2005;48(2):274–283.

Heller DS. Pathologist-clinician communication: The role of the pathologist as consultant to the minimally invasive gynecologic surgeon. *J Minim Invasive Gynecol.* 2007;14(1):4–8.

Powsner AM, Costa J, Homer RJ. Clinicians are from Mars and pathologists are from Venus. *Arch Pathol Lab Med.* 2000;124:1040–1046.

Silverberg SG. The endometrium. Pathologic principles and pitfalls. *Arch Pathol Lab Med.* 2007;131:372–382.

Tranbaloc P. Clinicien et pathologiste: un couple singulier et indissociable. *Gynecologie Obstetrique et Fertilite.* 2005;33:961–963.

Valenstein PV. Formatting Pathology Reports. Applying four principles to improve communication and patient. *Arch Pathol Lab Med.* 2008;132:84–94.

78

FROZEN SECTIONS: USE AND MISUSE

GABRIELA M. OPREA-ILIES, MD AND BHAGIRATH MAJMUDAR, MD

A 58-year-old woman is diagnosed with an ovarian tumor. Ultrasound examination is consistent with a mature cystic teratoma. During a 6-month follow-up, an increase in size is noted. Oophorectomy is performed. Gross examination shows the usual appearance of a mature cystic teratoma with abundant hair and sebaceous material. Histopathologic sections are submitted after formalin fixation: sections from a solid portion of the cyst wall show invasive squamous cell carcinoma.

FROZEN SECTIONS

Frozen sections are an important part of patient management and deserve special attention. The limits of frozen section diagnosis have to be understood. This is an area where the surgeon's expectations may run unreasonably high. Decisions based upon frozen sections in some instances have led to therapeutic mistakes. One may suggest residents in obstetrics-gynecology to take a rotation in pathology in order to really understand the requirements of tissue processing, for frozen and permanent sections, for a valid diagnosis.

Frozen section is a time-consuming and rather inaccurate procedure. It should be restricted to guide intraoperative decision making. Curiosities, wanting to tell the patient about the diagnosis, do not have any place in frozen section request. The understandable wish to tell the patient or the family the exact diagnosis at the end of the procedure may backfire, since many a time the final pathologic diagnosis will be worse than the intraoperative diagnosis. For instance, the patient having a large ovarian mass may have a benign diagnosis on frozen section and a malignant diagnosis upon adequate sampling of the tumor (one section for 1 cm of tumor).

Also, a frozen section is a separately billable procedure for the patient and therefore should be used for patient management and not for the curiosity of the surgeon. Any time a definitive surgical procedure is scheduled for the next 1 to 2 days, a "rush" processing should be requested rather than a frozen section. This will preserve tissue quality and allow for a more targeted sampling. The surgeon must know that not all tissues can be frozen and in some tissues, the quality of the frozen section is limited. Bones and adipose tissue cannot be cut as a frozen section. Large lesions as smooth muscle uterine tumors; large ovarian tumors in many instances cannot be adequately sampled and the frozen diagnosis should be kept open for correction after permanents.

Valid reasons for frozen sections may include when assessment of diagnostic tissue is critical to make a diagnosis that determines the extent of a procedure, determining tumor extension and margin evaluation, unexpected findings, and obtaining fresh tissue for ancillary testing. At the time of frozen section, proper communication between the surgeon and the pathologist is paramount for rendering an accurate and timely intraoperative report and avoiding misinterpretation. Orientation of margins should be explained to the pathologist by the surgeon.

Relevant clinical information, including serum markers, imaging studies, previous malignant history, and pathology reports, should be shared in the care team and help also in the interpretation of frozen sections. Keep in mind that a gross examination may be adequate as intraoperative consultation in certain selected cases.

OVARY

The most frequently misdiagnosed frozen sections are ovarian. Uniformly, thin-walled smooth cysts usually do not require frozen sections. Firm areas in ovarian cysts may be a justifiable target for frozen sections if the outcome determines the further course of the procedure. However, in the case of larger multicystic and solid tumors, the surgeon has to be aware of the limitations of sampling and diagnostic capability of frozen sections.

A frozen section request for an ovarian tumor should be accompanied by the age, clinical history and presentation, size, and bilaterality. Sampling of the specimen will be determined in correlations with the clinical presentation and gross appearance of the tumor. Although complex ovarian masses in an adult or in a postmenopausal woman are suspicious, 75% of those are benign.

Ovarian epithelial neoplasms, serous or mucinous, are the most common cause for oophorectomy. In any cystic lesion, after careful gross examination for intact wall and inking of both surface and margins, all the cysts should be opened and any solid area, avoiding necrosis, should be targeted for potential frozen section. If a tumor is papillary, sections from confluent growth should be frozen. Distinction among benign, borderline, and carcinoma can be attempted. Frank stromal invasion is diagnostic for malignancy while cytologic atypia is less reliable and most prone to frozen artifact. Considering the large size of the lesion and freezing artifact favors deferring to permanent diagnosis due to the limitation of the procedure and improves patient management by avoiding overcall and overtreatment. Apparently, benign epithelium with focal atypia should be deferred to rule out a borderline tumor. A tumor with architectural complexity and no frank invasion may be called "at least borderline" and deferred for further more extensive sampling in the permanents.

Differentiation of serous from mucinous neoplasms is important in patient management: when mucinous ovarian lesions are diagnosed, suggestion to the surgeon to inspect the colon and consider an appendectomy has to be kept in mind. While serous and clear cell carcinomas may be confused in frozen sections due to freezing artifact, the presence of squamous differentiation should raise the possibility of an endometrioid carcinoma even if endometriosis foci are no longer identifiable. This appearance is also useful in differentiating endometrioid carcinomas from a sex cord tumor (granulosa or Leydig cells).

When a sex cord tumor is in the differential, the finding of hemorrhage and necrosis in a mitotically active fibroma-like tumor may lead to a wide spectrum of differential diagnoses with the possibility of a fibrosarcoma but also may include a granulosa cell tumor with spindle cell areas. For such specimens, the frozen tissue interpretation would be deferred.

A high-grade ovarian neoplasm in a young patient may be either a poorly differentiated carcinoma or a germ cell tumor that requires different patient management. During gross examination, a solid tan lesion may indicate a dysgerminoma or a high-grade lymphoma. On frozen section evaluation, they both contain lymphocytes. Ancillary studies to include flow cytometry and serologic evaluation may occasionally be needed for the definitive diagnosis. A lesion with areas of necrosis and hemorrhage on gross examination may represent a yolk sac tumor or a granulosa cell tumor; they both have overlapping histopathologic characteristics, problematic in a limited frozen sample. Deferring such definitive diagnosis is a reasonable contribution to better patient management.

A mature cystic teratoma has a characteristic gross appearance. Careful gross examination has to be performed and suspicious nodules, necrotic and adjacent tissues, which may appear hemorrhagic or fleshy, will be sampled and may be submitted for frozen section to rule out malignancy. Most commonly, apparently mature teratomas may develop squamous cell carcinoma. Teratomas in older patients should always be submitted for frozen section to rule out malignancy.

Ovarian cysts also are sent for frozen section with the aim to preserve fertility. When there is a benign gross examination, a tentative diagnosis of benign cyst can be rendered intraoperatively. They most frequently represent nonfunctional cysts or endometriomas and no further surgery is necessary.

Hemorrhagic ovary is worrisome for both the surgeon and the pathologist. The most common cause will be a torsioned ovary. The torsion may occur secondary to a benign or malignant lesion. Grossly, a torsioned ovary will show a homogenous cut surface exuding a blood-tinged fluid. In making a definitive diagnosis, one should take into consideration all data, clinical, serologic, and gross appearance, into consideration. For example, the clinical presentation may suggest hormonal effect, a ruptured granulosa cell tumors maintain tan-yellow areas, and a choriocarcinoma, extremely rare, will have high levels of HCG while demonstrating the biphasic histo-pathologic appearance.

PREGNANCY-RELATED FROZEN SECTIONS

Ovarian lesions in a pregnant patient pose a uniquely challenging frozen section diagnosis with tremendous implication in patient management. To the problems of interpretation of ovarian lesions, in general, are added those induced by pregnancy changes. Nodules of ectopic decidua present on the ovarian surfaces and/or the peritoneum may be of concern for the surgeon and may be confused with a metastatic squamous cell carcinoma of the cervix. The history of current pregnancy may help in the correct diagnosis. Multiple nodules in the omentum may represent benign leiomyomatosis peritonealis disseminata.

Identification of chorionic villi in a curettage specimen to rule out an ectopic, potentially life-threatening, pregnancy may be required in a frozen section, although, when possible, these specimens should be processed in permanents as "rush." Histologic findings necessary for a positive diagno-sis are chorionic villi showing syncytio- and cytotrophoblast and/or fetal parts. Freezing may lead superficial fragments of endometrium to appear blown up and be misinterpreted as chorionic villi placing the patient at considerable risk for complications of an undiagnosed ectopic pregnancy. Still there is a high rate of concordance between frozen examination and permanents.

UTERINE CERVIX

As previously stated, and more so in cervical specimens, frozen section is indicated only if the diagnosis will change patient management. For example, a diagnosis of invasive squamous cell carcinoma will lead to a radical hyster-ectomy. A request to evaluate depth of invasion in a frozen section may be subject to sampling error and freezing artifact and further may compromise the permanently processed tissue. Such a request for frozen section could be made when a previous biopsy showed uncertain or equivocal invasion or when there are related reproductive issues. However, the surgeon should be aware that these parameters are better estimated on a permanently fixed, correctly sectioned tissue. A request to grade dysplasia on frozen section is strongly discouraged. Any results on frozen section should be checked with previous diagnosis and cytology, and in case of discordance, any radical treatment should be delayed until permanent sections can be evaluated.

Examining entire cone specimens on frozen section is practiced in some laboratories, with good results and up to 100% concordance rate with permanents in cases of squamous lesions. However, it is our opinion that cervical cone should preferably be processed as permanent section to ensure optimal tissue quality, avoid loss of material, and have enough tissue for additional deeper sections when the findings are equivocal. Also, the evaluation of glandular atypia and/or malignancy, which is seen not infrequently together with squamous lesions, is considerably better in permanent rather than in frozen sections. Permanent sections also allow the use of proliferation markers, which is not feasible in frozen sections, and avoid the loss of tissue occurring in preparation of the frozen section.

MYOMETRIUM

A rapidly enlarging "fibroid" or an unusual gross appearance is what prompts the surgeon to ask for a frozen section. While a gross examination is most frequently sufficient, a single frozen section may render the diagnosis of leiomyoma. However, in case of fleshy, infiltrating tumors with areas of hemorrhage or necrosis and cellular atypia, a single frozen section may not be sufficient for a definitive diagnosis and "smooth muscle tumor with atypical feature" will be called with the final diagnosis depending on adequate sampling. Rarely, the surgeon will be concerned about "wormlike" plugs in vascular channels in a patient with leiomyomata: Intravenous leiomyomatosis, a low-grade stromal sarcoma or leiomyosarcoma, may involve the large extrauterine vessels, which can be confirmed by frozen section. When a tan–yellow soft mass is present, a stromal sarcoma should be ruled out by frozen diagnosis.

ENDOMETRIUM

Dating of the endometrium is made very difficult by freezing and is often of questionable accuracy due to the significant freezing artifact in the late secretory phase tissue. A reason for a frozen section of the endometrium is diagnosis and staging of an endometrial carcinoma, leading to regional lymph node dissection in an advanced stage. While the literature shows good concordance, with upgrading in only 15% in the permanent specimen, a pitfall for overcalling is involvement of deep endometrial foci by adenocarcinoma. Although the depth of invasion and tumor grade may be difficult to interpret on frozen section, an attempt should be made, based on gross examination. There are problems and limitations in the frozen section examination on an intraoperatively obtained curettage specimen to make a primary diagnosis of endometrial adenocarcinoma: tissue fragmentation, distortion, and other artifacts will often make interpretation challenging.

VULVA

Frozen sections for margins in vulvar specimens for the diagnosis of Paget disease may be difficult due to nuclear changes secondary to freezing artifact. Vulvar lesion that can wait for a "rush diagnosis" should not be frozen. It is not common for the clinicians to obtain touch prep cytology for vulvar lesions, but the latter can be very useful in some instances.

LYMPH NODES

Sentinel lymph node is not frequently applied in gynecologic oncologic specimens. Recent evaluation speaks against frozen section (FS) evaluation of lymph nodes due to sampling and other artifacts. The surgeon may choose when in certain conditions to send lymph nodes for frozen examination or obtain pre-op fine needle aspiration (FNA) of inguinal nodes. All suspected cases of lymphoma should be sent to pathologists in fresh, unfixed state, to perform flow cytometry studies.

MISCELLANEOUS

Fallopian tubes are rarely submitted for frozen examination. When abnormal on gross examination, especially in older patients or carriers of BRCA mutation, a frozen examination, to rule out malignancy, should be performed. More frequently and in younger patients, examinations of fallopian tube for cystic lesion may find hydrosalpinx or pyosalpinx, frequently secondary to pelvic inflammatory disease (PID).

Vagina: A vaginal squamous cell carcinoma may need evaluation for margins.

Vaginal polyps: An important point has to be made: a history of hysterectomy should be clearly disclosed to the pathologist as an iatrogenically prolapsed fallopian tube with surrounding stromal reactive changes may be easily misinterpreted as adenocarcinoma during a frozen examination.

Peritoneal masses and sampling: The mistake of considering malignancy in a fragment of appendix epiploica should be avoided.

Benign mesothelial cysts raise the differential diagnosis of endometriosis and müllerian malignancies. Colonic or other GI tract carcinomas must be differentiated from ovarian and endometrial malignancies, which may be difficult in frozen sections and require use of clinical correlations followed by immunohistochemical techniques on permanent sections.

Open communication between the clinician and the gynecologist at the time of intraoperative consultation is essential. Direct communication would be ideal to avoid misinterpretation when communicating through multiple intermediaries. One may suggest having the operating physician repeat the diagnosis back to the pathologist to ensure that bit was correctly understood.

TAKE HOME POINTS

- Gross examination of properly oriented specimen will indicate the area for frozen section.
- Frozen sections have limited indications requiring a judicious use.
- Deferring for permanent is a reasonable step in patient management.
- "At least borderline" represents a valid intraoperative pathologic diagnosis.
- After opening of the uterus, a frozen section examination should be obtained from any suspicious lesion seen grossly.
- All ovarian teratomas in perimenopausal and postmenopausal patients should be submitted for frozen section diagnosis of suspicious areas.

SUGGESTED READINGS

Acs G. Intraoperative consultation in gynecologic pathology. *Semin Diagn Pathol.* 2002;19: 237–254.

Adib T, Barton DP. The sentinel lymph node: relevance in gynaecological cancers. *Eur J Surg Oncol.* 2006;32:866–874.

Baker P, Oliva E. Practical approach to intraoperative consultation in gynecological pathology. *Int J Gynecol Pathol.* 2008;27(3):353–365.

Chen RJ, Chen KY, Chang TC, et al. Prognosis and treatement of squamous cell carcinoma from a mature cystic teratoma of the ovary. *J Formos Med Assoc.* 2008;107(11):857–868.

Coffey D, Kaplan AL, Ramzy I. Intraoperative consultation in gynecologic pathology. *Arch Pathol Lab Med.* 2005;129:1544–1557.

Heller DS. Pathologist-clinician communication: The role of the pathologist as consultant to the minimally invasive gynecologic surgeon. *J Minim Invasive Gynecol.* 2007;14(1):4–8.

Kakawa F, Nawa A, Tamashik K, et al. Diagnosis of squamous cell carcinoma arising from mature cystic teratoma of ovary. *Cancer.* 1998;82:2249–2255.

Saglam EA, Usubütün A, Ayhan A, et al. Mistakes prevent mistakes: experience from intraoperative consultation with frozen section. *Eur J Obstet Gynecol Reprod Biol.* 2006;125:266–268.

Santwani PM, Trivedi DP, Vachhani JH, et al. Coexistence of squamous cell carcinoma with dermoid cyst ovary. *Indian J Pathol Microbiol.* 2008;51(1):81–82.

Wang KG, Chen TC, Wang TY, et al. Accuracy of frozen section diagnosis in gynecology. *Gynecol Oncol.* 1998;70:105–110.

79

THE PAP TEST: TO ERR IS HUMAN

GABRIELA M. OPREA-ILIES, MD AND BHAGIRATH MAJMUDAR, MD

A 31-year-old woman had a liquid-based Pap test showing high-grade, severe dysplasia with features suggestive of glandular involvement. Microinvasion could not be excluded. The patient had a normal, conventional Pap smear 8 years ago. The clinician called the cytopathologist who signed the case out with the clinical information that the patient is pregnant and the colposcopy is negative. He requested that the specimen be reviewed. The Pap test was reviewed by the original cytopathologist and two additional cytopathologists who concurred with the original diagnosis. The case was presented in the tumor board and a decision was made to re-call the patient for repeat colposcopic examination. Repeat biopsy showed carcinoma in situ (CIS) with no microinvasive component.

Establishing a relationship between the provider group and the pathology is essential in appropriate patient management. Too many times, the decision to have cytology and surgical specimen read by commercial labs, to meet financial bottom line, makes cytology/biopsy correlations and timely communication of discrepant results impossible. Although one of the aims of Bethesda reporting system was to underline the quality of consultant to the cytologist, this did not gain acceptance.

The Pap test is the most successful cancer screening test and has led to a remarkable reduction in cervical cancer morbidity and mortality in counties that have an organized screening program. Ironically, due to this very real success, the Pap test gave rise to unrealistic expectations and to widespread failure to communicate the limitations of this test to the patient. The limitations of the Pap test were described in the medical literature since the introduction of this test into clinical practice and were continuously investigated to improve its sensitivity, yet the inherent shortcomings of the Pap test were regarded as failures or errors, only to be negatively trumpeted in the lay literature. Every patient should know and every caregiver should understand that false-negative Pap tests may be caused by inadequacy of sampling including missing the area of the lesion by the Pap test taker (sampling error) or by missing the abnormal cells, which characteristically are few and represent <1% or even 1/1,000 of all cells present in the sample (screening error) or by misinterpreting the significance of the abnormal cells found (interpretation error). The latter are rare events but can result in serious consequences. The most important failure of screening for cervical cancer by Pap tests is, however, failure to obtain a Pap test at regular intervals.

In conventional Paps, frequently poorly smeared, thick, bloody smears, with inflammation obscuring cells, collected with a spatula that "kept" most of the specimen, screened by overworked cytotechnologists unrecognized dysplastic cells may lead to missed lesions and to a front page Wall Street story. On the other hand, some patients see the Pap test falsely as an insurance policy for cervical cancer.

This test was not proven effective in screening for adenocarcinoma of the cervix and yet missed adenocarcinomas, represent 80% of the lawsuits involving the Pap test. Despite >50 millions Pap tests now being performed annually in the United States and squamous carcinoma of the cervix having a natural history of long preinvasive disease, it never was eradicated and >10,000 women are still expected to develop and close to 4,000 to die of this disease in a single year.

A successful Pap screening requires a chain of events: the patient going to the care provider; the care provider obtaining an adequate, representative, well-prepared sample; the cytologist correctly identifying a dysplastic cell; the care giver appropriately treating and following the patient; and finally, the patient presenting for treatment or the next screening test. A failure in patient care will result if any of these links are broken. Mistakes resulting from lack of patient collaboration may be solved with persistent teaching, appropriate to different sensibilities and cultural levels. The accuracy of the self-reported Pap test or other clinical testings is very unreliable regardless of socioeconomic status.

From the clinician's point of view, offering and performing a correct collection of the Pap test will lead to an "adequate for interpretation" specimen containing sufficient representative cells and sampling of the cervical transitional zone. The sample should be obtained under direct visualization, the speculum should not be lubricated, and no attempts should be made to "clean" the cervix before sampling to avoid removal of pathologic areas. Direct visualization will also detect gross lesions.

In the face of a negative test, a history of a previous abnormal Pap should not be ignored. Mistakes in the management of cervical pathology are quite frequent. They include

- Failure to follow-up a positive Pap test.
- Failure to perform biopsy of suspicious areas. Colposcopy examination lacks sensitivity and should not be relied on to rule out a significant lesion: false-negative colposcopic examinations are frequent, 20% to 40% for squamous lesions and higher for glandular lesions.

- Failure to correlate with the clinical presentation: accepting a negative Pap test at face value and not correlating it with a previous abnormal test or with an abnormal clinical presentation.

For example, a mass lesion representing a keratinizing squamous cell carcinoma can have its Pap test interpreted as "hyperkeratosis." In such a case, the clinical impression has to override the false-negative test and lead to additional examinations. The use of the patient's past history is important because new management protocols for abnormal cervical cytology and pathology often depend upon the patient's extended Pap history, rather than simply the immediately preceding smear.

HPV testing is often heralded as having increased sensitivity; however, the specificity of the HPV test remains inferior to the Pap test. Co-testing with Pap and HPV in women older than 30 years of age is a strategy that was insufficiently tested and preliminary data show low yield.

From the pathologist/cytologist's part, meticulous examination and correct interpretation are, of course, necessary. However, one should keep in mind that no cytology department is free of errors and the sensitivity of a conventional Pap test is as low as 50%. Since the advent of the liquid preparations, this percentage has been improved, but lack of representative cellularity and presence of <10 dysplastic cells are still more likely to be interpreted as (false) negatives. While the Pap test has a bad reputation, tremendous progress has been made in improving the sample's quality, by using liquid preparation; in improving the screening by developing computer-assisted systems; and in improving the interpretation skills by cytologists and cytotechnologists participating in the proficiency testing.

The atrophic Pap represents one of the challenges cytologists/pathologists face in the interpretation of Paps: atypia can well hide in an atrophic smear showing cells with high nuclear-to-cytoplasmic ratio and irregular nuclear membranes. Either a challenge with local estrogen or determining the presence of high-risk HPV will lead to tipping the balance in the right direction.

For effective communication between pathologists and clinicians, a clear understanding and following of the guidelines of the newly revised Bethesda system is essential.

TAKE HOME POINTS

- Have a system-wide way of communicating severe or unexpected findings between the pathologist and the clinician, so no patient will fall "between the cracks."

- Correlate the diagnosis with the clinical examination; this is ideally done during colposcopy-cytology conferences.
- Hysterectomy, especially laparoscopic/morcellated and vaginal hysterectomy, should not be performed without Pap smear, endocervical sampling (ECS), and endometrial sampling (EMS) to rule out uterine malignancy. Although rare, an unsuspected malignancy in the uterus is found on routine hysterectomy.
- Obtain Pap smear in all patients pregnant and nonpregnant who do not have a previous Pap smear.
- Be well acquainted with the new guidelines issued by the American Society for Colposcopy and Cervical Pathology (ASCCP).
- Keep in mind that these guidelines should never substitute for clinical judgment.

SUGGESTED READINGS

Bowman JA, Sanson-Fisher R, Redman S. The accuracy of self-reported Pap smear utilization. *Soc Sci Med.* 1997;44(7):969–976.

DeMay RM. Cytopathology of false negatives preceding cervical carcinoma. *Am J Obstet Gynecol.* 1996;175(4 Pt 2):1110–1113.

DeMay RM. Common problems in Papanicolaou smear interpretation. *Arch Pathol Lab Med.* 1997;121(3):229–238.

DeMay RM. *The Pap Test.* Chicago, IL: ASCP Press; 2005.

Dworkin M, Killackey M, Johnson JC. Factors leading to delay in diagnosis of invasive cervical cancer. *Prim Care Update Ob Gyn.* 1998;5(4):158.

Koss LG. The Papanicolaou test for cervical cancer detection. A triumph and a tragedy. *JAMA.* 1989;261(5):737–743.

Newell S, Girgis A, Sanson-Fisher R. Accuracy of patients recall of Pap and cholesterol screening. *Am J Public Health.* 2000;90(9):1431–1435.

Nguyen HN, Nordqvist SR. The Bethesda system and evaluation of abnormal pap smears. *Semin Surg Oncol.* 1999;16(3):217–221.

Raab SS, Grzybicki DM, Zarbo RJ, et al. Frequency and outcome of cervical cancer prevention failures in the United States. *Am J Clin Pathol.* 2007;128(5):817–824.

Renshaw AA, Mody DR, Lozano RL, et al. Detection of adenocarcinoma in situ of the cervix in Papanicolaou Tests: Comparison of diagnostic accuracy with other high-. *Arch Pathol Lab Med.* 2004;128:153–157.

Wright TC, Massad S, Dunton CJ, et al. 2006 consensus guidelines for the management of women with abnormal cervical cancer screening. *J Low Genit Tract Dis.* 2007;11(4):201–222.

80

SORTING OUT HOOF BEATS!

GABRIELA M. OPREA-ILIES, MD AND BHAGIRATH MAJMUDAR, MD

A 23-year-old pregnant woman with preeclampsia delivers a healthy baby. After 2 years, during her second pregnancy, her preeclampsia is more severe, with severe hypertension leading to pulmonary edema. She delivers successfully a healthy baby. Clinical and imaging examinations followed by serologic and urinary tests diagnose a pheochromocytoma.

While frequent things are frequent, sometimes when you hear a hoof, think about zebras too. Stories are powerful mainly because human brain seems to be better able to process stories rather than numbers (statistics). When one shares with a resident or colleague such rare diagnosis, a connection with the storyteller makes this experience memorable. Such stories make us to easily imagine the dramatism of the particular "case" and may lead us to overestimate probabilities of rare events. However, they are compelling and make us think "outside the box."

Pregnant women frequently are diagnosed with ovarian masses. These are fortunately most frequently benign and most likely represent corpus luteum cysts. However, they may represent rare and serious pathologic processes. A decision to biopsy or excise is difficult one, as it may result in pregnancy loss. We recently encountered a squamous cell carcinoma arising in an ovarian mature cystic teratoma complicating the pregnancy of a 37-year-old woman. Ovarian mature cystic teratoma is the most common germ cell tumor of the ovary in women of reproductive age and it makes it also the most common tumor in pregnancy. While they are usually incidentally found during pregnancy, they also increase the risk of complication including torsion, rupture, infection, and possibly malignant degeneration. Rupture may mimic gynecologic malignancy, as they give rise to chemical peritonitis, extensive adhesions, granulomatous reactions, and possible gliomatosis. Malignant changes are described in 1% to 2% of these tumors, most frequently in the postmenopausal age. They have a dismal 5-year survival rate in the range of 21% to 34% in stage II and III. They are rarely diagnosed preoperatively, especially when no paraneoplastic syndrome is present. The histologic examination establishes the definitive diagnosis. While squamous cell carcinoma is the most common malignant component, any type of carcinoma, sarcoma, or hematologic malignancy may arise when malignant transformation of a teratoma does occur. Thyroid tissue in mature teratomas is quite frequent (struma ovarii and rare circumstances may even lead to hyperthyroidism and occasionally to malignant degeneration). When a teratomatous tumor is grossly multinodular, multicystic, and necrotic, a frozen section should be obtained to rule out immature teratoma or other malignant germ cell tumors.

Pregnancy is a physiologic state of a young woman and one expects ordinarily little if any significant pathology. However, malignancies may complicate pregnancies, as in nonpregnant state. The incidence is 1 in 1,000 pregnancies and the most common malignancies found during pregnancy are breast cancer, cervical cancer, Hodgkin lymphoma, malignant melanoma, and leukemias. The signs and symptoms of early pregnancy or late pregnancy, preeclampsia-like may mask an underlining malignancy. Some symptoms like bleeding gums, enlarging breasts, deepening moles, and gastrointestinal symptoms may be common to pregnancy and malignancy!

Clinicians should be aware of these possibilities and perform a thorough and complete physical examination at the time of presentation and during the follow-up visits. As the trend is to see pregnancy at a later reproductive age, one may expect to see more cases of cancer complicating pregnancy. The management of these patients is not standardized; the golden rules consist of benefit the mother, treat curable disease in pregnant women, protect the product of conception from effects of chemotherapy and radiation therapy, preserve the reproductive potential, and consult an expert from the appropriate specialty. Early diagnosis may lead to improved patient outcome, and it is the role of the clinician to think about these rare occurrences and order appropriate tests and follow-up. From the pathology point of view, one must not discard the possibility of a malignancy in a pregnant woman only because she is young and pregnant.

A few possible clinical presentations these authors encountered in their daily practice are summarized below:

- Pregnant woman presenting with irregularly enlarging breast; this was mistaken as appropriate pregnancy change. Diagnosis: breast cancer.
- Pregnant woman presenting with headaches and hypertension; these signs and symptoms were mistaken as preeclampsia. Diagnosis: Pheochromocytoma.
- Pregnant woman presenting with protracted nausea and vomiting; these signs and symptoms were mistaken for hyperemesis gravidarum. Diagnosis: gastric carcinoma.
- Pregnant woman presenting with bleeding gums, anemia, and fatigue; these signs and symptoms were mistaken as lack of proper nutrition due to pregnancy. Diagnosis: leukemia.

- Pregnant woman presenting with multiple nonspecific gastrointestinal symptoms and constipation; these signs and symptoms were mistaken as symptoms related solely to pregnancy. Diagnosis: colon cancer.
- Pregnant woman presenting with focal skin hyperpigmentation; the symptom was mistaken as a common pregnancy change. Diagnosis: melanoma.
- Pregnant woman presenting with headaches; the symptom was mistaken as related exclusively to pregnancy. Diagnosis: choriocarcinoma metastatic to the brain or primary brain tumor.
- Pregnant woman presenting with sinus mass and mild epistaxis; these signs and symptoms were mistaken as fungal sinusitis. Diagnosis: T-cell lymphoma.
- Pregnant woman with small cell carcinoma of the lung delivers a healthy appearing baby and a normal-appearing placenta. Diagnosis: metastatic small cell carcinoma to the placenta. Later: metastatic small cell carcinoma to the 8-month baby.

TAKE HOME POINTS

- Think of zebras: a thorough personal and family health history and physical examination may discover them early.
- Obtain a Pap smear in all patients pregnant and nonpregnant who do not have a previous Pap smear.
- Do not neglect any persistent symptoms during pregnancy, as only a consequence of pregnancy.

SUGGESTED READINGS

Chen RJ, Chen KY, Chang TC, et al. Prognosis and treatment of squamous cell carcinoma from a mature cystic teratoma of the ovary. *J Formos Med Assoc*. 2008;107(11):857–868.

Ioffe OB, Brooks SE, De Rezende RB, et al. Artifact in cervical LLETZ specimens: correlation with follow-up. *Int J Gynecol Pathol*. 1999;18:115–121.

Kakawa F, Nawa A, Tamashik K, et al. Diagnosis of squamous cell carcinoma arising from mature cystic teratoma of ovary. *Cancer*. 1998;82:2249–2255.

Newman TB. The power of stories over statistics. *Br Med J*. 2003;327:1424–1427.

Powsner AM, Costa J, Homer RJ. Clinicians are from mars and pathologists are from venus. *Arch Pathol Lab Med*. 2000;124:1040–1046.

Pavlidis AN. Coexistence of pregnancy and malignancy. *Oncologist*. 2002;7:279–287.

Rooksby J, Gerry RM. abd Smith AF. Incident reporting schemes and the need for a good story. *Int J Mer Inform*. 2007;76S:S205–S211.

Santwani PM, Trivedi DP, Vachhani JH, et al. Coexistence of squamous cell carcinoma with dermoid cyst ovary. *Indian J Pathol Microbiol*. 2008;51(1):81–82.

81

Metastatic mucinous carcinoma to the ovary simulating a primary ovarian mucinous neoplasm

Sanjay Logani, MD

A 40-year-old female was noted to have bilateral adnexal masses on an ultrasound performed to evaluate for uterine fibroids. On laparotomy, both ovaries were enlarged. The right ovary measured 10 × 8 × 6 cm and on sectioning, a multiloculated mass filled with mucinous material was noted. Frozen section diagnosis was mucinous cystadenoma. The left ovary measured 15 × 10 × 8 cm and was similar in appearance to the right ovary on gross examination at the time of frozen section. The left ovary was interpreted to represent a possible mucinous borderline tumor at the time of frozen section.

This case exemplified two important points that are very helpful in the correct interpretation of mucinous neoplasms involving the ovary. First, bilateral ovarian involvement by a mucinous tumor strongly favors the possibility of a metastatic tumor from the appendix, gastrointestinal tract, or the pancreas especially if there is peritoneal involvement by the mucin-producing tumor (clinically pseudomyxoma peritonei). Second, the morphologic appearance of the mucinous epithelium in a metastatic tumor can mimic a primary mucinous neoplasm and lead to an erroneous interpretation.

Pseudomyxoma peritonei was thought to originate from a mucinous ovarian neoplasm for the better part of the last century. In the last 20 years, morphologic studies backed by molecular analysis have suggested the source of almost all ovarian mucinous neoplasms associated with pseudomyxoma peritonei to be the appendix. Szych et al. showed identical genetic mutations in K-ras gene in the appendiceal and the ovarian tumors to provide the molecular link between the two tumors. Certain histologic criteria favor a diagnosis of metastatic tumor over primary ovarian mucinous neoplasm. Lee and Young showed that bilateral ovarian involvement, ovarian surface involvement and presence of an infiltrative pattern of invasion in the ovary were histologic features that favored a metastatic tumor rather than an ovarian primary. Pancreatic primary has the propensity to mimic a primary ovarian neoplasm (*Fig. 81.1*). A disassociation between the cytologic features and the architectural pattern of the mucinous epithelium is a helpful clue that one may be dealing with a metastatic tumor. In the patient described

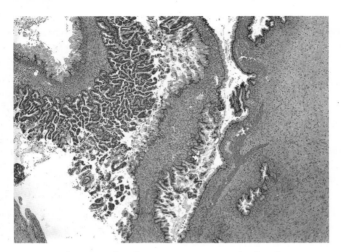

FIGURE 81.1. A pancreatic primary tumor metastasized to the ovary.

above, the presence of bilateral involvement prompted a search for an extra ovarian primary that was ultimately identified in the pancreas.

TAKE HOME POINTS

- Bilateral ovarian involvement by a mucinous neoplasm favors the possibility of a metastatic tumor to the ovary from the appendix, gastrointestinal tract, or the pancreas.
- Pseudomyxoma peritonei is a clinical term and tumors associated with this clinical syndrome most often arise in the appendix and secondarily involve the ovary and the peritoneum.
- Metastatic mucinous tumors, especially from the pancreas, can mimic a primary mucinous neoplasm on histologic examination.

SUGGESTED READINGS

Bradley RF, Stewart JH, Russell GB, et al. Pseudomyxoma peritonei of appendiceal origin: a clinicopathologic analysis of 101 patients uniformly treated at a single institution with literature review. *Am J Surg Pathol.* 2006;30:551–559.

Lee KR, Young RH. The distinction between primary and metastatic mucinous carcinoma of the ovary: gross and histologic findings in 50 cases. *Am J Surg Pathol.* 2003;27:281–292.

Szych C, Staebler A, Connolly DC, et al. Molecular genetic evidence supporting the clonality and appendiceal origin of pseudomyxoma peritonei in women. *Am J Pathol.* 1999;154:1849–1855.

Young RH, Scully REC. Metastatic tumors in the ovary: a problem-oriented approach and review of the recent literature. *Semin Diagn Pathol.* 1991;8:250–276.

Young RH. Pseudomyxoma peritonei and selected other aspects of the spread of appendiceal neoplasms. *Semin Diagn Pathol.* 2004;21:134–150.

82

HYDATIFORM MOLE: FAILURE OF FOLLOW-UP MANAGEMENT

MICHAEL OWOLABI, MD AND DIANA BROOMFIELD, MD, MBA, FACOG, FACS

A 20-year-old Asian woman presents to your office with vaginal pain and moderate vaginal bleeding 2 months after she delivered her first child. She states that 2 weeks prior to presentation she underwent a thyroidectomy for uncontrolled hyperthyroidism. She also states that she has seen several physicians (OB/GYN and internal medicine) for her symptoms, which have progressively worsened. Her blood pressure is 100/60 mm Hg, and her heart rate is 140 beats per minute. Her hemoglobin level is 10 g/dL, and her hematocrit value is 30%. Although she has recently delivered and denied sexual activity since delivery, you decide to check a pregnancy test. To everyone's surprise, the quantitative hCG is >120,000.

The spectrum of gestational trophoblastic disease (GTD) includes hydatidiform mole (complete or partial), invasive mole, choriocarcinoma, and placental site trophoblastic tumor. Nearly 90% of patients with a molar pregnancy present with vaginal bleeding. The widespread use of imaging in early pregnancy can be helpful in asymptomatic patients. Ultrasonography leads to accurate diagnosis of molar pregnancy in nearly 90% of cases demonstrating cysts that appear as "cluster of grapes" within the uterine cavity. These "cluster of grapes" are a mixture of trophoblastic tissue and intrauterine clots that may undergo oxidation and liquefaction, producing the pathognomonic fluid that resembles prune juice.

The definitive diagnosis of molar pregnancy is made at the time of dilatation and evacuation (D&E). The presence of systemic symptoms (e.g., hyperemesis gravidarum, preeclampsia, and thyroid storm) is rare. However, the presence of these symptoms coupled with an elevated human chorionic gonadotropin (hCG) level >100,000 mIU/mL or the presence of ovarian thecomas larger than 6 cm is associated with a 40% to 50% risk of persistent disease.

Treatment of choice is to have the patient undergo a D&E procedure. Once evacuation is complete, weekly serum hCG levels should be assessed until they have been within normal range for 3 weeks. Thereafter, serum hCG levels are determined monthly for the next 6 months. Because it is rare for postmolar GTD to result in reelevation of serum hCG levels after

>6 months of normal hCG levels without an intercurrent pregnancy, a minimum of 6 months of hCG remission typically is recommended for patients before they attempt a pregnancy after the evaluation of a molar pregnancy.

A common error in treating these patients is to disregard symptomatology of thyrotoxicosis. In addition to the molar pregnancy, some patients may also have an associated thyroid storm and do require treatment with a β-blocker. Fluid resuscitation is critical in the acute setting prior to the D&E procedure. Transfusion is reserved for a patient who is hemodynamically unstable after failure of fluid resuscitation with crystalloid and colloid. Hysterectomy may be the preferred treatment for women who do not desire retention of fertility. Adjuvant hysterectomy decreases the risk of postmolar sequelae and decreases the total dose of chemotherapy required to achieve primary remission in women who develop nonmetastatic, low-risk GTD.

TAKE HOME POINTS

- The most common presentation of molar pregnancy is abnormal vaginal bleeding.
- Suction curettage followed by sharp curettage is the primary mode of treatment for molar pregnancy.
- Intravenous administration of oxytocin should be started with dilation of the cervix and continued postoperatively to reduce the likelihood of hemorrhage.
- Postoperative contraception is recommended because a new pregnancy is indistinguishable in its early stages from recurrent GTD.
- As part of the mandatory follow-up care, serum β-hCG levels should be monitored weekly to identify the 5% of women with partial mole and the 20% of women with complete mole who develop malignant sequelae.
- Any postpartum patient with symptoms of thyrotoxicosis must be evaluated for GTD.

SUGGESTED READINGS

American College of Obstetricians and Gynecologists. ACOG Practice Bulletin No. 53: diagnosis and treatment of gestational trophoblastic disease. *Obstet Gynecol.* 2004;103: 1365–1377.
Benson CB, Genest DR, Bernstein MR, et al. Sonographic appearance of first trimester complete hydatidiform moles. *Ultrasound Obstet Gynecol.* 2000;16:188–191.
Gerner O, Segal S, Kopmar A, et al. The current clinical presentation of complete molar pregnancy. *Arch Gynecol Obstet.* 2000;264:33–34.

83

DO NOT GIVE ANTICHOLINERGIC MEDICATIONS TO PATIENTS WITH NARROW-ANGLE GLAUCOMA

SAMEENA AHMED, MD AND RONY ADAM MD

A 65-year-old gravida 2 para 2 female presents with symptoms of urgency and frequency. A complete history and physical examination are done. Urodynamic testing reveals spontaneous detrusor contractions during filling. Her past medical history is significant for hypertension and narrow-angle glaucoma. She is given a prescription for tolterodine. After beginning the medication, she develops acute-onset visual changes.

Overactive bladder is a syndrome consisting of urgency, with or without urge incontinence. It is also known as urge syndrome or urgency-frequency syndrome. Urgency is defined as the feeling that a patient must void immediately otherwise she will lose urine. Detrusor overactivity is defined as demonstrable involuntary detrusor contractions during filling cystometry during urodynamics. Overactive bladder is a clinical diagnosis and urodynamic testing is not necessary to make the diagnosis.

Initial treatment for overactive bladder includes lifestyle interventions, pelvic floor exercises (Kegel's), and bladder retraining. Lifestyle interventions include fluid reduction and avoiding caffeinated beverages. Bladder training involves feedback inhibition and patients are asked to postpone voiding and void according to a timetable. Patients initially void hourly and extend this to every 2.5 to 3 hours over a 6-week period.

Pharmacotherapy is the main treatment for overactive bladder. Anticholinergics are the first line in treatment. They target the main pathway controlling the detrusor contraction, focusing on the pathway in which acetylcholine is released by parasympathetic nerves, thus activating muscarinic receptors. There are five subtypes of muscarinic receptors. The M2 and M3 receptors are the main subtypes found in the bladder. Side effects include dry mouth, blurred vision, constipation, and urinary retention. Other less common side effects include headache, dizziness, and peripheral edema. Because of these side effects, noncompliance is a significant issue. This class of medications is contraindicated in patients with gastric retention, urinary retention, and narrow-angle glaucoma.

Tolterodine was introduced for the treatment of overactive bladder in 1997. It is metabolized by the cytochrome P-450 system. Dosage is recommended at 2 mg twice a day and 4 mg once a day for the timed-release preparation. Oxybutynin is another medication recommended for overactive bladder. It has both anticholinergic and smooth muscle relaxant properties. Dosage of this medication is 5, 10, or 15 mg and also comes in a transdermal form. Solifenacin and darifenacin are selective for the M3 receptor, so they target the bladder more selectively. This should decrease adverse side effects and help to improve compliance. They have been found to be at least as effective as tolterodine and better tolerated. Trospium is a quaternary amine that is hydrophilic and may not cross the blood–brain barrier. As a result, theoretically it should have fewer central nervous system effects. However, it has a short half-life and poor absorption from the gastrointestinal tract and has not been widely used.

Recently, botulinum toxin has been shown to be effective in treating overactive bladder. Botulinum toxin is derived from the organism *Clostridium botulinum*. Early studies show that it may be an effective treatment for overactive bladder.

TAKE HOME POINTS

- Overactive bladder is a syndrome consisting of urgency, with or without urge incontinence.
- Anticholinergics are the mainstay of pharmacologic treatment for overactive bladder.
- Side effects include dry mouth, blurred vision, constipation, and urinary retention and are often a cause of noncompliance.
- This class of medications is contraindicated in patients with gastric retention, urinary retention, and narrow-angle glaucoma.
- Solfenacin and darifenacin are selective for the M3 receptor, more commonly found in the bladder, thus leading to less side effects and increased compliance.

SUGGESTED READINGS

Abrams P, Cardozo L, Fall M, et al. The standardisation of terminology of lower urinary tract function: report from the Standardisation Sub-committee of the International Continence Society. *Neurourol Urodyn*. 2002;21:167.

Appell RA, Abrams P, Drutz HP, et al. Treatment of overactive bladder: long-term tolerability and efficacy of tolterodine. *World J Urol*. 2001;19:141–147.

Cannon TW, Chancellor MB. Pharmacotherapy of the overactive bladder and advances in drug delivery. *Clin Obstet Gynecol*. 2002;45:205.

Payne CK. Epidemiology, pathophysiology and evaluation of urinary incontinence and overactive bladder. *Urology*. 1998;51:3.

Wein AJ. Pharmacologic options for the overactive bladder. *Urology*. 1998;51:43.

84

DO NOT ASSUME ALL URINARY LEAKAGE IS STRESS URINARY INCONTINENCE

SAMEENA AHMED, MD AND RONY ADAM, MD

A 74-year-old gravida 5 para 4 female presents with a several-year history of leaking urine when she coughs or sneezes. She also describes occasional urgency, though she feels these symptoms are not as bothersome. Her history is significant for four spontaneous vaginal deliveries, the largest baby measuring 9 lb. Cough stress test in the office demonstrates stress incontinence and urodynamic testing confirms detrusor overactivity. The patient is diagnosed with mixed urinary incontinence.

Urinary incontinence is defined as the involuntary leakage of urine and is a common problem in the United States. The prevalence of stress urinary incontinence (SUI) is estimated to be 12% to 24%. It has significant economic impact and annual direct costs for treating these women are upwards of $12.4 billion. In addition, urinary incontinence has significant emotional impact on women and can affect their quality of life.

There are generally four types of urinary incontinence. These are stress incontinence, urge incontinence, mixed incontinence, and overflow incontinence. Stress incontinence is the complaint of involuntary leakage with effort, exertion, sneezing, or coughing. It occurs as a result of weakened pelvic floor muscles or urethral hypermobility. When intra-abdominal pressure exceeds urethral pressure, patients leak urine. Urge incontinence is the complaint of involuntary leakage of urine either preceded or followed by urgency. Mixed incontinence is the complaint of both stress and urge symptoms. Overflow incontinence is the dribbling and/or continuous leakage associated with incomplete bladder emptying, due to bladder outlet obstruction, or a neurological condition.

When evaluating patients with urinary incontinence, it is important to consider the reversible cause. Key reversible causes include urinary tract infections, atrophic vaginitis, and urethritis. Always remember to ask patients about other medications. Diuretics, alcohol, and caffeine can all cause incontinence. Patients may also have restricted mobility, dementia, or chronic illness that hampers their ability to reach the bathroom.

Taking a history and a physical examination is key to determining the nature of a patient's incontinence. The history should include voiding symptoms, gynecological and obstetrical history, coexistent medical conditions, current medications, and previous treatments. A bladder diary can be completed for 3 to 7 days. A 3-day diary has been shown to be as accurate as a 7-day diary. Patients are asked to record the frequency and volume of urine output as well as any episodes of urinary leakage. A physical examination should include a neurologic examination as well as a pelvic examination. Pelvic organ prolapse can sometimes mask lower urinary tract symptoms. A rectal examination will assess for rectal tone, masses, and fecal impaction.

Other testings done at the time of physical exam include the Q tip test, cough stress test, and measurement of a postvoid residual. The Q tip test is done by placing a lubricated cotton swab into the urethra to the level of the bladder neck. The patient should perform a Valsalva maneuver and the angle of deflection is measured. A 30-degree deflection or more indicates the presence of urethral hypermobility. A cough stress test involves having a patient cough or valsalva and observing for the loss of urine. Often, the bladder can be filled in a retrograde fashion with approximately 200 to 300 mL of sterile water. Measurement of a postvoid residual can also be done using either a bladder scanner or a bladder catheterization. Residuals of <50 mL are normal. Postvoid residuals measuring 100 to 200 mL or higher are indicative of inadequate bladder emptying. Pertinent laboratory testing includes a urine analysis and culture. This will screen for hematuria, glucosuria, pyuria, or bacteriuria. The role of urodynamic testing is controversial and can be used for patients who have failed conservative therapies or are going to undergo surgical intervention.

TAKE HOME POINTS

- The four major types of urinary incontinence are stress (involuntary leakage of urine with coughing, sneezing, or exertion), urge (leakage with urgency), mixed (both stress and urge symptoms), and overflow incontinence.
- When evaluating patients with urinary incontinence, a systematic approach should be used including a history, physical examination, and clinical testing.
- A cough stress test can determine the presence of SUI.
- Routine urodynamic testing is not recommended but may be useful prior to surgical intervention.

SUGGESTED READINGS

Abrams P, Cardozo L, Fall M, et al. The standardisation of terminology of lower urinary tract function: report from the Standardisation Sub-committee of the International Continence Society. *Neurourol Urodyn*. 2002;21:167.

American College of Obstetricians and Gynecologists. Urinary incontinence in women. *Obstet Gynecol*. 2005;105(6):1533–1545.

Scientific Committee of the First International Consultation on Incontinence. Assessment and treatment of urinary incontinence. *Lancet*. 2000;355:2153.

Sze EH, Jones WP, Ferguson JL, et al. Prevalence of urinary incontinence symptoms among black, white and Hispanic women. *Obstet Gynecol*. 2002;99:572–575.

Wilson L, Brown JS, Shin GP, et al. Annual direct cost of urinary incontinence. *Obstet Gynecol*. 2001;98:398–406.

85

DO NOT FORGET TO ASK PATIENTS ABOUT FECAL INCONTINENCE SYMPTOMS

SAMEENA AHMED, MD AND RONY ADAM, MD

A 24-year-old gravida 1 para 1 female undergoes a vacuum-assisted vaginal delivery. Her delivery is complicated by a fourth-degree laceration and subsequent wound breakdown. Postpartum, she develops fecal incontinence. At her postpartum visit, she is hesitant to talk about her complaints.

Fecal incontinence is often an underreported complaint by women and its prevalence is difficult to estimate. It has been defined as the continuous or recurrent uncontrolled passage of fecal material (>10 mL) for at least 1 month in an individual older than 3 years of age. Often women do not want to discuss fecal incontinence with their physicians and experience a great deal of anxiety from this condition.

The etiology of fecal incontinence is multifactorial. The majority of patients have undergone obstetric trauma and have injury to the anal sphincter. Vaginal delivery can also cause pudendal neuropathy; this loss of innervation leads to incomplete rectal evacuation, straining, and fecal incontinence. Other known etiologies of fecal incontinence include anorectal surgical trauma, neurological disorders (such as dementia, stroke, multiple sclerosis, diabetes mellitus, and fecal impaction), and smooth muscle dysfunction (such as proctitis from inflammatory bowel disease, radiation, and childhood encopresis).

All patients should undergo a thorough history and physical examination. Perianal sensation can be evaluated by evoking the anocutaneous reflex. The reflex is checked by gently stroking the skin immediately surrounding the anus and observing a reflexive contraction of the external anal sphincter. The anal wink assesses for nerve damage. A digital rectal examination will assess for masses and anal tone.

Diagnostic testing for fecal incontinence measures can also be performed. Anal manometry measures anal pressures including resting tone, squeeze pressure, the threshold of rectal sensation, and pressures during straining. Low sphincter pressures are indicative of a sphincter defect. Endoanal ultrasound can evaluate for structural abnormalities of the anal sphincter, the rectal wall, and puborectalis muscle. It is the simplest and most reliable test to detect injuries of the internal and external sphincters.

Defecography is done by instilling barium into the rectum while x-ray films are taken. It helps to delineate anorectal anatomy at rest and while straining. Its use in fecal incontinence is limited. Pudendal nerve terminal latency measures the time required, after stimulating the pudendal nerves with an electrode as it crosses the ischial spine, to induce a contraction of the external anal sphincter. Prolongation suggests nerve damage. Finally, electromyography activity of the sphincter can be done using either needle electrodes or surface electrodes. It can give information regarding neurogenic or myogenic damage.

Treatment options for fecal incontinence include medical therapy, behavioral therapy, and surgery. Initial therapy begins with dietary modification. Patients gradually increase their fiber intake in an effort to improve the consistency and volume of bowel movements. Constipating agents can also be used. Loperamide reduces bowel motility, but a common side effect is constipation. It has been found to be more effective than Lomotil in treating fecal incontinence. Tricyclic antidepressants such as amitriptyline and anticholinergics such as hyoscyamine can also be helpful.

Biofeedback therapy involves retraining the pelvic floor and abdominal wall musculature. Electromyographic surface electrodes are used to guide patients to improve muscle control. Patients experience improvement in their symptoms by improved contraction of the striated muscles of the pelvic floor and a better ability to perceive rectal distension.

Many different surgical interventions have been described to treat fecal incontinence. Surgical treatment can involve direct sphincter repair, implantation of an artificial sphincter, or plication of the posterior aspect of the sphincter. Long-term success rates of sphincteroplasty have been reported as 50% to 60%. Sacral neuromodulation has also been successfully described in a small number of patients. Colostomy is reserved for patients who have failed all other management options.

TAKE HOME POINTS

- Fecal incontinence is the continuous or recurrent uncontrolled passage of fecal material (>10 mL) for at least one month in an individual older than 3 years of age.
- The etiology of fecal incontinence is multifactorial. Common causes include obstetric trauma, anorectal surgical trauma, neurological disorders, and smooth muscle dysfunction.
- Endoanal ultrasound is the simplest and most reliable test to detect injuries of the internal and external sphincters.
- Treatment options include medical therapy, behavioral therapy, and surgery.

SUGGESTED READINGS

Drossman DA, Funch-Jensen P, Janssens J, et al. Identification of sub-groups of functional gastrointestinal disorders. *Gastroenterol Int*. 1990;3:159.

Falk PM, Blatchford GJ, Cali RL, et al. Transanal ultrasound and manometry in the management of patients with fecal incontinence? *Dis Colon Rectum*. 1997;40:896.

Rao SS. Diagnosis and management of fecal incontinence. *Am J Gastroenterol*. 2004;99:1585.

Wald A. Fecal incontinence in adults. *N Engl J Med*. 2007;356:1648–1655.

86

IN PATIENTS WITH MIXED INCONTINENCE, SURGICAL MANAGEMENT OF THEIR STRESS SYMPTOMS MAY WORSEN THEIR URGE SYMPTOMS

SAMEENA AHMED, MD AND RONY ADAM, MD

A 56-year-old female complains of a urinary incontinence for several years. She notes losing urine while exercising and coughing. She also describes occasional urgency and urge incontinence. Physical examination reveals a hypermobile urethra and a positive cough stress test. Urodynamic testing confirms stress incontinence and detrusor overactivity. She undergoes placement of a tension-free vaginal tape. Postoperatively, her urgency symptoms worsen.

Stress urinary incontinence (SUI) is the complaint of involuntary leakage of urine with effort, exertion, sneezing, or coughing as defined by the International Continence Society. Its main cause is weakened pelvic floor muscles or urethral hypermobility. When intra-abdominal pressure exceeds urethral pressure, patients lose urine.

Surgical treatment for SUI is common. Surgery is recommended for patients who have failed conservative measures including pelvic floor exercises, biofeedback, and pessary use. Current surgical techniques include retropubic colposuspension, midurethral slings, and suburethral fascial slings. Anterior colporrhaphy has not been shown to be effective in treating SUI.

Up to 30% of patients with stress incontinence can also have urge incontinence. Following surgery, 30% to 60% of patients can have improvement of their urge symptoms, while approximately 5% to 10% may experience worsening of their urge symptoms. In the remainder of the patients, their symptoms will be unchanged. Patients should be counseled appropriately prior to undergoing treatment.

In the Burch procedure, the endopelvic fascia adjacent to the mid and proximal urethra is attached to Cooper ligaments on the posterior aspect of the superior pubic ramus. Studies have shown that the Burch procedure is more effective than the Marshall-Marchetti-Krantz (MMK) procedure in which the endopelvic fascia next to the bladder neck is attached to the periosteum of the posterior pubic symphysis. The Burch procedure can be done via laparotomy or laparoscopy. The laparoscopic Burch technique has been found to be as effective as the open procedure. Robotic-assisted colposuspension is also becoming more common. Complications of the Burch include urinary retention, de novo urge incontinence, injury to the bladder or ureter, infection, and hemorrhage.

Several different sling techniques have been developed. Regardless of the type of sling, they all function as a hammock, supporting the bladder neck and urethra. A strip of material is placed under the urethra and passed upward and attached either to the rectus fascia or pubic bone. Different materials have been used for slings including autologous materials (rectus fascia or fascia lata), xenografts (porcine dermis, porcine small intestine), and synthetic materials (polypropylene, Mersilene, and Gore-Tex). In the autologous fascial sling, a strip of fascia is used. Sling tunnels are developed retropubically through the vagina. A 2×10-cm strip of fascia is then passed from the vagina to the abdomen and sutured to the rectus fascia via an abdominal incision. The sling is placed under no tension and correct placement is key. Common complications include postoperative voiding dysfunction and de novo irritative voiding symptoms.

Sling procedures have undergone significant advancement in recent years, and the tension-free vaginal tape (TVT) is somewhat different from traditional sling procedures. The TVT was developed in 1996 by Ulmstem et al. and has gained widespread popularity. Studies have shown that it is as effective as the Burch and other traditional sling procedures. The sling is placed under the midurethra using two trocars that are passed blindly from the vagina to the abdomen. The arms are made of polypropylene mesh and do not require any suturing. The sling remains in place through the collagen ingrowth. Variations of the TVT include the SPARC procedure in which trocars are passed from the abdomen down to the vagina. In the transobturator tape (TOT) technique, trocars are passed blindly through a transobturator approach. Complications of these procedures are similar to that of traditional sling procedures.

TAKE HOME POINTS

- Surgery is the most common treatment for SUI when patients have failed conservative management.
- Current surgical techniques for SUI include retropubic colposuspension, midurethral slings, and suburethral fascial slings.
- The TVT procedure has become widely popular and is as effective as the Burch colposuspension and traditional sling procedures.
- Following surgery for stress incontinence, patients with mixed incontinence may experience worsening, improvement, or no change in their urgency symptoms.

SUGGESTED READINGS

Carey MP, Goh JT, Rosamilia A, et al. Laparoscopic versus open Burch colposuspension: a randomized controlled trial. *BJOG*. 2006;113:999.

DeLancey JO. Structural support of the urethra as it relates to stress urinary incontinence: the hammock hypothesis. *Am J Obstet Gyencol*. 1994;170:1713.

Segal JL, Vassallo B, Leeman S, et al. Prevalence of persistent and de novo overactive bladder symptoms after the tension-free vaginal tape. *Obstet Gynecol*. 2004;104:1263–1269.

Ward KL, Hilton P. A prospective multicenter randomized trial of tension-free vaginal tape and colposuspension fro primary urodynamic stress incontinence: two-year follow-up. *Am J Obstet Gynecol*. 2004;190:324–331.

PEDIATRIC AND ADOLESCENT GYNECOLOGY

87

PEDIATRIC AND ADOLESCENT GYNECOLOGY

EDOM YARED, MD AND DIANA BROOMFIELD, MD, MBA, FACOG, FACS

An 11-year-old girl who is very apprehensive about visiting the gynecologist is escorted by her mother who wants her child examined after recent episodes of a thick, white, cloudy vaginal discharge and complaints of vaginal burning. The girl's mother insists that her daughter has an infection and therefore must have gotten it from someone. She becomes hysterical and proceeds to tell the gynecologist that she did not even know her daughter was sexually active and is ashamed of the situation. The mother wants an immediate pregnancy test.

After calming down the mother, you notice that the girl seems very distant and frightened by her mothers' reaction. You ask the mother to speak to the child alone. She agrees and as soon as she leaves the room, the girl begins to cry and discloses to you that she has been hiding a secret from her mother. She has been sexually abused by her mother's boyfriend for the past 3 years and does not know how to tell her. You reassure her that everything will be alright and that she did the right thing by telling someone.

ELEMENTS OF THE PEDIATRIC AND ADOLESCENT GYNECOLOGICAL EXAMINATION

The gynecologic examination of the adolescent requires time and patience. The first encounter will leave a lasting impression on the patient and will dictate the patient's future gynecological health care routine; therefore, it is of utmost importance to provide a comfortable environment for her.

Because the gynecological exam can be intimidating for a child or adolescent, you should begin each examination with routine care that they will be comfortable with. You may begin by plotting the height and weight on a growth chart. Starting with other portions of the exam, such as checking the heart and lungs, may help to reassure the child. The genital examination should be performed in a methodical manner with careful visualization of the genital structures and careful notation of abnormalities or variations. In older females, the focus of the examination is to evaluate the cervix and internal genital structures, but with the prepubertal female, the external visualization of the genitalia can diagnose the majority of the problems. The need to perform an internal examination is unnecessary for routine care; however, if there are specific complaints such as vaginal bleeding, recurrent or unresponsive vaginal discharge, suspected foreign body, or suspected vaginal tumor, further evaluation would be required. The preferred means to evaluate these problems is to do an examination under anesthesia using a fiberoptic vaginoscopy, hysteroscope, pediatric cystoscope, or endoscope with irrigating properties.

BENIGN VAGINITIS IN THE ADOLESCENT PATIENT

Vulvovaginitis is the most common gynecologic problem in prepubertal girls. In early puberty, physiologic leukorrhea begins in response to the increased levels of circulating estrogens. It develops weeks to months prior to the onset of menarche and may persist for several years. It can be described as a thick, clear-to-white colored, cloudy vaginal discharge and is composed of desquamated vaginal cells, vaginal transudate, and endocervical mucus. Many times, it is interpreted as an infection; however, this discharge is completely normal. Reassurance of the patient and her family is the only required treatment.

IRRITATION TO THE VULVA AND VAGINA

Vulva and vaginal irritation can result from trauma such as "straddle" injuries or accidental penetration (e.g., foreign bodies) or can be a result of sexual abuse. This vignette introduces child sexual abuse, which is an unfortunate event that is reported up to 80,000 times a year. The number of unreported cases is far greater, because the victims are afraid to tell anyone what has happened, and the legal procedure for validating an episode is difficult. Child sexual abuse is characterized by dynamics to which young, dependant children are particularly vulnerable. Victims are warned that should they disclose any information, consequences will ensue to themselves or other family members. The legal definition of child sexual abuse includes both sexual contact (either intrusion into body orifices, fondling, or requiring the child to fondle or fellate the perpetrator) and noncontact acts (such as exhibitionism, involvement in child pornography, and deliberate exposure of children to sexually explicit materials).

VAGINAL FOREIGN BODIES

Commonly children will insert a foreign body that will eventually cause irritation and a foul-smelling discharge. They will present to the emergency room with irritation and/or discharge; meanwhile, their parents have no idea what the cause is. While examining the child, sometimes the object can be visualized using a nasal speculum. Lost or forgotten tampons are also common and can be removed using vaginal forceps. In difficult cases, however, where sharp or large objects are involved, young patients may require general anesthesia in order to remove the object under direct vision. The key is to never ignore vaginal discharge in a pediatric patient. Although it may just be benign vaginitis, there are other more serious causes that should be investigated.

TAKE HOME POINTS

- Oftentimes, victims of sexual abuse do not disclose information about their abuse or about their abusers for fear of the ramifications.
- Documentation is key in cases of suspected sexual abuse; all information from a victim that is documented in the medical records is admissible in court.
- Vaginal discharge in a prepubertal or pubertal female is most often than not normal physiologic changes in response to increasing hormone levels.
- Vulva of vaginal irritations from sexual abuse can be easily mistaken for accidental trauma, consensual sexual activity, or normal physiological changes.
- Most adolescents hear about their peers' experiences with the gynecologist and from there form their first opinion, either positive or negative.

SUGGESTED READINGS

Buttaravoli PM, Stair TO. *Common Simple Emergencies.* Washington, DC: Longwood Information, LLC;1984.

Carpenter SE, Rock J. *Pediatric and Adolescent Gynecology.* 2nd ed. Philadelphia, PA: Lippincott Williams & Wilkins; 2000.

Kass-Wolff JH, Wilson E. Pediatric gynecology: assessment strategies and common problems. *Semin Reprod Med.* 2003;21(4):329–338.

88

ADRENAL INSUFFICIENCY AND HYPOTENSION IN THE PRETERM INFANT

ERIC I. FELNER, MD, MSCR

Arterial hypotension in preterm infants is associated with significant morbidity including an increased risk of intracranial hemorrhage and long-term neurologic sequelae. The management of severe hypotension resistant to volume expansion and inotropic administration is a difficult therapeutic problem. Many hypotensive, premature infants respond to glucocorticoid replacement therapy suggesting that an inadequate hypothalamic-pituitary-adrenal (HPA) axis is a contributing cause. Glucocorticoid replacement therapy is the treatment for preterm infants with refractory hypotension, but there is no consensus on when to discontinue therapy and how and when to reassess adrenal status. The central issue is whether or not the infant has a transient or permanent state of adrenal insufficiency. What is the ideal approach for determining when to provide and when to discontinue glucocorticoid therapy in the preterm infant with hypotension?

In the preterm infant with hypotension, the initial treatment is to increase fluid delivery to correct the fluid losses. If the blood pressure does not improve with volume expansion alone, inotropic support with dopamine, dobutamine, and/or epinephrine promotes alpha- and beta-adrenergic receptor stimulation that usually normalizes blood pressure. If these measures fail, adrenal insufficiency should be considered. After initiating therapy, the primary goal in the hypotensive preterm infant is to determine if the infant has transient adrenal insufficiency of prematurity (TAP) or a permanent form of adrenal insufficiency.

Although adrenal insufficiency is not uncommon in preterm infants, it is usually transient, as a result of the immaturity of the adrenal gland and the HPA axis. TAP is the term used to describe these infants because they require glucocorticoid replacement therapy but rarely need it for a prolonged period of time. In fact, most require less than a week of therapy and once discontinued, blood pressure remains in the appropriate range. Although many cases involving TAP and glucocorticoid therapy are reported, few systematic large-scale studies have been performed. Most preterm infants who are hypotensive, and refractory to volume expansion and inotropic support, have TAP. Some, however, have permanent adrenal insufficiency and require lifelong therapy.

The adrenal gland is a critical component of the body's response to stress. The inability to secrete cortisol, the glucocorticoid secreted by the adrenal gland, in response to stress, can be catastrophic, associated with hypotension, electrolyte disturbances, hypoglycemia, and marked shifts in body fluid. Baseline cortisol levels are variable shortly after birth in preterm and term infants. In healthy preterm or term infants, stress-induced cortisol levels generally triple baseline levels and/or reach an absolute level >18 µg/dL. The adrenal gland is not fully functional until after 40 weeks gestation placing preterm infants at risk for adrenal insufficiency. As baseline cortisol levels are variable in the preterm infant, only those who encounter a stressful event and are unable to produce a significant cortisol response are likely to have clinical evidence of adrenal insufficiency. Infants who may have adrenal insufficiency do not display evidence of it unless they encounter a stressful event. Those who fail to respond to adrenocorticotropic hormone (ACTH) stimulation with cortisol levels three times the baseline cortisol level and/ or >18 µg/dL have adrenal insufficiency.

A systematic approach to the diagnosis and treatment of disorders leading to adrenal insufficiency requires an understanding of the hormone production of the adrenal gland as well as the HPA axis. The most common causes of adrenal insufficiency of the newborn include disorders of steroid biosynthesis, hypopituitarism, adrenal gland immaturity, bilateral adrenal gland hemorrhage, and sepsis. If these entities are excluded, then consider a diagnosis of TAP.

Most preterm infants with resistant hypotension will respond to <7 days of glucocorticoid therapy. For those few infants who develop hypotension (and/or other clinical features consistent with adrenal insufficiency) after glucocorticoid discontinuation, an in-depth evaluation for permanent adrenal insufficiency should be undertaken.

Consider adrenal insufficiency in preterm infants with hypotension who fail to respond to volume expansion and inotropic support. Careful evaluation after discontinuation of glucocorticoid therapy involves monitoring the infant for symptoms of adrenal insufficiency and performing an ACTH stimulation test. The preterm infant who maintains appropriate baseline and ACTH-stimulated cortisol levels after a short course (≤7 days) of glucocorticoid therapy has TAP and does not require any further glucocorticoid therapy. On the other hand, the preterm infant who has an inappropriate ACTH-stimulated cortisol level 24 hours after discontinuation of glucocorticoid therapy requires reinstitution of glucocorticoid therapy. An evaluation for the causes of permanent adrenal insufficiency should ensue. Chronic glucocorticoid therapy along with increased dosage for stressful conditions should also be employed.

- The adrenal gland is not fully mature in the term infant; however, healthy term and preterm infants' adrenal glands produce appropriate physiologic and stress-needed glucocorticoid.
- Preterm infants with hypotension who are resistant to volume expansion and inotropic support likely have TAP.
- Preterm infants with TAP respond to a short course of glucocorticoid therapy.
- Preterm infants with TAP should receive no >1 week of glucocorticoid therapy, and their HPA axis should be evaluated with ACTH stimulation testing 24 hours after discontinuation of glucocorticoid therapy.
- Preterm infants with suspected TAP who cannot maintain normal blood pressure off glucocorticoid therapy or who do not secrete appropriate levels of cortisol (during ACTH stimulation testing) 24 hours after discontinuation of glucocorticoid therapy should be restarted on therapy and undergo evaluation for causes of permanent adrenal insufficiency.

SUGGESTED READINGS

Calixto C, Martinez FE, Jorge SM, et al. Correlation between plasma and salivary cortisol levels in preterm infants. *J Pediatr*. 2002;140:116–118.

Gaissmaier RE, Poblandt FP. Single dose dexamethasone treatment of hypotension in preterm infants. *J Pediatr*. 1999;134:701–705.

Ng PC, Lam CWK, Fok TF, et al. Refractory hypotension in preterm infants with adrenocortical insufficiency. *Arch Dis Child Fetal Neonatal Ed*. 2001;84:F122–F124.

Ng PC, Lee CH, Lam CWK, et al. Transient adrenocortical insufficiency of prematurity and systemic hypotension in very low birthweight infants. *Arch Dis Child Fetal Neonatal Ed*. 2004;89:F119–F126.

Pittinger TP, Sawin RS. Adrenocortical insufficiency in infants with congenital diaphragmatic hernia: a pilot study. *J Pediatr Surg*. 2000;35(2):223–226.

89

IS THE BABY A BOY OR GIRL?

ERIC I. FELNER, MD, MSCR

Almost immediately after a baby is born, the obstetrician proudly announces, "Congratulations, you have a beautiful baby boy (or girl)." For many families, the suspense has been removed with the prenatal ultrasound. This announcement is simply a confirmation of the expected. There are instances, however, when delivery room personnel are speechless, as in the baby with ambiguous genitalia. Although it only occurs in 1 in 4,000 live births, when it does occur, it is distressing for not only the immediate family members but also the medical personnel. The baby is rarely in danger of developing an acute medical crisis, but the psychological effects on the family make this condition an emergency. The speed with which gender assignment can be made is extremely important. Assignment of the baby's gender may be straightforward, but in some cases, it is controversial. What is the ideal approach for determining gender assignment?

The immediate goal is to determine what should be the most appropriate sex for rearing the child. The second goal, which may take longer to achieve, is to identify the definitive diagnosis. Knowledge of the specific diagnosis will allow therapeutic interventions to be planned and will enable genetic counseling for future pregnancies.

A systematic approach to the diagnosis and treatment of predisposing conditions that lead to the diagnosis of ambiguous genitalia requires an understanding of the processes involved in normal sexual differentiation. The most common causes of ambiguous genitalia include disorders involving gonadal differentiation, abnormal steroid biosynthesis, maternal hyperandrogenism, androgen sensitivity, hypogonadotropic hypogonadism, and müllerian duct abnormalities. Only the disorders involving steroid biosynthesis and hypogonadotropic hypogonadism require early hormone replacement therapy, and this may not be necessary in the first few days of life unless the baby experiences hypoglycemia. Therefore, there is time to obtain important test results and to discuss both the medical and the psychological aspects of gender assignment with the family. Allowing the parents to discuss their child's condition with each other and the medical team is essential. If they have input regarding the gender decision, the parents will be better prepared to promote their child's self-esteem.

The approach for determining gender assignment begins with the identification of the child's genotype and internal genitalia. Once these facts are known, appropriate medical specialists should be consulted, and management options should be discussed with the parents. In the past, gender assignment was based on how quickly a surgical intervention could be performed in order to create the appearance of normal genitalia. Other factors that were commonly used to determine gender assignment included (1) the least difficult surgical procedure, (2) a surgery that would favor the performance of normal gender-related activities (i.e., males — standing to urinate), (3) a surgery that would permit sexual intercourse and the possibility of reproduction, and (4) physician preference.

There have been several long-term studies of the psychological effects on adolescents and adults who were born with ambiguous genitalia. The best approach involves a medical team with the parents playing a major role in the gender assignment. The goal for caring for the baby with ambiguous genitalia involves both the gender assignment and preparing for the discussion with the parents. The parents may have guilt, and the interaction with the parents may be as important as with the child. The primary physician should explain to the family that the baby experienced a birth defect involving genital development. Reviewing diagrams of the internal and external genitalia of boys and girls and showing that these structures develop from the same structures may be helpful. Although this birth defect impedes the usual method of determining whether the infant is a boy or a girl, there is an appropriate sex of rearing for each child. Explaining to the parents that they will be instrumental in this process is imperative.

TAKE HOME POINTS

- For babies born with ambiguous genitalia a team approach should be utilized for determining gender assignment.
- The team should include the parents of the affected child, endocrinologists, urologists, neonatologists, and general pediatricians.
- The attitudes and practice of endocrinologists and urologists have changed in the past 20 years toward the baby born with ambiguous genitalia.
- The basis for the decision-making process of gender assignment should not be limited to the baby's appearance or the potential for reproduction.
- The baby's karyotype and internal genitalia should be determined as soon as possible in an effort to rule out a medically-treatable condition and help guide the team in making a decision on gender assignment.

SUGGESTED READINGS

American Academy of Pediatrics. Evaluation of the newborn with developmental anomalies of the external genitalia. *Pediatrics*. 2000;106:138–142.

Berenbaum SA, Korman Bryk K, Duck SC, et al. Psychological adjustment in children and adults with congenital adrenal hyperplasia. *J Pediatr*. 2004;144:741–746.

Diamond DA, Burns JP, Mitchell C, et al. Sex assignment for newborns with ambiguous genitalia and exposure to fetal testosterone: attitudes and practices of pediatric urologists. *J Pediatr*. 2006;148:445–449.

MacLaughlin DT, Donahoe PK. Sex determination and differentiation. *N Engl J Med*. 2004;350:367–378.

Meyer–Bahlburg HFL. Gender assignment in intersexuality. *J Psych Hum Sex*. 1998;10:1–21.

90

REPRODUCTIVE MILESTONES: ARE WE THERE YET?

LYDIA MAYIDA, MD AND DIANA BROOMFIELD, MD, MBA, FACOG, FACS

A 17-year-old girl presents to the office with her mother who reports she is concerned that her daughter has breast development but has not started having her periods yet. What is your list of differential diagnoses?

Primary amenorrhea is defined either as the absence of menses by age 14 in the absence of normal growth or other secondary sex characteristics or the absence of menses at age 16 in the presence of normal growth and secondary sex characteristics. Amenorrhea can be classified as primary when the patient has never had prior menses as above or secondary defined as absence of menses for more than three cycles (some experts require 6 months) in a woman who was previously menstruating. In addition, delayed puberty is considered when no breast development is evident by age 13.5 or when pubic hair is absent at 14 years. The most common cause of delayed puberty is constitutional.

Primary amenorrhea is a disorder that affects <1% of adolescent girls in the United States. The most common causes of primary amenorrhea include chromosomal or genetic disorders (such as Turner syndrome, Swyer syndrome, or Prader-Willi syndrome, androgen insensitivity), hypothalamic disorders (hypogonadotropic hypogonadism), pituitary disease (such as hyperprolactinemia), absence of or structural abnormalities of reproductive organs, adrenogenital syndrome, congenital heart disease (cyanotic), congenital adrenal hyperplasia, craniopharyngioma, chronic (long-term) illnesses (starvation, excessive exercise, depression, psychological stress, marijuana use, Crohn disease, Cushing disease, cystic fibrosis, sickle cell disease, thalassemia major, human immunodeficiency virus infection, renal disease, thyroid disease, diabetes mellitus, malnutrition, obesity, extreme weight loss, anorexia nervosa), gonadal dysgenesis, hypoglycemia, hypothyroidism and hyperthyroidism, pregnancy, polycystic ovarian disease, true hermaphroditism, and tumors of the CNS including the pituitary, adrenal glands, or ovaries.

Of these, the most common causes are chromosomal abnormalities leading to ovarian failure due to premature depletion of all oocytes and follicles. Examples of conditions associated with ovarian failure that results in an increase in FSH levels due to lack of feedback from estrogen and inhibin are Turner syndrome 45,XO, 46,XX gonadal dysgenesis, and 46,XY gonadal dysgenesis. In these patients, normal female external genitalia appear with a uterus but without ovaries or presence of rudimentary ovaries. Acquired causes of hypergonadotropic hypogonadism and gonadal failure include radiation therapy or high-dose alkylating chemotherapy, or autoimmune oophoritis.

Hypothalamic hypogonadism refers to functional hypothalamic amenorrhea, which may be due to anorexia nervosa, stress, or excessive exercise. Patients may also have a congenital GnRH deficiency that can be inherited; when this deficiency occurs with anosmia, it is known as Kallmann syndrome. Pathologic infiltration of the hypothalamus or the pituitary with tumor may also lead to pathological hypogonadism, for example, craniopharyngioma, germinoma, and Langerhans cell histiocytosis, which can be diagnosed on MRI imaging. Hyperprolactinemia may also cause amenorrhea and is usually accompanied with galactorrhea. Serum prolactin levels >15 to 20 ng/mL are considered abnormal in reproductive age women but this may also be due to stress, exercise, recent sexual intercourse, sleep, or meals; hence, it is recommended to repeat levels prior to ordering an MRI for elevated prolactin levels. Prolactin levels should be drawn during the follicular phase of the menstrual cycle and have the patient avoid any breast stimulation at least 24 hours prior to testing.

Absence of a vagina, vaginal agenesis also called müllerian agenesis, or the Mayer-Rokitansky-Kuster-Hauser (MRKH) syndrome may lead to primary amenorrhea and is the most common cause of primary amenorrhea secondary to gonadal dysgenesis. In most cases, it is associated with absence of the uterus and cervix, 7% to 10% of cases have a normal uterus though. For normal menstrual flow to occur, there is a need for an intact uterus, cervix, and vagina, so congenital anomalies with the uterus and cervix may also cause primary amenorrhea.

Occasionally, there is a transverse vaginal septum or imperforate hymen, which may obstruct the reproductive tract leading to the formation of a hematocolpos or collection of blood in the uterus. Consider this differential if there is primary amenorrhea associated with cyclical pelvic pain at ages 12 to 13. Diagnosis can be made by physical examination (palpable and tender uterus) and confirmed by an ultrasound.

Receptor and enzyme abnormalities are also associated with primary amenorrhea, for example, complete androgen insensitivity syndrome, with complete testosterone resistance, an X-linked recessive syndrome. Androgen insensitivity syndrome is a disorder of sex development caused by mutations of the gene encoding the androgen receptor. Affected patients develop female external genitalia with male internal organs, testes. At puberty, these patients do develop breasts, but their areola appears pale with sparse pubic and axillary hair. Diagnosis is consistent with lack of uterus and elevated testosterone levels and abnormal karyotype (46,XY). The internal gonads have potential for malignant change to dysgerminoma or gonadoblastoma and hence need to be surgically removed.

5-alpha-reductase deficiency is similar to complete androgen insensitivity; however, at puberty, there is an increased level of testosterone available so that there is evidence of virilization. These patients are unable to convert testosterone to dihydrotestosterone due to lack of 5-alpha reductase, and hence they fail to undergo DHT-dependent masculinization. Nevertheless, these patients undergo voice change (deepening), muscle enlargement, and male pattern hair growth with testosterone activity at puberty.

17-alpha-hydroxylase (CYP17) deficiency leads to overproduction of adrenocorticotropic hormone and inability to produce sex steroids. Affected individuals are phenotypic females with hypertension and lack pubertal development.

Absent testes–determining factor (TDF) is found on the short arm of the Y chromosome and its mutation or deletion causes the Ullrich–Turner syndrome; affected individuals do not produce testosterone or mullerian inhibiting substance and have female internal and external genitalia–associated primary gonadal failure. Y-DNA hybridization studies are necessary for diagnosis.

In view of the long list of possible etiological factors in patients with primary amenorrhea, it is important to obtain a complete history (including family history) and physical examination with height and weight and perform imaging studies such as pelvic ultrasound to determine the presence or absence of the uterus and ovaries, the internal female genitalia. Blood tests such as FSH, testosterone, prolactin levels, and thyroid function studies could be ordered. The most common cause of secondary amenorrhea is pregnancy. However, pregnancy is also a differential in patients with primary amenorrhea. A common error to be avoided is not considering pregnancy in your differential. Thus, a pregnancy test is important in both primary and secondary amenorrhea. An MRI of the brain and genetic studies looking at the karyotype may be necessary to clinch the diagnosis.

Full clinical evaluation is recommended for

- Patients with lack of breast development by age 14.
- Patients without menses by age 16.
- Secondary amenorrhea for three cycles or more.
- First Pap smear is not due until 3 years after the first intercourse.

Algorithm for Amenorrhea in the presence of delayed Puberty

- Check labs and x-ray for bone age:
  - If TSH levels are elevated and thyroxine (T4) levels are low, the diagnosis is hypothyroidism.
  - If the bone age is delayed, the cause is constitutional delay.
  - If the bone age is normal, check LH, FSH, and prolactin levels.
  - If LH and FSH levels are elevated, check the karyotype.
    - If the karyotype is 45,XO, the cause is gonadal dysgenesis (i.e., Turner syndrome).
    - If the karyotype is 46,XX, the primary etiology is ovarian failure (i.e., pure gonadal dysgenesis, autoimmune oophoritis, status postradiation therapy or chemotherapy, 17-alpha-hydroxylase deficiency, or resistant ovary syndrome) and rule out neurosensory loss (Kallmann's).
    - If the karyotype is 46,XY, the diagnosis is Swyer syndrome. Schedule gonadectomy.
  - If LH and FSH levels are low or within normal range and the bone age is normal, obtain a head MRI. Rule out pituitary tumor, pituitary destruction, or hypothalamic disease.
  - If prolactin levels are elevated, obtain a head MRI.
    - If head MRI findings are abnormal, the cause is pituitary tumor or a brain lesion disrupting the pituitary stalk.
    - If the MRI finding is normal, rule out marijuana use or psychiatric medicine (dopamine agonist).
    - If head MRI findings are normal with normal history and physical examination findings, the etiology may be drug use, an eating disorder, athleticism, or psychosocial stress.
    - If head MRI findings are normal but clinical evaluation and screening study findings are abnormal, chronic disease can be excluded.

Algorithm for evaluation of amenorrhea with normal puberty and the uterus present
Obtain a pregnancy test.

- If the pregnancy test result is positive, refer to an obstetrician.
- If the pregnancy test result is negative, obtain TSH, prolactin, FSH, and LH levels.
- If the FSH level is low, obtain a head MRI.
- If FSH is elevated, premature ovarian failure is the diagnosis. Obtain a karyotype.

- If TSH, prolactin, and FSH levels are within reference range, perform a progestin challenge test.
- If hirsutism and acne are present, check testosterone, DHEAS, and 17-OH progesterone level.

Algorithm for evaluation of amenorrhea with genital tract abnormalities

Obtain a pelvic sonography. If the uterus is absent and the vagina shortened, obtain a karyotype.

- If the karyotype is 46,XY, obtain testosterone levels.
  - If testosterone levels are elevated, the cause is androgen insensitivity or 5-alpha-reductase deficiency. Surgical gonad removal is recommended in patients with androgen insensitivity.
  - If testosterone levels are within normal limits or are low, the cause is testicular regression or gonadal enzyme deficiency. Surgical gonad removal is recommended.
- If the karyotype is 46,XX, the cause is müllerian agenesis (i.e., MRKH syndrome).

SUGGESTED READINGS

Bielak KM, Harris GS. http://emedicine.medscape.com

Stenchever MA, Droegemueller W, Herbst AL, et al. (eds) *Comprehensive Gynecology*, 4th ed., 2002, New York, NY, Elsevier.

First Aid for the Obstetrics and Gynecology Boards. A Resident to Resident Guide.

UpToDate.com

91

Do not miss polycystic ovary syndrome in the teenager

Ekta Vishwakarma, MD and Diana Broomfield, MD, MBA, FACOG, FACS

A 17-year-old nullipara, Ms. Smith, came with complaints of irregular menstruation (once every 3 to 4 months) and excessive facial hair for the past 3 years. She also complains of steadily putting on weight for the past 3 years. On examination, she was obese (BMI: 30) with excessive hair on chin and upper lip. Her abdomen and pelvic examination was normal. After a transvaginal ultrasound, she was found to have polycystic ovaries. She was reassured and started on low-dose oral contraceptive pill. It was not until 3 years later that she was given the diagnosis of polycystic ovary syndrome (PCOS).

Female factors are responsible for up to 40% of infertility cases, and of those, 25% are due to ovulatory problems. Among women with ovulatory dysfunction, PCOS must be considered and can be diagnosed with any two of the following three features: oligo–ovulation, hyperandrogenism/hyperandrogenemia, and polycystic ovaries by ultrasonography (12 or more follicles per ovary measuring 2 to 9 mm in diameter or a total ovarian volume of >10 cm^3).

PCOS is often undiagnosed or misdiagnosed because the presenting symptoms vary greatly and there is no specific diagnostic test for the disorder. It is a diagnosis of exclusion after Cushing disease, thyroid problems, late–onset congenital adrenal hyperplasia, androgen–secreting tumors, hyperprolactinemia, primary ovarian failure, and pregnancy have been ruled out. Biochemical and radiologic studies must be done to ascertain the diagnosis: testosterone, dehydroepiandrosterone sulfate, 2-hour oral glucose tolerance test, blood lipids, and a pelvic ultrasound.

PCOS is more likely to be undiagnosed in adolescents since menstrual irregularities, acne, or increased weight is believed to be a normal occurrence during puberty. Since adolescents rarely attempt to get pregnant, infertility problems are less likely to be noticed.

The failure to diagnose PCOS can result in complications such as type 2 diabetes, increased triglycerides, hypertension, decreased HDL cholesterol, cardiovascular disease, metabolic syndrome, uterine cancer, miscarriage, abnormal uterine bleeding, gestational diabetes, and gestational hypertension. The major biochemical feature of PCOS is insulin resistance accompanied by compensatory hyperinsulinemia. A considerably increased risk (relative risk of 7.4) of developing myocardial infarction was observed for women with PCOS compared to age-matched referents.

Often, even if PCOS is diagnosed, treatment is only offered for the symptoms that present (acne treatment and recommendation of the pill to control menstrual cycles, or fertility medication for infertility) rather than treating the whole syndrome. Antiandrogenic medications can treat hair growth, insulin-sensitizing agents can treat weight gain, and oral contraceptive pills can regulate the cycles. The administration of metformin improves clinical and biochemical features of PCOS and induces ovulatory cycles in anovulatory patients with PCOS.

TAKE HOME POINTS

- Because of varying presentations, PCOS is a commonly misdiagnosed condition especially in teens.
- The whole syndrome should be treated rather than just the symptoms.
- Metformin improves ovulation rate in PCOS.

SUGGESTED READINGS

American College of Obstetricians and Gynecologists Committee Opinion # 351. The Overweight Adolescent: Prevention, Treatment and OBstetric-Gynecologic Implications. Washington, DC, ACOG, 2006.

Dahlgren E, Janson PO, Johansson S, et al. Polycystic ovary syndrome and risk for myocardial infarction evaluated from a risk factor model based on a prospective population study of women. *Clin Endocrinol (Oxf)*. 1996;44(3):277–284.

Hughes E, Collins J, Vandekerckhove P, et al. Clomiphene citrate for ovulation induction in women with oligo-amenorrhoea. *Cochrane Database Syst Rev*. 2000;CD000056.

Jakubowicz DJ, Iuorno MJ, Jakubowicz S, et al. Effects of metformin on early pregnancy loss in the polycystic ovary syndrome. *J Clin Endocrinol Metab*. 2002;87:524–529.

Lord JM, Flight IHK, Norman RJ. Metformin in polycystic ovary syndrome: systematic review and meta-analysis. *Br Med J*. 2003;327(7421):951.

Rautio K, Tapanainen JS, Ruokonen A, et al. Effects of metformin and ethinyl estradiol–cyproterone acetate on lipid levels in obese and non-obese women with polycystic ovary syndrome. *Eur J Endocrinol*. 2005;152(2):269–275.

Rotterdam ESHRE/ASRM-Sponsored PCOS Consensus Workshop Group. Revised 2003 consensus on diagnostic criteria and long-term health risks related to polycystic ovary syndrome. *Fertil Steril*. 2004;81(1):19–25.

92

DYSGENETIC GONADS WITH Y CHROMOSOME

OSUEBI OKECHUKWU, MD AND DIANA BROOMFIELD, MD, MBA, FACOG, FACS

A 19-year-old female was brought to the gynecology clinic by her mother because she has "never had her menses." Her past medical and surgical histories were unremarkable. Physical exam revealed a phenotypic female with normal stature, while pelvic exam was unremarkable except for "scanty pubic hair." Initial laboratory workup was unremarkable, while a transvaginal ultrasound revealed a normal uterus with "atrophic ovaries" bilaterally. A chromosomal analysis showed a 46,XY karyotype.

Genes play a significant role in the early and late processes of sex differentiation and determination. Mutations in these genes can result in syndromes that can predispose to the development of malignancies. At approximately the 7th gestational week, the indifferent gonads differentiate into testis in the presence of Y chromosome or ovary in the presence of two X chromosomes. This differentiation is in response to the hormones produced by the ovary or testis.

GONADOBLASTOMAS

These are tumors that contain both germ cells and sex cord elements with a well-organized nest. They occur mostly in individuals with dysgenetic gonads and a Y chromosome.

In 1978, Page and colleagues suggested that the Y chromosome contains a gene (oncogene), which in the presence of dysgenetic gonads induces gonadoblastoma formation. This gene, in the normal testis, is involved in spermatogenesis.

SYNDROMES OF GONADAL DYSGENESIS

Patients with pure gonadal dysgenesis have a 46,XX or 46,XY karyotype and bilateral streak gonads. These gonads are small and fibrotic and lack the usual germ cells. This results from a mutation in the sex-determining region of the Y chromosome. These patients usually present with delayed puberty and amenorrhea.

Gonadal dysgenesis (Swyer syndrome) is characterized by "streak gonads" in a phenotypic female with a 46,XY karyotype. This condition results from a mutation which inhibits the function of the Y-borne determinant that would normally cause the indifferent embryonic gonad to differentiate into a testis. The streak gonad is nonfunctional and incapable of ovulation or estrogen secretion. The syndrome is sometimes called pure gonadal dysgenesis.

Mixed gonadal dysgenesis has extreme variability, which may extend from a Turner-like syndrome to a male phenotype. This disorder presents with dysgenetic and asymmetric gonads.

The 46,XY female karyotype is often discovered prepubertally when chromosomal studies are made in short girls or later when the patients fail to attain sexual maturation. The fallopian tubes and uterus are present as well as gonads of intra-abdominal undifferentiated streaks. Gonadal tumors, usually gonadoblastomas, occur in about 25% of these patients particularly in those with the more female phenotypes. It is often recommended as a precaution to remove the gonadal tissue in patients raised as females.

The condition is thought to occur because the SRY gene normally located on one arm of the Y chromosome is translocated to an X chromosome or it is not functional at the normal location on the Y chromosome. This gene is believed to be the testis-determining factor that triggers the undifferentiated gonadal tissue of the embryo to form testis. The presence of immature testicular tubules has been observed in female patients who have karyotype 46,XX with the normal SRY gene translocated to the X chromosome. These patients usually have small fibrotic gonads. Owing to the risk of malignancy, gonadectomy is recommended even at young age. The karyotypes are commonly 45,X/46,XY or 46,XY. *Turner syndrome*, which results from partial or total absence of one X chromosome, usually presents with short stature sexual infantilism, streak gonads, and primary amenorrhea. In some patients, there is an associated mosaicism with some cells containing the XY genotype. Gonadectomy is recommended in these patients due to the risk of malignant transformation.

Another condition of the mixed gonadal dysgenesis is the OX/XY male. The mechanism underlying this masochism is probably the result of a mitotic nondisjunction in an originally XY embryo causing XO/XY and XYY cell lines.

Neoplastic transformation of germ cells in dysgenetic gonads (the formation of gonadoblastoma and/or an invasive germ cell tumor) occurs in about 20% to 30% of cases and is associated with the presence of (part of) the Y chromosome in the patients' karyotype. It is usually diagnosed at a young age.

Early gonadectomy, often combined with gender reassignment and genital surgery, is recommended.

Management. Dysgenetic gonads with Y chromosome pose a risk of malignancy and gonadectomy is recommended. The preferred treatment approach is via laparoscopy. This is dependent on the operator's skill. Laparotomy is an equally viable option in gonadectomy if the laparoscopic approach is not feasible.

TAKE HOME POINTS

- Y chromosome–containing dysgenetic gonads are at an increased risk of malignant transformation.
- Gonadectomy is recommended in such patients.
- Laparoscopic gonadectomy is the preferred mode of management.

SUGGESTED READINGS

Cools M. Stoop H, Kersemaekers AM, et al. Gonadoblastoma arising in undifferentiated gonadal tissue within dysgenetic gonads. *J Clin Endocrinol Metab.* 2006;91(6):2404–2413.

Ding XL. Identification of potential neoplastic risk in gonadal development abnormality with Y chromosome of 79 cases. *Zhonghua Fu Chan Ke Za Zhi.* 2008;43(6):442.

Fallat ME, Donahoe PK. Intersex genetic anomalies with malignant potential. *Curr Opin Pediatr.* 2006;18(3):305–311.

Kliegman N. *Textbook of Pediatrics.* 18th ed. Philadelphia, PA: Saunders; 2007.

Page DC. Hypothesis: a Y-chromosomal gene causes gonadoblastoma in dysgenetic gonads. *Development.* 1987;(Suppl 101):151–155.

Saenger P. Clinical manifestations and diagnosis of Turner's syndrome. UpToDate, January, 2009.

Wein AJ. *Campbell–Walsh Urology.* 9th ed. Philadelphia, PA: Saunders; 2007.

93

ARE YOU SURE SHE HAS POLYCYSTIC OVARY SYNDROME?

JESSICA B. SPENCER, MD, MSc

A 23-year-old graduate student makes an annual appointment with you for the first time. She was previously seen by a gynecologist in another state where she went to college. Her past medical history includes polycystic ovary syndrome (PCOS) and she has been on oral contraceptive pills (OCPs) for the last 6 months for treatment. She has no records with her but when asked tells you that she has in fact had problems with acne and hair growth on her chin. Her periods are regular on OCPs but were previously irregular. Her BP is 140/90 and her BMI is 32 with a high waist-to-hip ratio. The diagnosis sounds reasonable enough, but are you really sure she has PCOS? PCOS is common, affecting approximately 5% to 8% of reproductive aged women. However, there are several endocrinopathies that have an indolent onset and often masquerade PCOS. While rare, they deserve consideration in any patient.

In general, the evaluation of irregular menses should include a gynecologic exam, BMI assessment, pregnancy test, TSH, prolactin, endometrial biopsy especially if the woman has additional risk factors for endometrial hyperplasia, and possibly an ultrasound or sonohystogram if you are looking for a structural cause. FSH and estradiol levels are of benefit if you are considering premature ovarian insufficiency (FSH high, estradiol low) or hypothalamic amenorrhea (FSH low, estradiol low). Psychosocial stressors such as depression and anxiety may also play a role. However, the following disorders are mentioned because they mimic the presentation of PCOS (in the absence of finding abnormalities of those above) and often are associated with hyperandrogenism.

Nonclassic, or late-onset, congenital adrenal hyperplasia (CAH) due to 21-hydroxylase deficiency usually presents after puberty, causing irregular menses and excess androgen production which leads to hirsutism, acne, balding, and cliteromegaly. This form of CAH is common, especially among certain ethnic subgroups, and is one of the most common autorecessive disorders. The diagnosis is made by a random 17-hydroxyprogesterone (17-OHP) assay and confirmed by an ACTH stimulation test with measurement of 17-OHP after 1 hour. Any women with irregular menses and hyperandrogenism after puberty should have a 17-OHP checked once. Treatment involves replacing their glucocorticoids and sometimes mineralocorticoids.

Cushing disease should be considered especially in women with central obesity and hypertension. A 24-hour urine collection for free cortisol will suggest this diagnosis.

Acromegaly, caused by growth hormone (GH) excess, often presents with such a slow onset that it is missed by many providers until the physical changes are too late. Often in women, the first sign is oligo or amenorrhea. An elevated IGF-1 (aka somatomedin C) level will make this diagnosis.

Androgen-secreting tumors of the adrenal gland or ovary usually have a more rapid onset than the androgen excess seen with PCOS, but there are exceptions. Generally, the testosterone level will be much higher than that seen in PCOS. If your patient does not improve with 6 months of treatment with oral contraceptives and/or another antiandrogen, and you have ruled out the disorders above, you may also want to consider an indolent tumor. A thin-section CT scan of the adrenals and an ultrasound of the ovaries will find many but not all of them. Rarely, selective venous catheterization with blood sampling is needed to find the very small ones.

TAKE HOME POINTS

- Consider the following in any woman with hyperandrogenism and irregular menses: nonclassic congenital adrenal hyperplasia, Cushing disease, acromegaly, and androgen-secreting tumors if the course is particularly severe and resistant to treatment.
- The following lab assessment is recommended in any woman with hyperandrogenism and irregular menses: pregnancy test, TSH, prolactin, total testosterone, and 17-OHP. Consider 24-hour urinary-free cortisol and IGF-1 if appropriate. If you suspect insulin resistance, check a 2-hour glucose tolerance test.
- PCOS is essentially a diagnosis of exclusion. If the above labs are normal, and the patient has irregular menses and hyperandrogenism (either clinical or serologic evidence), a diagnosis of PCOS can be made.

SUGGESTED READINGS

American College of Obstetricians and Gynecologists. ACOG Practice Bulletin No. 41. Clinical Management Guidelines for Obstetrician-Gynecologists. December 2002. *Obstet Gynecol.* 2002;100(6):1389–1402.

Azziz R, Carmina E, Dewailly D, et al. Androgen Excess Society. Positions statement: criteria for defining polycystic ovary syndrome as a predominantly hyperandrogenic syndrome: an Androgen Excess Society guideline. *J Clin Endocrinol Metab.* 2006;91(11):4237–4245.

94

POLYCYSTIC OVARIAN SYNDROME IN ADULTS

DONNA R. SESSION, MD

Polycystic ovarian syndrome (PCOS) affects approximately 6% of reproductive-aged women. The present diagnostic criteria for PCOS consists of clinical or biochemical hyperandrogenism and chronic anovulation excluding other endocrinopathies. Other endocrinopathies, such as adrenal disorders, hyperprolactinemia, and androgen-secreting neoplasms, can mimic the clinical and morphological findings of PCOS and must be ruled out. Chronic anovulation is defined as amenorrhea of 3 months' duration or oligomenorrhea (intermenstrual intervals >35 days). Clinical evidence of hyperandrogenism may include hirsutism as defined as a modified Ferriman-Gallwey score >7, male pattern hair loss, and acne. Patients with insulin resistance may demonstrate acanthosis nigricans. PCOS patients usually have slightly elevated testosterone, androstenedione, and dehydroepiandrosterone sulphate (DHEAS), although some patients may have levels in the normal range. This lack of specificity has led to the challenge of establishing accurate diagnostic criteria. The Rotterdam Consensus Workshop on PCOS in 2003 changed diagnostic guidelines by adding ultrasonographic criteria of a mean follicle number per ovary of ≥12 and/or ovarian volume >10 cm^3 to the criteria for hyperandrogenism and oligo-ovulation. Two out of three criteria are required to make the diagnosis. Since patients with hyperandrogenism of diverse etiologies have polycystic ovarian morphology on ultrasound and vice versa, and since many normoandrogenic, normovulatory women have ≥12 follicles per ovary, the Rotterdam criteria overdiagnose PCOS. The Androgen Excess Society has proposed that PCOS should be diagnosed by the presence of three features: (a) androgen excess (clinical and/or biochemical hyperandrogenism), (b) ovarian dysfunction (oligo-anovulation and/or polycystic ovarian morphology), and (c) exclusion of other androgen excess or ovulatory disorders.

Sonographic findings of polycystic ovaries occur in over 80% of women with PCOS. Most of these women have ultrasound evidence of ovaries enlarged beyond the upper limit of normal, which is a volume of 10 cm^3. Within these ovaries, the preovulatory follicle does not develop and multiple small subcapsular follicles accumulate. The polycystic ovary has been defined either by the presence of ten or more follicles, 2 to

18 mm in diameter by transabdominal sonography, arranged peripherally around an increased stroma or by multiple follicles 2 to 4 mm in diameter distributed throughout an increased stroma. The ovary is enlarged due to both arrested follicular growth and increased stroma. While no universally accepted sonographic criteria exist, abundant ovarian stroma may be suspected if the stromal volume or echogenicity is increased or the stroma/total ovarian area is >0.34. Three-dimensional ultrasound diagnostic thresholds for PCOS with 100% specificity are >20 mean follicle number per ovary, >10 maximum follicles in a single plane, and >13 cm^3 for ovarian volume.

An LH/FSH ratio above 3.2 is suggestive of PCOS but is not a reliable diagnostic tool. Serum antimüllerian hormone (AMH) is elevated in women with PCOS. A morning serum 17-hydroxyprogesterone >200 ng/dL in the early follicular phase suggests congenital adrenal hyperplasia. Since 17-hydroxyprogesterone is elevated in the luteal phase, a serum progesterone should be performed in patients with oligomenorrhea to rule out ovulation. Cushing syndrome may be evaluated with an overnight dexamethasone suppression test and a 24-hour urine test for cortisol or salivary cortisol. Ovarian and adrenal tumors are considered when the serum testosterone is above 200 ng/dL and are unlikely if the level is under 150 ng/dL. Adrenal tumors usually have serum dehydroepiandrosterone sulfate twice the normal level for age. Serum LH levels are low in the setting of such tumors.

Lipid abnormalities are common in women with PCOS, particularly high triglycerides. This may be clinically significant when considering the type of contraceptive and risk of pancreatitis in pregnancy. Both lean and obese women with PCOS may have insulin resistance. A 2-hour oral glucose tolerance test (OGTT) should be used to make the diagnosis. Fasting glucose and glycosylated hemoglobin lack sensitivity.

Signs of virilization, including deepening of the voice, frontal balding, increased muscle mass, severe acne, and clitoromegaly, are suggestive of androgen-producing neoplasms. Short duration and rapidly worsening symptoms are also suggestive of androgen-producing neoplasms and warrant greater vigilance.

A progesterone withdrawal test has been shown to predictably induce a withdrawal bleed if the circulating serum estradiol level is at least 50 pg/mL. However, the progesterone withdrawal test can provide inappropriately reassuring information that may delay the diagnosis of serious conditions such as hypothalamic hypogonadism due to a CNS tumor as up to 50% of women with premature ovarian failure have a withdrawal bleed in response to progestin.

TAKE HOME POINTS

- Exclude other endocrinopathies when diagnosing PCOS.
- Patients with hyperandrogenism of any source will have PCOS morphology on ultrasound and the source of androgens should be investigated.
- An LH/FSH ratio above 3.2 is not a reliable diagnostic tool.
- A positive progesterone withdrawal test does not rule out other causes of anovulation.
- Virilization and rapidly progressing symptoms suggest an androgen-producing neoplasm.

SUGGESTED READINGS

Adams J, Franks S, Polson DW, et al. Multifollicular ovaries: clinical and endocrine features and response to pulsatile gonadotropin releasing hormone. *Lancet.* 1985;2:1375–1379.

Allemand MC, Tummon IS, Phy JL, et al. Diagnosis of polycystic ovaries by three-dimensional transvaginal ultrasound. *Fertil Steril.* 2006;85(1):214–219.

Azziz R, Carmina E, Dewailly D, et al. Positions statement: criteria for defining polycystic ovary syndrome as a predominantly hyperandrogenic syndrome: an Androgen Excess Society guideline. *J Clin Endocrinol Metab.* 2006;91:4237–4245.

Ferriman D, Gallwey JD. Clinical assessment of body hair growth in women. *J Clin Endocrinol Metab.* 1961;21:1440–1447.

Fulghesu AM, Ciampelli M, Belosi C, et al. A new ultrasound criterion for the diagnosis of polycystic ovary syndrome: the ovarian stroma/total area ratio. *Fertil Steril.* 2001;76(2): 326–331.

Laven JS, Mulders AG, Visser JA, et al. Anti-Mullerian hormone serum concentrations in normoovulatory and anovulatory women of reproductive age. *J Clin Endocrinol Metab.* 2004;89:318–323.

Lobo RA, Kletzky OA, Campeau JD, et al. Elevated bioactive luteinizing hormone in women with the polycystic ovary syndrome. *Fertil Steril.* 1983;39(5):674–678.

Polson DW, Adams J, Wadsworth J, et al. Polycystic ovaries—a common finding in normal women. *Lancet.* 1988;1(8590):870–872.

Rebar RW, Connolly HV. Clinical features of young women with hypergonadotropic amenorrhea. *Fertil Steril.* 1990;53(5):804–810.

The Rotterdam ESHRE/ASRM-sponsored PCOS consensus workshop group, Revised 2003 consensus on diagnostic criteria and long-term health risks related to polycystic ovary syndrome (PCOS). *Hum Rep.* 2004;19:41–47.

Zawadski JK, Dunaif A. Diagnostic criteria for polycystic ovary syndrome: towards a rational approach. In: Dunaif A, Givens JR, Haseltine F, Merriam GR, eds. *Polycystic Ovary Syndrome.* Boston, MA: Blackwell Scientific; 1992:377–384.

95

"HOW HAIRY IS TOO HAIRY?" DIAGNOSIS AND EVALUATION OF HIRSUTISM

CHARLENE EMMANUEL, MD

In our society and culture, hairiness is often associated with "maleness" and is considered "unladylike." The hair removal industry, which ranges from plucking and waxing to the extremes of electrolysis and laser hair removal, is a million dollar industry here in the United States. In fact, a woman is more likely to present to a beautician for assistance with hirsutism prior to seeking the advice of a physician.

Hirsutism is defined as the presence of coarse hair in a malelike distribution and occurs in 5% to 15% of the female population. One of the earliest measures of hirsutism was a scoring system developed by Ferriman and Gallwey in 1961. The Ferriman and Gallwey scoring system employs 11 body sites where there are male predilection toward developing body hair. These include upper lip, chin, chest, upper back, lower back, upper abdomen, lower abdomen, arm, forearm, thigh, and lower leg.

In terms of causative factors, polycystic ovary syndrome (PCOS) accounts for vast majority of cases and affects 70% to 80% of hirsute women. Common findings that comprise this syndrome include an increased LH:FSH ratio, decreased fasting glucose: insulin ratio, polycystic ovaries on ultrasound that appear as a "string of pearls," and obesity. Initial treatment usually begins with the recommendation of weight loss. Adjunctively, medical treatment and surgical treatment in the form of ovarian wedge resection may be employed depending on a woman's present and future reproductive desires.

Other causes of PCOS are less common and include 21-hydroxylase deficiency, androgen-secreting tumors, drug induced, and hyperandrogenic insulin–resistant acanthosis nigricans syndrome. In 10% of cases, the hirsutism is idiopathic and evaluations reveal a normal hormonal profile.

The evaluation of a hirsute woman begins as all good medical workups do—with a thorough history. Important inquiries to make during the history include characterization of the patient's menstrual cycle, discussion of the onset and progression of the hirsutism, medical history including medications, and family history. Next, proceed to the physical exam, paying particular attention to the coarseness and distribution of the hair growth, body habitus, thyromegaly, or other signs of an underlying endocrine disorder.

Laboratory evaluation may also aid in diagnosis. In women who report normal menstrual cycles, anovulatory cycles representing PCOS may be the culprit underlying hirsutism. This may be evaluated by asking the patient to perform a basal body temperature chart in conjunction with a serum progesterone level in the latter or luteal phase of the menstrual cycle. Low levels of progesterone may indicate either PCOS or insulin–resistant acanthosis nigricans, and the patient should, therefore, be evaluated for glucose intolerance and diabetes. Adrenal hyperplasia may be determined by obtaining a 17-HP level, measured soon after menses has been completed. If this test is positive, the patient should then undergo a corticosteroid stimulation test to rule out 21-OH deficiency. A 24–hour urine free cortisol can be used to evaluate a patient for Cushing syndrome. Finally, androgen levels (DHEA sulfate; total and free testosterone) can be used to diagnosis androgen access and anovulatory cycles and, rarely, indicate the presence of androgen-secreting neoplasms.

Hirsutism is most successfully treated when a concert of treatments are employed tailored to the patient's underlying disorder and reproductive needs. Hormonal suppression (i.e., OCPs, GnRH agonists), insulin sensitizers, and peripheral androgen blockade (spironolactone, flutamide, cyproterone acetate, finasteride) are all suitable options. It is important to emphasize to the hirsute woman that it often takes 6 to 12 months after the initiation of therapy to see results, and consequently, medical treatment may be used in conjunction with cosmetic means of hair removal including electrolysis, laser hair removal, and waxing to mitigate the appearance of unwanted hair.

TAKE HOME POINTS

- "Normal" pattern of hair growth differs by race and varies throughout the lifetime of an individual.
- Hirsutism is a common disorder that has the potential to be extremely devastating psychologically, emotionally, and socially.
- The most common instigator of hirsutism is PCOS.
- Very often hirsutism is an indicator of an underlying endocrine disorder.
- A multifaceted approach to the treatment of hirsutism is most successful.

SUGGESTED READINGS

Azziz R. The Evaluation and management of hirsutism. *Obstet Gynecol.* 2003;101:995–1007.
Azziz R, Carmina E, Sawaya ME. Idiopathic hirsutism. *Endocr Rev.* 2000;21:347–362.
Ferriman D, Gallwey JD. Clinical Assessment of body hair growth in women. *J Clin Endocrinol Metab.* 1961;21:1440–1447.
Hatch R, Rosenfield RL, Kim MH, et al. Hirsutism: implications, etiology, and management. *Am J Obstet Gynecol.* 1981;140:815–830.

96

WHERE IS THE VAGINA? DISTINGUISHING BETWEEN DIFFERENT CAUSES OF PRIMARY AMENORRHEA

AIMEE S. BROWNE, MD, MSc

A 17-year-old female presents to your clinic because she has never had a period. She was referred by her family doctor and was told that she had an anatomical defect. She denies any cyclic pelvic pain. She has no medical problems and has never had any surgeries. You perform a thorough history and physical exam. The patient has essentially normal secondary sex characteristics and a blind vaginal pouch. No uterus is identified on pelvic ultrasound. You are unsure whether the patient has müllerian agenesis or androgen insensitivity. How will you tell the difference between the two disorders and how would the management be different for each one?

Evaluation of primary amenorrhea is indicated when there has been no menstruation by the age of 15 in the presence of normal secondary sexual characteristics or within 5 years after breast development. This clinical scenario represents a classic question regarding primary amenorrhea. This patient presents for evaluation of amenorrhea and an anatomical defect. A complete history and physical exam will help distinguish between congenital anomalies, and an abdominal ultrasound may be performed to check for the presence of a uterus.

Unfortunately, müllerian agenesis, complete androgen insensitivity syndrome (AIS), vaginal septum, and imperforate hymen can present with similar symptoms. In all of these cases, a young patient will present with normal secondary sexual characteristics and may have what appears to be a blind vaginal pouch. In contrast to müllerian agenesis and complete AIS, patients with a vaginal septum or imperforate hymen often have a normal uterus and present with cyclic pelvic pain. Patients without a uterus will not have cyclic pain and will lack a uterus on exam, ultrasound, or MRI.

Müllerian agenesis results from failure of the müllerian structures to form, whereas AIS is due to the androgen receptor being insensitive to androgens that are produced. A karyotype and a testosterone level can easily distinguish between these two disorders. Müllerian agenesis is seen in chromosomal females (46,XX) with normal female testosterone levels. AIS is seen in chromosomal males (46,XY) who have normal male testosterone levels. Despite the similar presentation, these disorders are treated differently.

Müllerian agenesis accounts for 10% of cases of primary amenorrhea. Müllerian agenesis results from failure of the müllerian structures to form. There is a range of abnormalities that may be seen with this anomaly ranging from no uterine tissue to persistent uterine anlagen with functional endometrial tissue. If functional uterine tissue causing cyclic pelvic pain is identified, it can be resected laparoscopically. Creation of the vagina can be done using vaginal dilators or can be done surgically. These women also have associated urogenital malformations, so renal ultrasound should be performed to evaluate for unilateral renal agenesis, pelvic kidney, horseshoe kidney, hydronephrosis, or ureteral duplication.

Complete androgen insensitivity accounts for approximately 5% of cases of primary amenorrhea. On physical exam, these women will likely have normal breast development but lack pubic or axillary hair. There may also be presence of inguinal masses. Management will differ in this case as the gonads should be removed following breast development and adult statures. Gonadectomy is performed because the chance of malignancy in these gonads is 22%.

Other anatomical defects including imperforate hymen, transverse vaginal septum, and isolated absence of vagina or cervix will more likely present with cyclic pain and an accumulation of blood behind the obstruction.

TAKE HOME POINTS

- Amenorrhea should be evaluated by age 16 in the absence of secondary sexual characteristics.
- Patients with an imperforate hymen or vaginal septum, with a normal functioning uterus, often present with cyclic pelvic pain.
- Müllerian agenesis and complete AIS can be distinguished by a karyotype and a testosterone level.
- A vagina can be created either through the use of vaginal dilators or surgical creation of a neovagina.

SUGGESTED READINGS

Practice committee of the American Society for Reproductive Medicine. Current evaluation of amenorrhea. *Fert Steril*. 2004;82:266–272.
Schulman L. Mullerian anomalies. *Clin Obstet Gynecol*. 2008;51:214–222.

97

KARYOTYPE AND HORMONES HELP TO DIFFERENTIATE MÜLLERIAN AGENESIS FROM COMPLETE ANDROGEN INSENSITIVITY

VITALY A. KUSHNIR, MD

A 17-year-old female presents with primary amenorrhea and pelvic pain. On exam, secondary sexual characteristics including hair and breasts are normal; a short blind vagina is noted. Differential diagnosis includes androgen insensitivity, müllerian agenesis, low-lying transverse vaginal septum, and imperforate hymen. Testosterone level is in the normal female range and karyotype is 46,XX. Müllerian agenesis is diagnosed. MRI reveals a rudimentary uterine horn and absence of the left kidney. A laparoscopic removal of uterine horn is performed with subsequent improvement of pelvic pain. The patient attempts unsuccessfully to create a functional vagina using dilators. At age 22, a McIndoe vaginoplasty is performed; the patient reports successful intercourse 1 year later.

For patients presenting with primary amenorrhea, anatomic causes including androgen insensitivity, müllerian agenesis, and obstructive lesions of the reproductive tract should be considered, as well as gonadal dysgenesis and endocrine causes (not discussed here). *Table 97.1* outlines the most important clinical features of müllerian agenesis and androgen insensitivity syndrome (AIS).

Women with müllerian agenesis also known as Mayer-Rokitansky-Küster-Hauser syndrome have normal ovarian function, and therefore, they develop normal secondary sexual characteristics. Ultrasound or MRI can be used to evaluate the kidneys and confirm the presence of ovaries and rudimentary uterus. A functional vagina can be created with self-dilation, which is the preferred first-line therapy; satisfactory intercourse is most often achieved. A number of vaginoplasty procedures are available for patients who fail first-line treatment with dilatation. Psychosocial support particularly for adolescents plays a critical role in the correction of this abnormality. Reproduction may be achieved with the help of a gestational carrier.

AIS is characterized by a range of phenotypes. Patients with complete AIS typically present at puberty with primary amenorrhea; some cases are identified in phenotypic female infants with inguinal hernias. Abdominal or inguinal testes produce high levels of testosterone and antimüllerian hormone leading to variable wolffian development and regression of müllerian structures. The key clinical features are outlined in *Table 97.1*. Pubic and

TABLE 97.1	MÜLLERIAN AGENESIS VERSUS ANDROGEN INSENSITIVITY	
	MÜLLERIAN AGENESIS	**COMPLETE ANDROGEN INSENSITIVITY**
Karyotype	46,XX	46,XY
Testosterone level	Normal female	High, normal male
Pubic and axillary hair	Normal female	Scant
Breast development	Normal female	Normal female
Uterus	Absent	Absent
Vagina	Blind	Blind
Associated findings	Renal and skeletal anomalies	Gonadal neoplasia

axillary hair which is sensitive to androgens is absent or minimal. Height, breast development and bone growth are usually normal. Physical exam and imaging studies reveal abdominal testes and the absence of müllerian structures. Due to an increased risk of gonadal neoplasia, the testes are generally surgically removed after puberty. Patients with partial AIS usually present in infancy with some degree of virilization and should have an immediate gonadectomy. The patient's self-identity is female and should not be challenged. Creation of a functional vagina is initially attempted through self-dilation with vaginoplasty procedures reserved for patients who fail this approach. AIS patients are infertile. It is also important to consider 5α-reductase deficiency in the differential diagnosis for AIS.

TAKE HOME POINTS

- Patients with AIS have an increased risk of gonadal neoplasia; the testes should be surgically removed after puberty.
- In patients with congenital absence of vagina, self-dilation is the preferred initial treatment with vaginoplasty procedures reserved for patients who fail initial therapy.

SUGGESTED READINGS

Rock JA, Azziz R. Genital anomalies in childhood. *Clin Obstet Gynecol.* 1987;30:682.
Sultan C, Lumbroso S, Paris F, et al. Disorders of androgen action. *Semin Reprod Med.* 2002;20(3):217–228.

98

IMPERFORATE HYMEN VERSUS TRANSVERSE VAGINAL SEPTUM: HOW ARE THEY CORRECTED?

VITALY A. KUSHNIR, MD

A 14-year-old female presents to the emergency department with cyclic pelvic pain that has become worse. She reports primary amenorrhea. There is no history of in utero DES exposure. Imaging studies suggest hematocolpos and hematometra. Differential diagnosis includes imperforate hymen, transverse vaginal septum, obstructed hemivagina, and cervical agenesis. A bulging membrane is noted and a cruciate incision is made in the operating room with the resultant drainage of blood. At a follow-up visit, the patient reports resolution of pain and normal menses.

Imperforate hymen and transverse vaginal septum are the most common conditions leading to obstruction of menses. Imperforate hymen is a translucent thin membrane just inferior to the urethral meatus that bulges with the Valsalva maneuver. When hematocolpos is present, a bluish discoloration can be seen behind the membrane. Imperforate hymen can be diagnosed at birth or in early childhood and occasionally may lead to bladder outlet obstruction due to hydrocolpos or mucocolpos. A cruciate incision typically corrects the obstruction.

Failure of fusion or canalization of the müllerian tubercle and sinovaginal bulb leads to transverse vaginal septum. Mucocolpos may develop in children; but a more common presentation is with hematocolpos or pyo-hematocolpos due to an ascending infection through a small perforation in adolescents. A mass may be palpable in a rectoabdominal exam. Ultrasound and MRI are the most helpful studies in determining the location and thickness of the septum. Imaging can also help to differentiate between a high septum and cervical agenesis. Resection of the septum followed by an end-to-end anastomosis of vaginal mucosa can be performed by an experienced vaginal surgeon. Pregnancies have been reported in women with corrected transverse septa.

An obstructed hemivagina is associated with ipsilateral renal agenesis. Patients typically present with pain, retrograde menstruation, and ascending infections. Ultrasound and MRI are the most useful studies. Surgical correction can be achieved by resecting the tissue between the two vaginas.

Cervical agenesis is a rare condition that is typically recognized at menarche. Most patients have a cervical hypoplasia rather than complete agenesis. Adolescents may present with primary amenorrhea and pelvic pain from hematometra and retrograde menstruation. Ultrasound and MRI are the most useful studies. In the past, hysterectomy was the only treatment option. Several procedures utilizing skin or mucosal grafts to create a vagina–cervical tract have been described. These procedures carry the risk of ascending infection. Another treatment approach involves the use of medications to suppress menstruation in order to prevent hematometra and pelvic pain. Pregnancy may be achieved through assisted reproductive techniques; cesarean delivery is required.

TAKE HOME POINTS

- Congenital anomalies of the female reproductive tract are a result of disruption of normal embryologic development. The main mechanisms are agenesis, failure of fusion, and failure of canalization.
- Genital tract anomalies are often associated with anomalies of the urinary system.
- 3D ultrasonography and MRI are preferred imaging modalities for müllerian anomalies.
- Treatment of anomalies that lead to menstrual obstruction is typically surgical.

SUGGESTED READINGS

Acien P. Reproductive performance of women with uterine malformations. *Hum Reprod.* 1993;8:122.

The American Fertility Society. The American Fertility Society classifications of adnexal adhesions, distal tubal occlusion, tubal occlusion secondary to tubal ligation, tubal pregnancies, mullerian anomalies and intrauterine adhesions. *Fertil Steril.* 1988;49:944.

Deffarges JV, Haddad B, Musset R, et al. Utero-vaginal anastomosis in women with uterine cervix atresia: long-term follow-up and reproductive performance. A study of 18 cases. *Hum Reprod.* 2001;16:1722.

Rock JA, Azziz R. Genital anomalies in childhood. *Clin Obstet Gynecol.* 1987;30:682.

99

SECONDARY AMENORRHEA: SOMETIMES IT IS ALL IN THE HEAD

AIMEE S. BROWNE, MD, MSc

A 27-year-old female presents to your office complaining of amenorrhea over the last 6 months. The patient states she has been on oral contraceptive pills for 8 years and has had regular monthly withdrawal bleeds. The patient stopped the pill approximately 6 months ago to give herself "a break" from the pill, and she has had no bleeding since that time.

In addition to your history and physical exam, your initial labs reveal a normal TSH and an elevated prolactin (144 ng/mL). Pregnancy test is negative. You immediately order an MRI of the brain, which shows a 7-mm pituitary microadenoma. During your follow-up visit, the patient asks you to describe her treatment plan and her long-term follow-up.

This patient has a prolactin-secreting microadenoma based on her hyperprolactinemia and evidence of pituitary tumor on MRI. Prolactinomas are the most common functioning pituitary tumors and often are diagnosed by gynecologists due to their disruption of the reproductive axis. The management of a patient with a prolactin-secreting microadenoma is dependent on the characteristics of the patient and her desire for fertility.

Although this patient has symptomatic menstrual dysfunction presenting as amenorrhea, many women with pituitary tumors are completely asymptomatic and are found incidentally. In autopsy studies, pituitary tumors are present in approximately 10% of women. To effectively treat and counsel patients, it is important to know the benign natural history of microadenomas. Less than 10% of prolactin-secreting microadenomas will enlarge over a 5-year period of follow-up. With such a low rate of progression, these tumors should not be treated solely to prevent growth. In an asymptomatic patient, it is reasonable to offer conservative management with occasional monitoring for progression. Serial prolactin levels and 1 to 2 follow-up imaging studies may be all that is needed to follow patients long-term. Any development of symptoms including vision changes, headaches, amenorrhea, or galactorrhea should prompt immediate evaluation for tumor growth with a repeat imaging study.

In contrast to an asymptomatic patient, this scenario presents a symptomatic patient with microadenoma and amenorrhea. Women may present with decreased libido, sexual or menstrual dysfunction, infertility, galactorrhea, hirsutism, or osteoporosis. Symptomatic patients warrant therapy over conservative management, yet the type of treatment is based mainly on the patient's desire for pregnancy.

If the patient actively wants to pursue pregnancy, treatment of the microadenoma and lowering of the prolactin level usually will restore reproductive function. Hyperprolactinemia suppresses the hypothalaimic-pituitary-gonadal axis through inhibition of the pulsatile gonadotropin-releasing hormone, as well as decreased luteinizing hormone, follicle-stimulating hormone, and suppression of gonadal steroidogenesis. A dopamine agonist is the most effective way of lowering the prolactin and resuming ovulation. Dopamine agonists lower prolactin by binding to the dopamine receptors and mimicking dopamine's inhibitory effect on pituitary prolactin secretion. DNA synthesis, prolactin mRNA production, cell multiplication, and tumor growth are all reduced. Mechanisms of action are similar among the dopamine agonists, but they differ in side effect profile and dosing. Of the dopamine agonists, cabergoline is often touted as the first-line treatment due to its superior effectiveness and limited side effects; however, when fertility is the major reason for treatment or during pregnancy, current guidelines recommend the use of bromocriptine. With treatment, normalization of prolactin levels and return of regular menses occur in >80% of patients with microadenomas. In these patients, prolactin levels should be checked after 1 to 2 months of therapy and monitored periodically thereafter.

In a patient who does not desire pregnancy and has no bothersome symptoms, the lack of estrogen may be the only true concern. These patients can be safely treated with estrogen replacement or oral contraceptive pills. Although rare, case reports have documented prolactinoma growth during estrogen treatment, and periodic measurement of prolactin levels are indicated. MRI may be repeated to assure stability and should be performed with an increase in prolactin levels or appearance of symptoms.

Another clinical situation encountered by obstetricians is microadenoma in pregnancy. Normal pregnancy physiology causes an increase in estrogen, which leads to an increase in prolactin synthesis and lactotroph hyperplasia leading to pituitary enlargement. Although prolactinomas may also increase in size, it has been well established that the tumor growth is unlikely to be clinically significant and the overall risk for clinically significant growth of microprolactinoma is 2.6%. In women requiring dopamine agonist treatment for fertility, bromocriptine is the most widely studied dopamine agonist in pregnancy. There have been no increases in spontaneous abortion, ectopic pregnancy, or congenital malformations with the use of bromocriptine. However, since it has not been well studied when taken throughout pregnancy, it is advised to limit fetal exposure to bromocriptine as much as possible and stop treatment with confirmation of pregnancy.

Of note, prolactin levels are unreliable during pregnancy and do not give additional information. Patients with microadenomas should only be subjected to repeat imaging if they become symptomatic and should only be retreated with dopamine agonists for significant tumor growth.

TAKE HOME POINTS

- Prolactin-secreting microadenomas are the most common functional pituitary tumor.
- The natural history of microadenomas is benign with low chance for significant progression.
- Treatment of hyperprolactinemia associated with microadenoma depends on patient characteristics and desires for fertility.
- Dopamine agonists are effective in restoring normal reproductive function in women with prolactin-secreting microadenomas.
- Although the pituitary normally increases in size during pregnancy, significant progression of microadenomas is rare during pregnancy.

SUGGESTED READINGS

Mancini T, Casanueva F, Giustina A. Hyperprolactinemia and Prolactinomas. *Endocrinol Metab Clin North Am*. 2008;37:67–99.

Molitch M. Medical management of prolactin-secreting pituitary adenomas. *Pituitary*. 2002;5:55–65.

Schlechte J. Approach to the patient. Long-term management of prolactinomas. *J Clin Endocrinol Metab*. 2007;92:2861–2865.

100

IDENTIFY THE SHAPE OF THE FUNDUS TO DETERMINE A SEPTATE UTERUS

VITALY A. KUSHNIR, MD

A 34-year-old Caucasian G3P0030 is undergoing evaluation for recurrent first trimester pregnancy loss. A hysterosalpingogram (HSG) reveals a uterine septum versus a bicornuate uterus. A 3D sonohysterogram is performed and a diagnosis of partial septate uterus is reached; the fundal contour is convex. An ultrasound-guided hysteroscopic resection of the uterine septum is performed. The next pregnancy results in a term delivery.

Women with history of recurrent pregnancy loss have a 5% to 10% incidence of uterine anomalies versus 3% to 4% in the general population, while women with preterm deliveries have a 25% incidence. Development of the female genital tract involves a series of events including cellular differentiation, migration, fusion, and canalization. Failure of any of these processes can lead to an anomaly. Female reproductive tract anomalies are categorized according to American Fertility Society (AFS) classification system. A basic understanding of embryology is the key to evaluating and treating patients with anomalies. Additionally, identification of associated renal and skeletal anomalies is important prior to initiating treatment.

Müllerian anomalies arise through three mechanisms:

1. Failure of organogenesis of one or both müllerian ducts
2. Failure or fusion of müllerian ducts in the midline or to the urogenital sinus
3. Failure of resorption of the uterine septum or central vaginal cells (canalization)

A number of studies are available to evaluate the reproductive tract for possible anomalies. HSG is the traditional study that involves injection of contrast through cervix followed by fluoroscopy. It allows mapping of the uterine cavity and fallopian tubes; however, the external contour of the uterus is not evaluated with this study. 3D ultrasound with contrast enhancing solution is the study of choice for evaluation of uterine malformations. MRI can be useful in complex cases to help delineate the anatomy.

Concomitant hysteroscopy and laparoscopy remains the gold standard for diagnosis and, in some cases, treatment of müllerian anomalies; however, with recent advances in ultrasound, this should not be the primary modality for evaluation. Normal and arcuate uteri have a uniformly straight or convex external contour with an indentation <10 mm. In a bicornuate uterus, the external contour has an indentation >10 mm.

Treatment of uterine septum is most often achieved though a hysteroscopic resection with either laparoscopic or ultrasound guidance. Multiple studies have documented improvement in pregnancy outcome after resection of a uterine septum. Several techniques of metroplasty have been described to reconstruct a "normal" uterine cavity; however, there are limited data on outcomes, and this approach should be reserved for patients with history of poor obstetrical outcomes.

TAKE HOME POINTS

- Congenital anomalies of the female reproductive tract are a result of disruption of normal embryologic development. The main mechanisms are agenesis, failure of fusion, and failure of canalization.
- 3D ultrasonography and MRI are preferred imaging modalities for müllerian anomalies.
- In women with recurrent abortion, a hysteroscopic resection of a septum can improve pregnancy outcome.

SUGGESTED READINGS

Acien P. Reproductive performance of women with uterine malformations. *Hum Reprod.* 1993;8:122.

The American Fertility Society. The American Fertility Society classifications of adnexal adhesions, distal tubal occlusion, tubal occlusion secondary to tubal ligation, tubal pregnancies, mullerian anomalies and intrauterine adhesions. *Fertil Steril.* 1988;49:944.

Goldenberg M, Sivan E, Sharabi Z, et al. Reproductive outcome following hysteroscopic management of intrauterine septum and adhesions. *Hum Reprod.* 1995;10(10):2663–2665.

Rock JA, Azziz R. Genital anomalies in childhood. *Clin Obstet Gynecol.* 1987;30:682.

101

IMAGING THE ADNEXA

DONNA R. SESSION, MD

For improved visualization and patient comfort, the patient's bladder should be empty prior to performing a transvaginal ultrasound. If transvaginal visualization of the ovaries is difficult, gentle downward pressure over the lower abdominal wall may guide a mobile ovary toward the vaginal probe. If proper transvaginal imaging of the ovaries is still not possible, a transabdominal scan may be helpful.

Signs of ovulation may include a decrease in size of the follicle, loss of sharp borders, peritoneal fluid, and echoes in the follicle. After ovulation, the follicle becomes a corpus luteum. Sonographically, the corpus luteum typically has an echogenic appearance from an admixture of luteinized granulosa cells with blood although it can be sonolucent. The blood within the corpus luteum organizes and then degenerates into a pattern resembling spider webs as the clot retracts from the walls of the follicle. Retracted clot may also appear as a solid component of the cyst. The variable appearance makes the corpus luteum difficult to differentiate from an endometrioma, a neoplasm, or an ectopic pregnancy. However, the corpus luteum usually lasts for about 2 weeks and then involutes in the absence of pregnancy.

An adnexal mass is usually present in the case of adnexal torsion and Doppler flow to the adnexa may be useful in ruling this out. Doppler is useful in identifying blood flow; however, if the color priority is not set high enough relative to gray scale imaging setting, an impression of lack of flow may be falsely created. Thus, it is important to perform color imaging of the contralateral ovary to confirm the sensitivity of the settings.

Visualization of either pelvic blood vessels or hydrosalpinges in a cross-sectional plane may mimic the appearance of a large follicle or cyst. Rotating the probe to a longitudinal plane will change the spherical appearance of these structures to an oblong shape but will not affect the round appearance of a follicle. Incomplete septi may distinguish the tube from a septated ovarian cyst, in which the septa transverse the entire length of the cyst. Color Doppler may also be useful to rule out a vascular structure. A paraovarian cyst remains spherical despite changing the position of the sonographic probe but is easily identified by its location outside the ovary.

TAKE HOME POINTS

- The corpus luteum's appearance is variable and may be mistaken for an endometrioma or neoplasm, but it generally regresses within 2 weeks. Most functional cysts resolve within 6 weeks.
- Doppler is useful in identifying blood flow; however, if the color priority is not set high enough relative to gray scale imaging setting, an impression of lack of flow may be falsely created.

SUGGESTED READINGS

Fleischer AC, Cullinan JA, Jones HW III, et al., Serial assessment of adnexal masses with transvaginal color Doppler sonography. *Ultrasound Med Biol* 1995;21:435-441.

Hackeloer BJ, Sallam HN. Ultrasound scanning of ovarian follicles. *Clinics in Obstet Gynaecol* 1983;10:603-20.

Timor-Tritsch IE, Lerner JP, Monteagudo A et al., Transvaginal sonographic markers of tubal inflammatory disease. *Ultrasound Obstet Gynecol* 1998;12:56–66.

102

IMAGING THE UTERUS

DONNA R. SESSION, MD

During the menses, the endometrium is shed to the basalis layer. At this time, on ultrasound, the endometrium appears as a single, thin, echogenic line. If the patient is actively menstruating, blood may be identified as both echolucenies and more echogenic clot. If sonohysterography is performed during this time, blood clots may appear similar to polyps; however, clots are more mobile. Bleeding may also cause thin fibrin bands, which appear similar to uterine synechiae; however, these also are very mobile and may be disrupted with the sonohysterography catheter.

Endometrial thickness is measured transvaginally. Transabdominally, pressure from a full bladder may compress the endometrium making it appear thinner. The thickness is measured anterior to posterior with the uterus in the sagittal plane (long axis). The sagittal plane may be confirmed by identifying the cervix in the same plane to prevent falsely increased measurements through an oblique plane. The thickest area is measured from basalis to basalis, excluding any fluid. The hypoechoic inner myometrium is also excluded in order to not overestimate the thickness.

Polyps, which appear as well-circumscribed echogenic masses, should have a definite pedicle between the polyp and the endometrium when viewed during sonohysterography. Polyps usually have a single vessel identified with color Doppler. Polyps are best visualized in the follicular phase as the echogenicity may be similar to luteal phase endometrium. The hyperechoic pattern progresses from the basalis inward and usually becomes homogeneous by 7 days postovulation. Polyps are usually more echogenic than fibroids, typically do not indent the adjacent endometrium, and do not have an intramural component.

Transvaginal ultrasound demonstrates leiomyomas to be generally spherical, solid, and heterogeneous. They are well circumscribed and may appear to be encapsulated. Encapsulation and heterogeneity distinguish the leiomyoma from the surrounding myometrium. Their appearance may be altered by infarction, hemorrhage, necrosis, or calcification. Infarction, hemorrhage, and necrosis may appear sonolucent. Keep in mind several pitfalls when imaging leiomyomas as noncontrast sonography has been reported to miss 30% to 40% of leiomyomata. They are often multiple and become quite large. If the uterus is large, a transvaginal scan may be limited. In this case, an additional transabdominal scan is helpful, particularly if the leiomyoma are fundal and pedunculated. In addition, a fundal myoma may not be detected with a transvaginal scan due to the distance from the probe. Shadowing may partially obscure the image resulting in difficulty evaluating the endometrium, adnexa, or additional fibroids. Myometrial contractions can be misinterpreted as leiomyomata. A myometrial contraction can be distinguished from a leiomyoma as it is transient, usually homogeneous, and does not shadow.

The incidence of congenital uterine anomalies is estimated to be 1 in 400 women of reproductive age. Sonohysterography can accurately diagnose a septate uterus. In a septate uterus, the conformity of the fundus does not change when scanned longitudinally from left to right or vice versa. Two cavities are evident in the transverse plane. A bicornuate uterus will have a heart shape of both the external contour and the endometrial contour. A unicornuate uterus is usually deviated laterally and maintains a circular structure, internally and externally, from the cervix to the fundus in the transverse view. The normal uterus is circular in the lower portion and becomes oval at the fundus.

An axial uterus may be difficult to image. Gentle downward pressure over the lower abdominal wall may change the position to retroverted improving the image.

TAKE HOME POINTS

- The endometrial thickness is measured transvaginally, anterior to posterior in the sagittal plane, excluding any fluid, with the cervix in the same plane to prevent falsely increased measurements.
- A transabdominal scan is helpful when leiomyomata are suspected.
- A myometrial contraction can be distinguished from a leiomyoma as it is transient, usually homogeneous, and does not shadow.
- Blood may mimic polyps and synechiae, but blood is usually mobile and easily disrupted with a sonohysterogram catheter. Repeating the exam when the patient is not bleeding may also be helpful.

SUGGESTED READINGS

Green LK, Harris RE. Uterine anomalies. Frequency of diagnosis and associated obstetrical complications. *Obstet Gynecol*. 1976;47:427–429.

Gross BH, Silver TM, Jaffe MH. Sonographic features of uterine leiomyomas: analysis of 41 proven cases. *J Ultrasound Med*. 1983;2:401–406.

Grunfeld L, Walker B, Bergh PA, et al. High resolution endovaginal ultrasonography of the endometrium: a noninvasive test for endometrial adequacy. *Obstet Gynecol*. 1991;78: 200–204.

Randolph JR, Ying YK, Maier DB, et al. Comparison of real-time ultrasonography, hysterosalpingography, and laparoscopy/hysteroscopy in the evaluation of uterine abnormalities and tubal patency. *Fertil Steril*. 1986;46:828–832.

103

DO NOT DELAY AN INFERTILITY EVALUATION

SPENCER S. RICHLIN, MD AND MARK P. LEONDIRES, MD

Infertility is defined as 1 year of unprotected intercourse without conception. Pregnancy rates depend mostly upon the female partner's age. A couple's chance of conceiving declines with increasing age and duration of infertility. In general, cycle fecundability is 20%. Eighty-five percent of young couples conceive within 1 year. Women under 35 years of age should seek care after 1 year of unprotected intercourse, while those over 35 should be offered evaluation immediately. A common error is to delay the initial evaluation, especially if a factor for infertility is suspected (male factor, anovulation, pelvic factor, or advanced age above 35).

The advancements in the field of reproductive medicine have allowed couples to become pregnant who in the past could not. The development of assisted reproductive technologies (ART) and in vitro fertilization (IVF) has opened the door to family building for many couples. While the perception is that IVF is associated with a very high incidence of higher order multiples, the reality is that ovulation induction with insemination is more the culprit than IVF.

EVALUATION

The causes of infertility can be categorized into five broad causes. They include ovulatory dysfunction (15%), peritoneal and tubal pathologies (35%), male factor (35%), unexplained (10%), and unusual causes (5%) of infertility. The initial infertility evaluation addresses these etiologies. Evaluation should include confirmation of ovulation, hysterosalpingography (HSG), a baseline transvaginal ultrasound (note the position of ovaries, integrity of the uterine stripe, and an evaluation for myomas), semen analysis, menstrual cycle day 3 follicle-stimulating hormone (FSH) and estradiol (E2) level, and screening blood work. The results of these studies, in concert with the history and physical exam, will direct the treatment plan. It would be an error not to initiate a complete evaluation when consulting a patient or couple for infertility. Even if your working diagnosis is ovulatory dysfunction and the treatment plan is clomiphene citrate, by not completing the evaluation, a pelvic or a male factor may be missed. Couples who are trying to become pregnant deserve a complete evaluation as time is of the essence. If many months are spent in treatment with an errant or incomplete diagnosis, patients feel frustrated and may not return to your practice for obstetrical care.

Unexplained infertility is diagnosed when the infertility evaluation reveals no obvious abnormalities. Couples who are unexplained have a normal uterine cavity and patent tubes, are ovulatory, and have a normal semen analysis and ovarian reserve testing. Couples older than 35 years by definition most likely have age-related subfertility and are not unexplained. In the past, many couples diagnosed with unexplained infertility underwent diagnostic laparoscopy. With the advent of ovulation induction and IVF, the majority of couples do not pursue diagnostic laparoscopy. Moderate and severe pelvic diseases are treated with IVF. The treatment of unexplained infertility is empiric and includes ovulation induction and IVF.

Screening blood work is done at the initial office visit. It includes serology for STDs, rubella, cystic fibrosis, and genetic studies based on the patient's ethnicity. Parvovirus titer and varicella zoster titer should also be considered. A thyroid-stimulating hormone (TSH) and a prolactin are part of a basic evaluation. If the prolactin is elevated (based on your laboratory criteria), it needs to be repeated fasting. A common error is not to repeat it fasting. Prolactin can be falsely elevated by eating, intercourse, nipple stimulation, and exercise. In order to avoid a falsely elevated prolactin, we tell patients to repeat their prolactin fasting in the early morning. If the repeat is elevated, a brain MRI may be warranted prior to starting a prolactin-lowering agent. TSH and free thyroxine (FT4) need to be normal before attempting pregnancy. Hypothyroidism can cause ovulatory dysfunction, lead to pregnancy complications, and will affect the health and development of the fetus and newborn. Subclinical hypothyroidism (elevated TSH and a normal FT4) has been associated with pregnancy loss and even recurrent pregnancy loss. TSH levels should range from 0.45 to 3.0 mIU/L while attempting pregnancy. Patients with primary hypothyroidism can have secondary hyperprolactinemia from the stimulatory effects of thyrotropin-releasing hormone at the lactotroph. Treatment with levothyroxine sodium (Synthroid) will correct the hypothyroidism and normalize the prolactin level. Referral for thyroid management and evaluation for a low TSH (i.e., hyperthyroidism) should be a regular practice.

TAKE HOME POINTS

- Complete a complete infertility evaluation on all patients who desire pregnancy.
- Prolactin can be falsely elevated by eating, intercourse, nipple stimulation, and exercise.
- Hyperprolactinemia with hypothyroidism is treated with a thyroid replacement medication, such as Synthroid, not prolactin-lowering agents.

SUGGESTED READINGS

Balasch J. Investigation of the infertile couple: investigation of the infertile couple in the era of assisted reproductive technology: a time for reappraisal. *Hum Reprod.* 2000;15(11): 2251–2257.

Gleicher N, Barad D. Unexplained infertility: does it really exist? *Hum Reprod.* 2006;21(8): 1951–1955.

Raber W, Nowotny P, Vytiska–Binstorfer E, et al. Thyroxine treatment modified in infertile women according to thyroxine-releasing hormone testing: 5 year follow-up of 283 women referred after exclusion of absolute causes of infertility. *Hum Reprod.* 2003;18(4):707–714.

104

TRANSVAGINAL ULTRASOUND: TAKE A LOOK!

SPENCER S. RICHLIN, MD AND MARK P. LEONDIRES, MD

Transvaginal ultrasound is an integral part of the infertility evaluation. It is noninvasive and allows evaluation of the uterus, ovaries, and pelvis. Day 3 is the best time to ultrasound the pelvis as the ovaries are suppressed. Prior to treatment, all patients should have a baseline ultrasound. The uterine myometrium is evaluated for fibroids and uterine malformations. It is very important to image and measure the endometrial stripe for contour and uniformity of echo. A deviation may represent a polyp, fibroid, or adhesion. Intracavitary lesions decrease implantation and pregnancy rates. Any hint of an intracavitary lesion should prompt an evaluation with a saline infusion sonogram (SIS). The SIS allows accurate visualization of the uterine cavity. Polyps, intracavitary fibroids, and adhesions are accurately seen with SIS. Prior to operative hysteroscopy, SIS allows the surgeon map out a surgical plan based on the location of the lesion. Polyps and submucous fibroids need to be removed, as they decrease implantation and pregnancy rates. The removal of intramural fibroids is controversial. Some reproductive surgeons remove intramural fibroids if they are larger than 5 cm. Before any infertility treatment, all patients should have some form of a cavity evaluation. This can be accomplished with an SIS or HSG. It would be an error to assume that a transvaginal ultrasound could accurately detect a lesion within the cavity.

Ovarian position, volume, antral follicle count, and appearance are noted at the initial visit. The ovary should be positioned above the iliac vessels. The ovary should not have complex cysts and the presence of a smooth echo textured cyst can be a sign of endometriosis. If the ovary is out of position or seemingly adhesed to the uterine fundus, the relationship between the ovary and the fallopian tube may be compromised leading to poor oocyte pick up. Ovarian volumes and antral follicle counts are used in conjunction with ovarian reserve testing (day 3 follicle stimulating hormone (FSH) or clomiphene citrate challenge test (CCCT)). An ovarian volume <3 cm^3 or an antral follicle count <6 connotes a poor response to superovulation, lower pregnancy rates, and a high cancellation rate with IVF. Ovarian volume and antral follicle counts are measured in the early follicular phase usually along with day 3 FSH testing. Other abnormalities may warrant a diagnostic laparoscopy.

Patients with malpositioned ovaries, persistent cysts, or a low antral follicle count need further evaluation. These patients have a low chance of pregnancy on their own or with clomiphene citrate. Suspect endometriosis and pelvic factor infertility in a patient with endometriomas.

TAKE HOME POINTS

- Complete a complete infertility evaluation on all patients who desire pregnancy.
- All patients should have a cavity evaluation (either an SIS or HSG).
- On day 3, obtain an E2, FSH, and antral follicle count. A single elevated FSH is a poor prognostic indicator even if subsequent levels return normal.

SUGGESTED READINGS

Dumesic DA, Damario MA, Session DA, et al. Ovarian morphology and serum hormone markers as predictors of ovarian follicle recruitment by gonadotropins for *in vitro* fertilization. *J Clin Endocrinol Metab*. 2001;86(6):2538–2543.

Lass A, Skull J, McVeigh E, et al. Measurement of ovarian volume by transvaginal sonography before ovulation induction with human menopausal gonadotrophin in-vitro fertilization can predict poor response. *Hum Reprod*. 1997;12:220–223.

Tomas C, Nuojua-Huttunen S, Martikainen H. Pretreatment transvaginal ultrasound examination predicts ovarian responsiveness to gonadotrophins in in-vitro fertilization. *Hum Reprod*. 1997;12:294–297.

105

INFERTILITY TREATMENT: KNOW THE OPTIONS

SPENCER S. RICHLIN, MD AND MARK P. LEONDIRES, MD

Clomiphene citrate (CC) is the initial agent of choice for the anovulatory or oligo-ovulatory patient. Over 75% of patients will ovulate. Patients who may not respond to CC include those with polycystic ovary syndrome (PCOS), elevated body mass index, and older age. Pregnancy rates in the anovulatory patient are 15% per cycle. In PCOS, the goal is monofollicular development. Multifollicular development in the anovulatory patient increases the risk for multiple pregnancy. At least one midfollicular transvaginal ultrasound should be completed in this patient to evaluate follicle number. Up to 75% of anovulatory patients treated with clomiphene will be pregnant within nine treatment cycles. The PCOS patient who is not ovulatory with CC may become ovulatory with weight loss or the addition of metformin. It is a common error to assume that all PCOS patients are overweight; in fact, 40% will have normal weights. Studies utilizing letrozole in the CC-resistant PCOS patients are promising. Letrozole is being used for this indication and superovulation but is not yet FDA approved. Anovulatory patients who do not respond to CC will respond to gonadotropins but their risk for higher order multiple gestations increases.

Patients with unexplained infertility by definition are ovulatory. CC and intrauterine insemination (IUI) is the initial treatment in the properly selected patient but is associated with pregnancy rates of only 5% to 8% per cycle. In general, patients under 35 are good candidates for CC. Patients over 35, or the patient with suspected age factor infertility, may need IVF. An error would be to use CC in patients with an elevated follicle-stimulating hormone (FSH), suspected pelvic factor, or in the patient who is above 35 and wants more aggressive treatment.

CC is meant to superovulate the patient with unexplained infertility. The goal of superovulation is to produce between two and four follicles, and a midfollicular ultrasound is needed to confirm an adequate response. With multiple follicles and oocytes produced, there is a higher probability that an oocyte will be picked up by the fallopian tube. The addition of IUI places a higher concentration of sperm into the uterine cavity. With intercourse, approximately 10% of the sperm swim to the uterine cavity. The majority die in the acidity of the vagina or within the cervix. Thus, superovulation and IUI bring the gametes closer together.

The couple with unexplained infertility has a monthly fecundity rate of 4.1% (*Table 105.1*). With CC and IUI, the monthly pregnancy rate increases to 8.3% (multiple pregnancy rate 8% to 10%). There is a limited role CC or insemination alone for the unexplained patient. Gonadotropins (FSH) and IUI give monthly pregnancy rates of 15% to 25%. The practitioner must be careful with gonadotropins; the multiple pregnancy rate can approach 30%. An error would be to have the unexplained patient do more than four CC with IUI cycles. The vast majority of pregnancies occur in the first four CC cycles. Subsequent cycles offer low pregnancy rates and lead to a higher degree of patient frustration and drop out from therapy. After four well-managed CC with IUI cycles, ovulation induction with gonadotropin or IVF is indicated.

When to refer your patients for IVF:

1. Four failed CC cycles
2. Unexplained infertility in a patient older than 35
3. Male factor infertility (i.e., <5 million motile sperm at time of IUI)
4. Diminished ovarian reserve
5. Tubal factor, endometriosis, pelvic adhesive disease, or multiple pelvic surgeries
6. Cancer patient prior to radiation or chemotherapy treatment
7. Couples who have sex-linked or autosomal-recessive disorders, or carry a balanced chromosomal translocation are candidates for IVF with pre-implantation diagnosis

TABLE 105.1	PREGNANCY RATES PER TREATMENT CYCLE: UNEXPLAINED INFERTILITY	
No treatment		4.1%
IUI alone		3.8%
CC alone		5.6%
CC + IUI		8.3%
Gonadotropins alone		7.7%
Gonadotropins + IUI		17.1%
IVF→ Pregnancy rates are center dependent. Individual center rates are available from the Society for Assisted Reproductive Technology (SART). Web site: www.SART.org		Age dependent

- Complete a complete infertility evaluation on all patients who desire pregnancy.
- In the unexplained patient, do not exceed four cycles of CC and IUI.
- In PCOS, the goal is monofollicular development.
- The goal of superovulation is to produce between two and four follicles, and a midfollicular ultrasound is needed to confirm an adequate response.

SUGGESTED READINGS

Hughes EG. The effectiveness of ovulation induction and intrauterine insemination in the treatment of persistent infertility: a meta-analysis. *Hum Reprod.* 1977;12:1865–1872.
Mitwally M. Use of an aromatase inhibitor for induction of ovulation in patients with an inadequate response to clomiphene citrate. *Fertil Steril.* 2001;75(2):305–309.

106

PRESENCE OF A MENSTRUAL CYCLE EQUALS FERTILITY

DIANA BROOMFIELD, MD, MBA, FACOG, FACS

Annie is a G1P0010 44-year-old female with a long history of secondary infertility. After graduating from law school at the age of 24 years, she landed a coveted job on Capitol Hill as a lobbyist. After 10 years, she met her husband, Frank a second-term senator who had two children ages 15 and 18. Although she and Frank had not used any form of contraception for the past 10 years, she never conceived despite many rendezvous of "timed intercourse." Annie was convinced that although she was almost 45, since she was "healthy," was a nonsmoker, did not use illicit drugs or alcohol, exercised regularly, and still had cycles (although lighter and less predictable), she must be fertile!

INSIGHT INTO INFERTILITY AND REPRODUCTIVE HEALTH

There are many myths and misconceptions surrounding infertility beginning with its true definition. Medically, infertility is the lack of conception after 1 year of unprotected intercourse if the woman is under 35 years old or 6 months of unprotected intercourse without conception if the female partner is over 35 years old. Infertility is not the inability to get pregnant after a set time of "attempting pregnancy"; it is simply unprotected intercourse without conception. There are over 61 million people of reproductive age living in the United States. Infertility affects nearly 25% of that population, roughly 15 million of them. Infertility is a chronic disease that affects not only the individual but also his or her family. This translates into an affected community of at least 90 million Americans. In fact, infertility impacts the entire social culture of America and has a significant impact on the reduction in the average number of children per family and can prove to be a significant setback with regard to family planning.

A RACE AGAINST THE CLOCK

In Annie's case, egg quality was one of the most important hurdles to conception, at least by the time she was in her mid to late 30s and certainly after age 40. Biologically, a female has the greatest amount of eggs at roughly 20 weeks old (in utero)—approximately 7 million eggs at that time.

By the time that she is born (20 weeks later), her egg quantity would have been reduced to only 2 million eggs, and by the time of puberty and her first menstrual cycle (usually by ages 12 to 13), a female's germ cell mass has been reduced to roughly 300,000 to 500,000 eggs. Although under the complex sequence of the hypothalaimic–pituitary–ovarian axis most of these primary follicles are lost to atresia or apoptosis, some of the primordial follicles will mature in response to FSH (and ovarian steroids and autocrine and paracrine factors) and as a result throughout her reproductive life a woman will ovulate nearly 450 oocytes. So from birth to menopause (cessation of menses), a woman will continuously lose hundreds of thousands of primary follicles. The primary physiologic factor that causes the eggs to diminish in quantity and quality is AGE and accelerated FSH levels (secondary to decreased inhibin B)! As a woman gets older, the rate of her oocyte loss increases. In the 10 to 15 years preceding menopause, there is acceleration of follicular loss. This loss is associated with increases in FSH and decreases in inhibin B and insulin-like growth factor (IGF-I).

For most women, there is a period of about 2 to 8 years (mean of 5 years) prior to menopause (the perimenopause) that is characterized by anovulation and cycle irregularities.

During this time, there is accelerated follicular loss that is typically ushered in when there are about 25,000 follicles remaining; this correlates to the woman's age of 37 to 38 and menopause usually occurs about 13 years later, average age of 51 in the United States. The depletion of follicular development is associated with decreased ovarian volume, egg quantity, and egg quality. During the perimenopausal transitional years, LH remains normal, but the FSH level is frequently >20 IU/L despite continued menstrual bleeding. Menopause is defined as permanent cessation of menstrual cycles and is ushered in when the total follicular number is <1,000 (regardless of age).

A woman is at her reproductive peak by age 25 and starts to decline ever so slightly around age 29. By the time a woman is 35 years old, there is an increased risk of compromise of her ovarian reserve. Thus, if a woman over 34 years of age is having unprotected intercourse for 6 or more months with no resulting pregnancy, she is deemed infertile and she should seek professional evaluation. When women approach age 37 to 38, there is a significant risk of ovarian compromise or dysfunction, thus, certainly as women approach age 40, it is imperative that they seek a fertility specialist immediately because time is of the essence! Having menstrual cycles, maintaining a good diet, exercising, and having a normal BMI do not predict normal ovarian function.

TAKE HOME POINTS

- Total number of eggs available for ovulation during the reproductive years is about 450.
- LH and Estradiol may remain within the normal range until menopause.
- FSH increases (probably because of decreasing inhibin B) as follicular atresia and apoptosis occur.
- The accelerated rate of follicular atresia begins when the number of follicles reaches about 25,000, which is typically as early as age 37 to 38.
- The perimenopausal period begins about 2 to 8 years before menopause and is usually associated with menstrual changes in cycle length and more frequent anovulatory cycles.
- The presence of menstrual cycles is not synonymous with fertility or egg quality, especially during the perimenopausal period.

SUGGESTED READINGS

Baker TG. A quantitative and cytological study of germ cells in human ovaries. *Proc Roy Soc Lond.* 1963;158:417.

Block E. Quantitative morphological investigations of the follicular system in women. *Acta Anat.* 1952;14:108.

Faddy MJ, Gosden RG, Gougeon A, et al. Accelerated disappearance of ovarian follicles in mid-life; implications for forecasting menopause. *Hum Reprod.* 1992;7:1342.

Gougeon A, Ecochard R, Thalabard JC. Age-related changes of the population of human ovarian follicles: increase in the disappearance rate of non-growing and early growing follicles in aging women. *Biol Reprod.* 1994;50:653.

Metcalf MG, Livesay JH. Gonadotropin excretion in fertile women: effect of age and the onset of the menopausal transition. *J Endocrinol.* 1985;105:357.

Treloar AE, Boynton RE, Behn BG, et al. Variation of the human menstrual cycle through reproductive life. *Int J Fertil.* 1967;12:77.

107

Understanding ovulatory dysfunction

Spencer S. Richlin, MD and Mark P. Leondires, MD

Ovulatory dysfunction is usually manifested by irregular menstruation. Women who are ovulatory will have a history of regular predictable menses. Anovulatory patients will be irregular and often cycle at an interval of 37 to 60 days. Basal body temperature (BBT) monitoring and urinary LH kits are best reserved for regular cycling patients. In the patient with ovulatory dysfunction or irregular cycles, these tests are tedious and unreliable. In this circumstance, 1 or 2 luteal progesterone levels are the most diagnostic and helpful. Anovulatory patients should be evaluated and then placed on an appropriate ovulatory induction agent (clomiphene citrate or gonadotropins). The urinary LH kit is especially helpful for timing intercourse and artificial inseminations in ovulatory cycles. A positive LH surge predicts ovulation within 14 to 26 hours. Couples should have intercourse the day of the positive surge and the following 2 days.

Serum progesterone levels above 10 ng/mL on day 21 of the cycle signify adequate levels and ovulation. Since progesterone is a pulsatile hormone, a single measurement has variability and is not a perfect indicator of ovulation. Nevertheless, we use progesterone levels (10 ng/mL and above) as a loose indication of ovulation in both natural and ovulation induction cycles.

The endometrial biopsy is no longer used as a test to confirm ovulation. Urinary LH testing, BBT, and serum progesterone are as accurate while not being as invasive and painful as a biopsy. Historically, a luteal deficiency was diagnosed with an endometrial biopsy. Histological and sampling dates in the luteal phase that were >2 days out of phase signified a luteal phase defect and were thought to cause infertility and pregnancy loss. Out of phase biopsies poorly discriminate between fertile and infertile women and 20% to 30% of these biopsies are found in normal cycles. The endometrial biopsy to diagnose ovulation or a luteal phase defect has fallen out of favor and is rarely used by reproductive endocrinologists.

A luteal phase of <12 days, measured from the LH surge to the onset on menstruation, may represent a luteal phase defect. A short luteal phase reflects poor corpus luteum progesterone production. The luteal phase defect as a cause of infertility is controversial. The etiology of a shortened luteal phase includes abnormal pituitary LH and FSH secretion, hyperprolactinemia, and hypothyroidism. Correction of thyroid disease and treatment of hyperprolactinemia will correct the defect and lengthen the luteal phase. Couples with a shortened luteal phase and normal thyroid and prolactin levels can be treated with clomiphene citrate or vaginal progesterone suppositories.

TAKE HOME POINTS

- Complete a complete infertility evaluation on all patients who desire pregnancy.
- On day 3, obtain an E2, FSH, and antral follicle count. A single elevated FSH is a poor prognostic indicator even if subsequent levels return to normal.
- Couples with a shortened luteal phase and normal thyroid and prolactin levels can be treated with clomiphene citrate or vaginal progesterone suppositories.
- The endometrial biopsy is no longer used as a test to confirm ovulation. Urinary LH testing, BBT, and serum progesterone are as accurate while not being as invasive and painful as a biopsy.
- Serum progesterone levels above 10 ng/mL on day 21 of the cycle signify adequate levels and ovulation.

SUGGESTED READINGS

Hammond MG, Talbert LM. Clomiphene citrate therapy of infertile women with low luteal phase progesterone levels. *Obstet Gynecol.* 1982;59:275–279.
Sherman BM, Korenman SG. Measurement of plasma LH, FSH, estradiol and progesterone in disorders of the human menstrual cycle: the short luteal phase. *Obstet Gynecol Surv.* 1974;29:820–822.

"DOES AMH HOLD VALUE?": OVARIAN RESERVE TESTING

A. JASON VAUGHT, MD

There are recent data to suggest that Antimüllerian hormone (AMH) may be used for ovarian reserve testing. Unlike follicle-stimulating hormone (FSH), AMH can be measured at anytime in the female cycle, because AMH concentration is gonadotropin and hormone independent. This means it is thought to be unaffected by oral contraception and other exogenous hormones.

AMH is produced by the preantral follicle and small antral follicle. AMH production actually starts when the follicles differentiate from the primordial to the primary stage, and AMH stops after the follicles become recruited and reach a diameter of >8 mm. Therefore, the AMH level is correlated to the primordial pool, which means the higher the AMH, the better the ovarian reserve.

Although the actual role of AMH in the female is unclear, data suggest that it may be a modulator of follicular recruiter. It is also known to have inhibitory effects on the population of primordial follicles, acting on pregranulosa limiting the number of follicles being recruited. Therefore, it is hypothesized that AMH actually decreases the sensitivity of the primordial follicle to FSH.

An AMH level >2.7 ng/mL is associated with high level of occurrence of implantation and pregnancy.

TAKE HOME POINTS

- AMH is a new serologic test.
- It is an excellent marker for ovarian reserve.
- One does not have to wait on a particular cycle day.
- One can be taking exogenous gonadotropins or hormones and AMH will not be affected.

SUGGESTED READINGS

De Carvalho BR, Rosa e Silva AC, Rosa e Silva JC, et al. Ovarian reserve evaluation: state of the art. *J Assist Reprod Genet*. 2008;25:311–322.

Kwee J, Schats R, McDonnell J, et al. Evaluation of anti-Mullerian hormone as a test for the prediction of ovarian reserve. *Fertil Steril*. 2008;90:737–743.

"DO NOT PUT ALL YOUR EGGS IN ONE BASKET!": SONOGRAPHIC TESTING FOR OVARIAN RESERVE

A. JASON VAUGHT, MD

"WHERE DID ALL OF MY FOLLICLES GO?"

Early follicular phase antral follicle counts (AFCs) have also come into use for ovarian reserve. An ultrasonographer counts follicles in each ovary. Generally, a value from 10 to 20 is associated with good reserve. The AFC is often done on day 3 with FSH and estriadol because the patient is usually already in the office. It is thought that the greater the number of antral follicles, the better the ovarian reserve.

It is known that the AFC decreases with age, allowing us to believe that the lower the AFC, the lower the fecundability. Women with AFC less than five follicles per ovary are thought to be poor responders to controlled ovarian hyperstimulation and are thought to have decreased ovarian reserve.

Ovarian volume has also been thought to be a predictor of ovarian reserve. It is believed that the lower the ovarian volume, the lower the ovarian reserve. However, recent studies have concluded that this marker has little clinical applicability for the predictor of poor pregnancy response. However, ovarian measurements could be included in the preparatory protocols and for providing data for future research.

In conclusion, AFC is an excellent way to assess ovarian reserve. However, its downfalls are observed cycle differences and intraobserver differences. Also, if there is an AFC that is too high, such as >50 for both ovaries, it is thought that the person may have polycystic ovary syndrome (PCOS), which is associated with anovulatory cycles. If PCO–like ovaries are seen on ultrasound, the patient may need to have the appropriate workup.

TAKE HOME POINTS

- AFC is a recognized way to assess ovarian reserve and should be done on day 2 to 5 of the cycle.
- Be sure to correlate AFC with hormonal testing as well.
- Sonographic testing is both cycle and observer dependent.
- Having an AFC that is too high, that is, >25 per ovary or >50 for both ovaries, can be a sign of PCOS.

SUGGESTED READINGS

De Carvalho BR, Rose e Silva AC, Rose e Silva JC, et al. Ovarian reserve evaluation: state of the art. *J Assist Reprod Genet*. 2008;25:311–322.

Coccia ME, Rizzelo F. Ovarian reserve. *Ann NY Acad Sci*. 2008;1127:27–30.

110

"Wow, my FSH is high: That is great, Right?"

A. Jason Vaught, MD

The FSH Value

The purpose of ovarian testing is to assess the likelihood of pregnancy with assisted reproductive technology or with future in vitro fertilization (IVF) cycles. These tests are testing the "ovarian reserve," which describes the size and the quality of the remaining follicular pool.

The most widely accepted tool for testing ovarian reserve is the day 3 (day 2 to 5) FSH. With age comes decreased fertility and elevated serum FSH levels, which is why it is widely believed day 3 FSH is an excellent tool for assessing ovarian reserve. It is thought that in most laboratories a day 3 FSH of 10 to 15 is abnormal.

However, it should be noted that different laboratories use different assay systems with different antibodies and thus FSH values can vary between different labs. Therefore, if a patient has an outside hospital FSH level, it may be worth your while to redo the test in your own lab or lab that you currently use for all of your patients.

Along with a day 3 FSH, one can also use a day 3 estradiol. It is thought that a level >80 can be associated with decreased fecundability. Higher cycle day 3 estradiol levels reflect advanced follicular development and *too* early of a selection of a dominant follicle, which is observed in older cycling women and is driven by heightened FSH levels.

However, it should be noted that an increased level of estradiol can cause a decrease in serum FSH level, masking a level that would otherwise reflect a low ovarian reserve. This would give you a false-negative test.

The clomiphene citrate test is another way to assess ovarian reserve by measuring gonadotropin levels under both basal and stimulated conditions before cycle day 3 and after cycle day 10. The clomid or clomiphene citrate is given from cycle days 5 to 9. In normal, fertile cycling women, there is a transient rise in gonadotropin levels where LH will be greater than FSH. However, in women with low ovarian reserve, the pattern may be reversed with FSH greater than LH. The day 10 estradiol has no prognostic value. The clomiphene citrate test can identify women who might otherwise have gone unrecognized by basal FSH levels alone.

- Make sure to measure a day 3 or day 2 to 5 FSH for accurate diagnosis.
- Be sure to also obtain a day 3 or day 2 to 5 estradiol level to correlate with the FSH.
- If the estradiol is too high, it can cause a decrease in FSH, giving you a false-negative test.
- Clomiphene citrate test can identify women with low ovarian reserve who would have gone unidentified on basal FSH alone.
- Day 10 estradiol of a clomiphene citrate test is not diagnostic.

SUGGESTED READING

Speroff L, Fritz MA, eds. *Clinical Gynecologic Endocrinology and Infertility.* 7th ed. Philadelphia, PA: Lippincott Williams & Wilkins; 2005.

111

OVARIAN RESERVE TESTING: FINDING THE EGG

SPENCER S. RICHLIN, MD AND MARK P. LEONDIRES, MD

Ovarian reserve is a barometer of a woman's reproductive potential. It represents oocyte number and quality and is a prognostic indicator for future pregnancy. The first measure of reproductive fitness is age. A patient's age, follicle-stimulating hormone (FSH), and basal antral follicle counts have become the screening triad for a potential pregnancy. Ovarian reserve testing is performed by measuring a menstrual cycle day 3 FSH and an estradiol (can be done on days 2 to 4). A normal day 3 FSH is under 10 mIU/mL and the estradiol needs to be under 80 pg/mL. A common error is not to order the concomitant estradiol as a high estradiol negates the predictive value of the test. A baseline ultrasound should be performed in conjunction with the day 3 FSH to count antral follicles (follicles <10 mm). A normal antral follicle count is above 6. Counts below 6 predict a higher cancellation rate and decreased pregnancy rates with ART cycles. An elevated FSH level is an independent predictor for poor reproductive performance. At the level of the follicle, levels of inhibin B decrease and FSH levels increase signifying a diminished ovarian reserve. This is most often seen in women above 35 as fertility begins to decline. In general, with increasing age, we see FSH levels rise. An error would be to tell a couple with an elevated FSH that they cannot become pregnant. An elevated FSH does not preclude pregnancy but will decrease pregnancy rates below a patient's age-expected rate. This should trigger counseling and aggressive treatment for subfertility.

Clinicians need to be familiar with their laboratory's FSH assay and its cut point for poor reproductive performance. There is a threshold level of FSH, above which conception is unlikely. In most laboratories, an FSH above 10 mIU/mL is considered abnormal and predicts a pregnancy rate of 5%. An elevated FSH is likely correlated with increased embryo aneuploidy and pregnancy loss. Therefore, if a level above 10 IU/L is noted, it should be addressed and a referral for fertility treatment should be strongly considered. It is important to note that there is intercycle variability of FSH levels. If a day 3 FSH level is elevated above 10, you cannot ignore it. A single elevated FSH is a poor prognostic indicator. If it is repeated and becomes <10, the patient still has the diagnosis of diminished ovarian reserve. Assume that your patient will have differing day 3 FSH values from month to month.

Even though ovarian reserve testing predicts success with advanced reproductive technologies (ART) and in vitro fertilization (IVF), basal FSH testing can be extrapolated to the general infertility patients in your practice. Who should be tested:

1. Couples regardless of age with unexplained infertility
2. Women 30 years of age and older
3. Patients with recurrent pregnancy loss
4. Patients with poor response to gonadotropin stimulation
5. Patients with a family history of early menopause
6. Patients who smoke or have had adnexal surgery

TAKE HOME POINTS

- Complete a complete infertility evaluation on all patients who desire pregnancy.
- On day 3, obtain an E_2, FSH, and antral follicle count. A single elevated FSH is a poor prognostic indicator even if subsequent levels return to normal.
- An elevated FSH is likely correlated with increased embryo aneuploidy and pregnancy loss.

SUGGESTED READINGS

Chang M. Use of the antral follicle count to predict the outcome of assisted reproductive technologies. *Fertil Steril*. 1998;69:505–510.

Navot D, Drews MR, Bergh PA, et al. Age related decline in female fertility is not due to diminished capacity of the uterus to sustain embryo implantation. *Fertil Steril*. 1994;61:97–101.

Navot D, Rosenwaks A, Mergalioth EJ. Prognostic assessment of female fecundity. Lancet 1987;332:645–647.

Tietze C. Reproductive span and rate of reproduction among Hutterite women. *Fertil Steril*. 8:89–97.

SEMEN ANALYSIS: DO NOT FORGET THE BOYS!

SPENCER S. RICHLIN, MD AND MARK P. LEONDIRES, MD

The semen analysis (SA) is the first step in evaluating the male partner. Abstinence for 2 to 3 days is recommended. A common error is not to get this at the beginning of discussions about subfertility as it represents one third of infertility problems and is usually easily overcome. The World Health Organization (WHO) has established normal reference ranges: volume 1.5 to 5.0 mL, sperm concentration >20 million/mL, motility >50%, morphology >50%, forward progression >2 (0 to 4 scale). The probability of male factor infertility increases with worsening sperm parameters. Collection is by masturbation without any lubricants and should be analyzed within 1 hour of collection. Two samples are needed, 1 month apart, in order to obtain an accurate count.

A common error is not to refer the male to a reproductive urologist when the concentration is below 10 million/mL. The goal of this referral is to identify correctable conditions, irreversible conditions (the couple may need IVF or donor sperm), genetic abnormalities, or even life-threatening conditions (testicular cancer or pituitary abnormality). Additionally, if the count is normal and the morphology or motility is below the normal range, a referral should be initiated. Oftentimes, the addition of intrauterine insemination can overcome male factor infertility.

TAKE HOME POINTS

- Complete a complete infertility evaluation on all patients who desire pregnancy. This includes the SA.
- Obtain two semen analyses on a male. If parameters are abnormal, a urologic consultation is warranted to identify correctable causes.

SUGGESTED READINGS

Cooper TG, Noonan E, von Eckardstein S, et al. World Health Organization reference values for human semen characteristics. *Hum Reprod.* Update, December 4, 2009; Human Reproduction Update, doi:10.1093/humupd/dmp048

Guzick DS, Overstreet JW, Factor-Litvak P, et al. Sperm morphology, motility, and concentration in fertile and infertile men. *N Eng J Med.* 2001;345(19):1388–1393.

Smith KD, Rodriguez-Rigau LJ, Steinberger E. Relation between indices of semen analysis and pregnancy rate in infertile couples. *Fertil Steril.* 1977;28(12):1314–1319.

DO NOT FORGET THE TUBES!

SPENCER S. RICHLIN, MD AND MARK P. LEONDIRES, MD

Tubal factor infertility is a common cause of infertility. Risk factors for tubal pathology include pelvic inflammatory disease, appendicitis, ectopic pregnancy, and prior pelvic or abdominal surgery. The hysterosalpingogram (HSG) is the gold standard test to image the uterine cavity and evaluate tubal patency, architecture, and position. HSGs are scheduled 5 to 10 days after menses begins. Patients should take 800 mg of ibuprofen 1 hour prior to their appointment to minimize discomfort. The risk of a pelvic infection after an HSG is uncommon (1.4% to 3.4%) if there is normal anatomy. Antibiotics are indicated for HSG if there is a history of pelvic infection or the study reveals an abnormality such as dilated tubes or peritubal adhesions. A common error is to not administer doxycycline 100 mg twice daily for 5 days in the patient who had dilated tubes on an HSG. These patients have an infection rate up to 11% and should be treated.

Hysterosalpingography has a very important limitation. As a study, it reveals tubal patency but does not allow visualization of the tubo–ovarian relationship. A common error would be to assume that the relationship between the ovary and the tube is normal based on a normal HSG. A couple with a long duration of infertility and a normal evaluation may have an unsuspected pelvic factor (poor relationship between the tube and the ovary) and will benefit from a diagnostic laparoscopy or IVF.

Distal tubal occlusion can be corrected by laparoscopic fimbrioplasty or neosalpingostomy. Successful pregnancies after repair are based on the severity of disease before surgery and the result after. Patients are advised to attempt pregnancy immediately after any tubal surgery as their chances are best in the first 6 months. In addition, they should be counseled about the risk of an ectopic pregnancy. In vitro fertilization is the treatment of choice in patients with distal occlusion or dense pelvic adhesive disease. Pregnancy rates with IVF far exceed rates with distal tubal surgery.

The hydrosalpinx (fluid-filled tube) is a unique type of distal tubal occlusion. The distal end of a hydrosalpinx is often damaged and not amenable to surgical reconstruction or neosalpingostomy. Prospective studies show that hydrosalpinges decrease pregnancy rates 40% with IVF when compared to patients who do not have hydrosalpinges. The hydrosalpinx fluid either mechanically disrupts early implantation or is directly toxic to the endometrium or embryo. It would be an error at laparoscopy to leave a hydrosalpinx in situ and not remove it. All patients who are having laparoscopy for tubal and peritoneal infertility should be counseled that a hydrosalpinx will be removed or interrupted at its proximal attachment to the uterus. Hydrosalpinx should be recognized at the time of HSG.

Proximal tubal obstruction noted on an HSG is often a false positive. Up to 40% of the time, the tube is in fact open. Tubal ostia can spasm due to the contrast dye acting as an irritant. Besides tubal spasm, proximal obstruction can be caused by prior infection, mucous plugs, and chronic salpingitis. Hysteroscopic tubal cannulation utilizing a balloon catheter can aid in diagnosis and even open the ostia or alternatively tubal recanalization can be done by an interventional radiologist.

TAKE HOME POINTS

- Complete a complete infertility evaluation on all patients who desire pregnancy.
- Remove a hydrosalpinx at laparoscopy.
- Patients with tubal factor infertility should consider IVF.
- All patients should have a cavity evaluation (either an SIS or HSG).

SUGGESTED READINGS

Hurst BS, Tucker KE, Awoniyi CA, et al. Hydrosalpinx treated with extended doxycycline does not compromise the success of in vitro fertilization. *Fertil. Steril.* 2001;75(5):1017–1019.

Mol BWJ, Collins JA, Burrows EA, et al. Comparison of hysterosalpingography and laparoscopy in predicting fertility outcome. *Hum Reprod.* 1999;14(5):1237–1242.

Strandell A, Lindhard A. Why does hydrosalpinx reduce fertility? The importance of hydrosalpinx fluid. *Hum Reprod.* 2002;17(5):1141–1145.

114

HYDROSALPINGES AND INFERTILITY: DILATED AND DANGEROUS

ALBERT ASSANTE, MD

M.H. is a 30-year-old woman with 14 months of primary infertility. She has had regular 28- to 30-day menstrual cycle since menarche. Her only relevant gynecological history is an episode of laparoscopically proven PID 10 years ago. Cervical swabs at the time diagnosed Chlamydia. She was treated with broad-spectrum antibiotics and doxycycline. Abdominal and pelvic examination is unremarkable.

Blood taken on cycle day 21 for serum progesterone confirmed ovulation. Normal spermatogenesis was confirmed in M.H.'s partner. The need to establish the condition of the fallopian tubes, using laparoscopy with dye studies versus hysterosalpingogram, was discussed with the couple. M.H. opted to have a laparoscopy with dye studies because she decided that she wanted to have as much information about what had happened to her fallopian tubes as possible.

The laparoscopy demonstrated bilateral hydrosalpinges with extensive peritubular and periovarian adhesions. Bilaterally, there was passage of dye into the pelvis through pinhole ostia. At the postoperative visit, the irreversible nature of the damage was explained and the option for IVF was introduced.

Tubal and peritoneal pathologies are among the most common causes of infertility and the primary diagnosis in approximately 30% to 35% of infertile couples. Hydrosalpinx (a fallopian tube closed at the end and distended with fluid) is usually a consequence of pelvic infectious/inflammatory disease spreading into the fallopian tubes and pelvis via the cervix and uterus. The diagnosis of hydrosalpinx can be made by ultrasound alone, by hysterosalpingography and/or laparoscopy, or by any one of these three examinations.

Several retrospective and prospective studies have demonstrated the negative effect of hydrosalpinges on IVF success rates. Suggested mechanisms include a direct embryotoxic effect, mechanical flushing during implantation, and changes in endometrial receptivity.

Comprehensive meta-analyses have concluded that the likelihood for IVF success in women with hydrosalpinges is reduced by approximately half. Two treatment options are available for patients suffering from tubal infertility due to hydrosalpinges: IVF after removal of the tube or closure of the connection from the hydrosalpinx into the uterus or a surgical repair of the hydrosalpinx.

Results of a large multicenter randomized clinical trial have confirmed that salpingectomy is beneficial, most dramatically so in women with large hydrosalpinges visible by transvaginal ultrasound examination. However, not every woman with large hydrosalpinges should undergo salpingectomy as some fallopian tubes may be amenable to surgical repair. Preserved tubal mucosa indicates a good prognosis for tubal surgery; therefore, an appropriate mucosal assessment should be routine prior to deciding upon further management.

Discriminating between a hydrosalpinx that should be removed and one that is suitable for surgical repair is a difficult task; tubal endoscopy is the most advanced and appropriate tool for selecting patients to undergo either salpingectomy or salpingostomy.

In women for whom the risks of surgery are high, (e.g., marked obesity or dense pelvic adhesions), a less invasive alternative to surgical removal of the hydrosalpinges, placement of the Essure hysteroscopic sterilization device to block the tubes proximally, should be strongly considered.

TAKE HOME POINTS

- Even when the history is strongly suggestive of tubal factors as responsible for a patient's infertility, the routine investigations should be done first to confirm ovulation and normal spermatogenesis.
- Hysterosalpingogram would confirm tubal occlusion but not help to show the extent of the damage and the possible need for further surgery (either reconstructive or salpingectomy). Hysteroscopy, laparoscopy, and dye studies whilst more invasive provide more information that is useful in planning further management.
- A salpingectomy is indicated for infertility patients prior to in vitro fertilization if they have a documented hydrosalpinx on ultrasonography.
- Surgical distal tubal repair is appropriate only for patients with preserved tubal mucosa.
- Unnecessary salpingectomies should, of course, not be performed, and they may easily be avoided by appropriate evaluation of the tubal mucosa at laparoscopy before any final decision of salpingectomy is made.
- There is no comparative study of restorative tubal surgery versus salpingectomy and in vitro fertilization in selected women with hydrosalpinges.

SUGGESTED READINGS

Kontoravdis A, Makrakis E, Pantos K, et al. Proximal tubal occlusion and salpingectomy result in similar improvement in in vitro fertilization outcome in patients with hydrosalpinx. *Fertil Steril.* 2006;86(6):1642–1649.

Sabatini L, Davis C. The management of hydrosalpinges: tubal surgery or salpingectomy? *Curr Opin Obstet Gynecol.* 2005;17(4):323–328.

Strandell A. How to treat hydrosalpinges: IVF as the treatment of choice. *Reprod Biomed Online.* 2002;4(Suppl 3):37–39.

Strandell A, Lindhard A. Hydrosalpinx and ART. Salpingectomy prior to IVF can be recommended to a well-defined subgroup of patients. *Hum Reprod.* 2000;15(10): 2072–2074.

Strandell A, Lindhard A. Why does hydrosalpinx reduce fertility? The importance of hydrosalpinx fluid. *Hum Reprod.* 2002;17:1141–1145.

115

YOU HAVE GOT TO LOOK: PRETREATMENT WORKUP AND THE PITFALLS OF UNMONITORED CYCLES

SAMUEL A. PAULI, MD

One of the most frequent treatments offered to the infertile couple is ovulation induction. Infertility has been defined as the inability of a couple to conceive after 12 months of unprotected and frequent intercourse. In practice, patients may present with the inability to achieve pregnancy before 12 months and desire treatment options. Earlier evaluation and treatment may be warranted in women older than 35 years, as fecundity decreases with increasing maternal age. In addition, earlier evaluation is indicated in patients with amenorrhea or oligomenorrhea, tubal disease, endometriosis, or a history of chemotherapy.

A thorough evaluation for the cause of infertility should be completed before treatment is initiated to direct treatment strategy. Basic evaluation should include an assessment of ovulatory function by history, basal body temperatures, ovulation predictor kits, or an appropriately timed progesterone level. Fallopian tube patency can be confirmed by hysterosalpingogram or at the time of laparoscopy by chromopertubation. Ovarian reserve testing may be performed by measuring a day 3 follicle stimulating hormone and estradiol level, antimullerian hormone level, or a day 3 antral follicle count by ultrasound. A semen analysis should also be performed to rule out male factor infertility. Additional laboratory testing, as well as evaluation of the uterine cavity and abdomen, may be performed if clinically relevant.

The goal of ovulation induction is to stimulate multifollicular development to increase the chance of pregnancy or make a woman with oligomenorrhea ovulatory. To maximize the chance of success, treatment selection should take into account the reason for infertility. While the acumen of medications and protocols available to the clinician to achieve ovulation inductions is vast, the most widely utilized medication is clomiphene citrate (Clomid). Ovulation can be detected by the use of ovulation predictor kits or achieved by administration of recombinant or urinary-derived human chorionic gonadotropin (hCG) and coupled with timed intercourse or intrauterine inseminations.

Clomiphene is typically initiated between cycle days 2 and 6 and given for 5 days after a spontaneous or induced bleed. Minor side effects of clomiphene are common and include hot flashes, emotional lability, and headaches. Rarely, clomiphene can cause visual changes including halos and blurry vision. Pooled case-control studies have failed to demonstrate a relationship between clomiphene and ovarian cancer; however, one small retrospective case cohort study by Rossing et al. showed an increase in ovarian cancer in women who took >12 cycles of clomiphene. Studies have shown that the risk of congenital anomalies and rates of miscarriage are similar in patients taking clomiphene when compared to women who conceived naturally.

Most patients are typically started with an empiric dose of 50 mg and titrated up to a maximum dose of 150 mg. An ovulatory response to treatment can be demonstrated by a change of basal body temperatures from uniphasic to biphasic, detection of the LH surge, or an appropriately timed progesterone level. Alternatively, follicular development and an ovulatory response can be assessed by transvaginal monitoring. In patients with a minimal or no response to the first cycle of clomiphene, ultrasound monitoring allows for quicker titration of the dosage to establish the minimal effective dose to induce follicular development. This may also minimize the risk of ovarian hyperstimulation syndrome. In addition, monitoring allows for intracycle counseling regarding the risk of a multiple pregnancy giving patients the option to forgo intercourse or inseminations in the event of an exaggerated response. While ultrasound monitoring can aid in defining the optimal period for timed intercourse, it is essential in monitoring follicular development for the timing of hCG administration in anovulatory women.

Clomiphene administration with concomitant transvaginal monitoring offers additional benefits other than monitoring follicular development, aiding in triggering ovulation, and timing of coitus or inseminations. Ultrasound can assess endometrial thickness after clomiphene administration, as clomiphene has an antiestrogenic effect on the uterus. In the event of poor endometrial growth with a preovulatory endometrial thickness <6 mm, a clinician may wish to change his or her treatment approach. Monitoring also carries the added benefit of screening for ovarian cysts, which if functional may alter the ability to conceive during the concurrent cycle. Alternatively, if stimulated, ovarian cysts may enlarge and place the patient at risk for ovarian torsion. While torsion is rare, emergency surgical correction is necessary and there is a potential risk of loss of the ovary if not detected and treated in a timely fashion.

A study by Imani et al. demonstrated that approximately 78% of patients will ovulate with clomiphene treatment. Another study by the same group showed cumulative pregnancy rates as high as 73% after nine cycles of clomiphene. Success rates are lower in ovulatory women with unexplained infertility. If pregnancy is not achieved after three to six cycles of treatment, other causes of infertility should be evaluated and other treatment options explored.

TAKE HOME POINTS

- Basic evaluation should include an assessment of ovulatory function, confirmation of fallopian tube patency, and ovarian reserve testing.
- Clomiphene is given for 5 days starting between cycle days 2 and 6.
- Clomiphene has mild antiestrogenic side effects.
- The risks of birth defects and miscarriages in pregnancies conceived with clomiphene are similar to those observed in spontaneous pregnancies.
- Most studies have failed to demonstrate a risk of ovarian cancer with the use of clomiphene; however, one small study demonstrated increased risk with >12 cycles.
- Transvaginal ultrasound monitoring may be beneficial in determining response to treatment and minimize treatment risks.

SUGGESTED READINGS

Fauser BC, Macklon NS. Medical approaches to ovarian stimulation for infertility. In: Straus JF III, Barbieri RL, eds. *Yen and Jaffe's Reproductive Endocrinology: Physiology, Pathophysiology, and Clinical Management.* 5th ed. Philadelphia, PA: Elsevier; 2004.

Imani B, Eijkemans MJ, te Velde ER, et al. Predictors of patients remaining anovulatory during clomiphene citrate induction of ovulation in normogonadotropic oligoamenorrheic infertility. *J Clin Endocrinol Metab.* 1998;83(7):2361–2365.

Imani B, Eijkemans MJ, te Velde ER, et al. Predictors of chances to conceive in ovulatory patients during clomiphene citrate induction of ovulation in normogonadotrophic oligoamenorrheic infertility. *J Clin Endocrinol Metab.* 1999;84(5):1617–1622.

Rossing MA, Daling JR, Weiss NS, et al. Ovarian tumors in a cohort of infertile women. *N Engl J Med.* 1994;331(12):771–776.

Speroff L, Fritz MA. *Clinical Gynecologic Endocrinology and Infertility.* 7th ed. Philadelphia, PA: Lippincott Williams & Wilkins; 2005.

116

SOMETIMES HOT = FSH

PENNY CASTELLANO, MD, FACOG

A 48-year-old female, gravida 3, para 3, presents to her gynecologist's office stating that she has missed five menstrual periods in a row. She is sexually active and she uses barrier contraception (condoms). The patient also reports hot flashes and night sweats for the last 3 months. The provider notes the patient's age and symptoms and counsels her that she is "probably menopausal." FSH and estradiol levels are ordered. Results are 50 mIU/mL and 25 pg/mL, respectively. The patient is given her results and told that "menopause is confirmed." The patient begins to self-educate via the internet.

The diagnosis of menopause can be a point of confusion for both the patient and the provider. The definition of menopause is retrospective and clinical, requiring 1 year of elapsed time since the final menstrual period, accompanied by other signs of permanent ovarian failure. In many cases, patients present, and providers need to intervene and treat, before these definitive criteria have been met. The patient's status is unclear and the patient may be treated as being postmenopausal, when in fact she is not. Additionally, the symptoms that are attributed to menopause are various, with only a small subset having evidence to link them with the estrogen deficiency and hormonal fluctuations accompanying the menopausal transition.

Understanding of the physiology of the menopause transition has expanded in recent years. The transition itself is best viewed as a dynamic process that can take several years to complete. Several large studies have outlined the transition characteristics from the early subtle changes along the hypothalamic-pituitary-ovarian axis to early symptoms, such as irregular bleeding and vasomotor symptoms. It is important to understand that there is not a level of FSH or estradiol that can (in isolation) be considered diagnostic of menopause.

Ovarian aging is a slow transition that sets the stage for understanding the menopause transition overall. The currently recommended nomenclature was adopted from the Stages in Reproductive Aging Workshop (STRAW) from 2001 and does provide clarity. The menopause transition is defined as the entire evolution of reproductive status from full reproductive function to absence of reproductive function. The term "premenopause" is eliminated. Perimenopause spans the start of ovarian dysfunction (usually heralded by a change in menstrual bleeding pattern) to the point of defined menopause (1 year after the final menstrual period). The final menstrual period is defined only in retrospect, 1 year after its occurrence.

During the perimenopause, most patients will describe changes in the character or amount of menstrual flow, with possible abnormal bleeding. As the follicular population in the ovaries continues to decline in responsiveness and number, menses may change more dramatically (menometrorrhagia, oligomenorrhea, amenorrhea). Poorly functioning follicles produce fluctuating levels of estrogen, with some periods of relative estrogen excess. The overall effect can result in episodes of estrogen deficiency, alternating endogenous periods of unopposed estrogen. Sporadically, ovarian function may synchronize, resulting in an ovulatory cycle. This possibility raises the question of pregnancy as a part of the differential diagnosis in the patient presented here.

As the menopausal transition proceeds, the ovarian follicle population eventually is exhausted. There is eventually negligible further production of estrogen from the ovarian follicles, resulting in prolonged amenorrhea. Once the full year of amenorrhea has transpired, the diagnosis of postmenopausal status is appropriate and the patient can be considered infertile. It is crucial to remember that until this point in time, ovarian activity can sporadically occur and may be accompanied by even more sporadic ovulatory activity. Women in this age group should be carefully counseled regarding the need for continued contraception. The perimenopausal age group is the second highest incidence group for unplanned/unwanted pregnancy. The patient described here should have counseling regarding future contraceptive needs and/or satisfaction with current needs.

Lastly, the fact that this patient is presenting with a combination of amenorrhea and vasomotor symptoms is suggestive of the stage of the transition known as "late perimenopause." She is having some symptoms that may warrant treatment, if they are bothersome to her. This patient should be assessed for symptom severity, and baseline risks that could affect desire and recommendations for hormonal therapy. Based on the contraceptive need and medical history, she could be a candidate for low-dose oral contraceptives. She may also be a candidate for hormone replacement therapy. In fact, her needs may fluctuate as her stage of transition changes. The most important step is understanding her risks, benefits, and perceived needs. This will require a consultative approach that includes patient education. Information obtained from non–peer-reviewed sources (e.g., the Internet) may not be medically accurate and should be approached with caution.

TAKE HOME POINTS

- Menopause can only be diagnosed retrospectively, 1 year after the final menstrual period.
- There is not a lab test(s) that, in isolation, can diagnose menopause.
- Pregnancy should always be ruled out when a women presents with missed menses, if she is at risk for pregnancy.
- Understanding of the physiology of the menopause transition is critical to being able to appropriately counsel and care for women who are progressing through these stages of reproductive function.
- There are many levels of misunderstanding and misinformation related to menopause. Women frequently require education and individual counseling to understand their individual clinical situation.

SUGGESTED READING

Burger HG, Hale GE, Robertson DM, et al. A review of hormonal changes during the menopausal transition: focus on fi ndings from the Melbourne Women's Midlife Health Project. *Hum Reprod Update*. 2007;13(6):559–565 [Epub 2007 Jul 14].

Freeman EW, Sammel MD, Lin H, et al. Symptoms associated with menopausal transition and reproductive hormones in midlife women. *Obstet Gynecol*. 2007;110(2 Pt 1):230–240.

Gracia CR, Sammel MD, Freeman EW, et al. Defining menopause status: creation of a new defi nition to identify the early changes of the menopausal transition. *Menopause*. 2005;12(2):128–135.

Hale GE, Zhao X, Hughes CL, et al. Endocrine features of menstrual cycles in middle and late reproductive age and the menopausal transition classifi ed according to the Staging of Reproductive Aging Workshop (STRAW) staging system. *J Clin Endocrinol Metab*. 2007;92(8):3060–3067 [Epub 2007 Jun 5].

Harlow SD, Mitchell ES, Crawford S, Nan B, Little R, Taffe J for the ReSTAGE Collaboration. The ReSTAGE Collaboration: defi ning optimal bleeding criteria for onset of early menopausal transition. *Fertil Steril*. 2008;89(1):129–140 [Epub 2007 Aug 6].

NIH. NIH State-of-the-Science Conference Statement on management of menopause-related symptoms. *NIH Consens State Sci Statements* (pp. 22(1):1–38). Bethesda: US government; (2005 Mar 21–23).

Prior J. Ovarian aging and the perimenopausal transition: the paradox of endogenous ovarian hyperstimulation. *Endocrine*. 2005;26(3):297–300.

Santoro N. The menopausal transition. *Am J of Med*. 2005;188(12B):8S–13S.

Santoro N, Crawford SL, Lasley WL, et al. Factors related to declining luteal function in women during the menopausal transition. *J Clin Endocrinol Metab*, (2008 Feb 19) [Epub ahead of print].

Soules MR, Sherman S, Parrott E, et al. Executive summary: Stages of Repoductive Aging Workshop (STRAW) Park City, Utah, July 2001. Menopause. 2001;8:402–407.

Soules MR, Sherman S, Parrott E, et al. Executive summary: Stages of Reproductive Aging Workshop. Climacteric. 2001;4:267–272.

Williams JK. Contraceptive needs of the perimenopausal woman. *Obstet Gynecol Clin North Am*. 2002;29(3):575–588, ix.

117

CAN MY MECHANIC FIX THESE VASOMOTOR SYMPTOMS?

PENNY CASTELLANO, MD, FACOG

A 52-year-old female, gravida 4, para 3, presents to her primary care provider complaining of "menopause symptoms." The patient's complaints include mild hot flashes and moderate sleep disturbances (including multiple episodes of wakening during the night). She is also having symptoms of depression and fatigue. She reports feeling overwhelmed and somewhat hopeless, and she has a lack of interest in most of her usual activities. Her last menstrual period was 16 months ago. She is not using hormone therapy. She is not sexually active, and she has noted no vaginal symptoms.

There is a growing body of evidence regarding the symptoms that are clearly related to declining estrogen levels during the menopausal transition. From the beginning of the perimenopause through postmenopause, ovarian production of estrogen and progesterone continues to decline (reflecting continued degradation of the follicular population), and estrogen deficiency symptoms may present. Vasomotor symptoms (VMS) include hot flushes, hot flashes, and night sweats, any of which may be followed by a chill. The triggers and mechanisms for these symptoms are still only partially understood but are believed to involve a portion of the central nervous system that governs thermoregulation. The result, in the face of estrogen deficiency, is inappropriate heat loss. Studies have suggested an alpha adrenergic event set that involves a narrowing of the thermoneutral zone. Small fluctuations in core body temperature can trigger the response, which includes surface vasodilation. Although these symptoms have been demonstrated to be significantly disturbing to some women, not all women complain of VMS. The link between these symptoms and sleep disturbances has been discussed but is not entirely clear in studies. Menopausal VMS can vary by individual, are known to follow circadian rhythms, and tend to resolve or improve over time, even if untreated.

Opportunities for errors in managing VMS occur because other medical conditions can be associated with hot flashes, poor temperature control, heat sensitivity, and night sweats. It is important that other possible causes for VMS (especially night sweats) are ruled out prior to making the assumption that ovarian failure is to blame. Sleep disturbances should trigger an investigation of primary sleep disorders which are common in this patient population and include sleep apnea.

In addition to VMS, there are other symptoms associated with menopause. Urogenital atrophy symptoms result from atrophic changes in the vaginal and vulvar epithelium, causing a decline in normal functioning. This can lead to a lack of normal lubrication of the vagina during intercourse, resulting in dyspareunia. Dyspareunia can lead to decline in libido, as pleasure from intercourse becomes less, and pain becomes more common. Additionally, the normal vaginal environment may be altered as lactobacilli populations decline, and more pathogenic bacteria from the GI tract begin to establish in the vagina. Vaginal pH rises and this further interferes with the normal vaginal flora. This can result in vaginal symptoms that are bothersome outside of intercourse. In this arena of menopausal therapy, errors can be made in the assumption that symptoms are simply due to atrophic changes, when, in fact, antimicrobial therapy may be in order. Recurrent symptoms may simply represent advancing atrophic changes, and local estrogen therapy may be indicated.

In addition to the evidence-based vasomotor and urogenital atrophy symptoms, there are other common complaints reported with menopause. In many cases, there is not strong evidence to support an association with the hormonal changes of menopause. Depression, weight gain, fatigue, and anxiety are among the reported complaints. There is currently insufficient evidence to directly associate these symptoms with the estrogen deficiency of postmenopause. In some women, anxiety and depression may be exacerbated during the perimenopause, but these symptoms are not clearly associated with the postmenopausal state. It is important to recognize the possible complexity of symptoms in the menopausal patient. While there is some evidence that mood disorders can surface during the perimenopause, there is less evidence that the postmenopausal state is associated with depression and/or mood disorders. In this patient complaining of feeling "overwhelmed" or having a loss of interest in normal activities, the possibility of depression must be considered. Additionally, other sources for the symptom of fatigue must be acknowledged. Patients in this age group may be at risk for multifactorial emotional symptoms. It is, thus, important for providers to properly categorize a patient's symptoms as related or unrelated to menopause. Hormone replacement therapy can be very useful for treatment of VMS and UGA. It may be nonhelpful, or even harmful, if used for symptoms that are actually related to another etiology, if for no other reason than lack of attention to the true underlying cause. In the patient presented here, a psychological evaluation should be a part of her assessment. While some of her symptoms (hot flashes) are most likely related to menopause (she does meet the clinical criteria for postmenopausal status), she has other symptoms suggestive of a psychological etiology. Comprehensive evaluation, possibly including a referral for psychiatric evaluation, would provide a complete plan of care.

TAKE HOME POINTS

- Vasomotor symptoms and urogenital atrophy symptoms have been demonstrated to be associated with declining estrogen levels in menopausal patients.
- There is some evidence that suggests the perimenopausal phase of the transition may be a point in time at which some patients are at risk for emotional symptoms.
- Symptoms that have insufficient evidence relating them to estrogen deficiency and/or menopause should be evaluated individually in patients presenting for treatment of menopausal symptoms.
- Care of menopausal patients requires individual counseling regarding therapeutic option assessment.

SUGGESTED READINGS

Freedman RR. Hot flashes: behavioral treatments, mechanisms, and relation to sleep. *Am J Med*. 2005;118(12B):124S–130S.

Freedman RR, Roehrs TA. Sleep disturbance in menopause. *Menopause*. 2007;14(5): 826–829.

Nelson HD. Menopause. Lancet. 2008;371(9614):760–770.

NIH Consens State Sci Statements. NIH State-of-the-Science Conference Statement on Management of Menopause Related Symptoms. *NIH Consens State Sci Statements. Bethesda*. 2005;22(1):1–38.

Pabich WL, Fihn SD, Stamm WE, et al. Prevalence and determinants of vaginal fl ora alterations in postmenopausal women. *J Infect Dis*. 2003;188(7):1054–1058.

Reed SD, Newton KM, LaCroix AZ, et al. Night sweats, sleep disturbance, and depression associated with diminished libido in late menopausal transition and early postmenopause: baseline data from the Herbal Alternatives for Menopause Trial (HALT). *Am J Obstet Gynecol*. 2007;196(6):593.e1–7.

Schmidt PJ. Mood, depression, and reproductive hormones in the menopausal transition. *Am J Med*. 2005;118(12B);54S–58S.

Van Voorhis BJ. Genitourinary Symptoms in the Menopausal Transition. *Am J Med*. 2005;118(12B):47S–53S.

Williams RE, Kalilani L, DiBenedetti DB, et al. Frequency and severity of vasomotor symptoms among peri-and postmenopausal women in the United States. Climacteric. 2008;11(1):32–43.

118

BREAST MASSES

EKTA VISHWAKARMA, MD AND DIANA BROOMFIELD, MD

A 32-year-old nullipara, Ms. Jones, presented with a palpable painless lump in her left breast for a few days. There was no family history of breast cancer. She was not using any contraception. On examination, there was a smooth, firm, mobile 2 × 2-cm lump in the outer quadrant of the left breast. It was not tender and the overlying skin was normal. The doctor took history and did complete physical examination. The screening mammogram was normal. The patient was reassured and sent home. She came back after 3 years with a larger lump, which was diagnosed as breast cancer.

A thorough patient history is necessary to arrive at the correct diagnosis and to identify the risk factors for breast cancer in any patient with a breast mass (*Table 118.1*). A complete clinical breast examination (CBE) should be done in the week following menstruation. CBE by itself is not enough and it must be combined with cytological/histological diagnosis and imaging. Any abnormal CBE in the presence of even a negative mammogram requires further follow-up. The false-negative rate of mammography in the detection of breast cancer has been consistently reported to be approximately 10%.

Fine-needle aspiration (FNA), core biopsy, or excision biopsy is required for a definitive diagnosis of any breast mass. Any lesion that completely resolves after FNA does not require any further diagnostic workup. A cyst that recurs more than twice within 4 to 6 weeks, contains bloody fluid, or leaves a residual palpable mass postaspiration should have a diagnostic imaging evaluation. Nonpalpable cysts detected by mammography and confirmed by ultrasound need not be aspirated unless symptomatic and causing pain.

A triple test is the combination of results from CBE, imaging, and tissue sampling. With concordant results, the triple test diagnostic accuracy approaches 100%. In any pregnant patient, a diagnosis can be confirmed or ruled out by FNA or ultrasound. Breast cancer tends to present in more advanced stages in pregnancy due to the difficulties in diagnosis and more rapid growth.

Figure 118.1 summarizes the comprehensive diagnostic approach to any patient with a palpable breast mass.

TABLE 118.1	**COMMON CAUSES OF A BENIGN BREAST MASS**	
CONDITION	**PRESENTATION**	**MANAGEMENT**
Fibrocystic disease	Breast discomfort and heaviness are worse just before menstruation. The breasts feel dense, irregular, and multiple masses with bumpy "cobblestone" consistency especially in the outer upper part of the breast tissue.	Ultrasound identifies the cystic changes and FNA may be therapeutic. Rarely, a biopsy is required to rule out cancer. Restrict dietary fat and caffeine and use well–fitting bra. Birth control pill or tamoxifen (in severe cases) help too.
Fibroadenoma	Rubbery, movable mass in a woman in her teens and 20s and in postmenopausal women who are taking hormone replacement therapy.	Needs no management but can be surgically removed. In case of doubt about diagnosis, we must do a biopsy.
Breast infection: includes engorgement, mastitis, and abscess (during lactation).	They present with localized breast edema, erythema, warmth, and pain. Symptoms of fever, vomiting, and spontaneous drainage from the mass or nipple.	Continue with breast-feeding, antibiotics, and rarely incision and drainage for abscess. Inflammatory cancer is a differential diagnosis for mastitis (the former is painless and more diffuse mass).
Fat necrosis	Firm, round, painless lumps in women with very large breasts or in response to a bruise or blow to the breast or after a lumpectomy and radiation treatment.	Watchful expectancy though some may require a mammogram. They do not become cancer.
Cystosarcoma phyllodes	Firm, mobile, well–circumscribed, nontender breast mass rapidly increasing in size.	Benign in 85%–90% of cases. The confirmatory test is biopsy. Treated by wide local excision with a 2–5-cm rim of normal tissue.

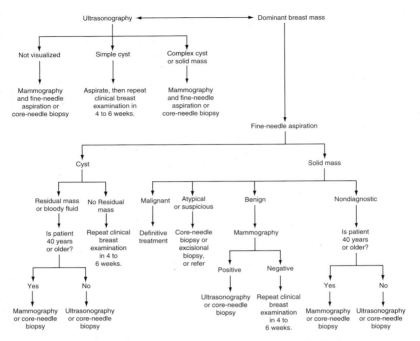

FIGURE 118.1 Diagnostic algorithm for patients with palpable breast masses. Adapted or Reprinted with permission from 'Evaluation of Palpable Breast Masses,' May 1, 2005, American Family Physician. Copyright © 2005 American Academy of Family Physicians. All Rights Reserved.

Imaging modalities such as ultrasonography, MRI, and screening and diagnostic mammography are required for routine health maintenance as well. In women 40 years and older who are at average risk, a mammographic screening is recommended every 1 to 2 years and every year after age 50 as long as the woman is healthy. For women at high risk, routine screening should be initiated sooner. For those with breast cancer genetic mutations, mammography should begin at age 25 or at an age 10 years younger than the youngest case diagnosed in the family.

TAKE HOME POINTS

- Triple test (CBE, imaging, and tissue sampling) when concordant has an accuracy close to 100% in picking up breast cancer.
- Mammogram can miss up to 10% of cancers due to difficulty in interpretation. It must always be supported by some imaging modalities.

- Women with a family history of breast cancer should have screening studies from a much younger age.
- After the treatment of breast cancer, there is a risk of recurrence so an ongoing lifelong surveillance is very important.

SUGGESTED READINGS

American Cancer Society. Detailed guide: breast cancer. Can breast cancer be found early? Last revised: 03/02/2009.

Mincey BA, Perez EA. Advances in screening, diagnosis, and treatment of breast cancer. *Mayo Clin Proc.* 2004;79:810–816.

Morris A, Pommier RF, Schmidt WA, et al. Accurate evaluation of palpable breast masses by the triple test score. *Arch Surg.* 1998;133:930–934.

119

ALL POSTMENOPAUSAL BLEEDING IS CANCER UNTIL PROVEN OTHERWISE

MARTINA BADELL, MD

Postmenopausal bleeding (PMB) is any vaginal bleeding in a menopausal woman. PMB accounts for approximately 5% of gynecology clinic visits annually. The most common cause of PMB is vaginal or endometrial atrophy and endometrial polyps. In addition, other common etiologies in early menopause include submucosal fibroids, endometrial hyperplasia, endometrial cancer, hormonal effects, and cervical cancer. The incidence of endometrial cancer is approximately 10% in women with PMB; however, as endometrial cancer is a potentially lethal disease, it should be investigated in all women presenting with PMB.

A full history and physical exam are required when evaluating PMB. Important information from the patient's history includes when the bleeding started, how much she is bleeding and when it is occurring, precipitating factors, associated symptoms, obstetrical and gynecologic history, medical history, family history, and any current medications. Risk factors for endometrial cancer include nulliparity, family history, tamoxifen use, hereditary nonpolyposis colorectal carcinoma, obesity, diabetes, and endogenous or exogenous increase in estrogens.

A thorough physical examination should initially evaluate general features such as the patient's weight, general appearance, and hair pattern and then focus on the gynecologic exam. First, evaluate the external female genitalia for any suspicious lesions/lacerations and then an internal exam is necessary. Visually inspect the vulva, vagina, and cervix for any lesions using a speculum. In addition, it is important to feel the cervix, uterus, and ovaries on bimanual exam for any abnormalities.

A Pap smear should be performed on all women per screening protocol. If any visible lesion is noted, a biopsy is warranted. An endometrial biopsy should be done as the initial diagnostic test for all postmenopausal women with bleeding. This is a relatively simple test done in the office with a low complication rate and high sensitivity. If for some reason an endometrial biopsy is not possible, a transvaginal ultrasound is an acceptable alternative. Endometrial cancer can be reasonably excluded if a thin, homogeneous endometrial stripe is seen. Endometrial thickness <5 mm without any heterogeneity has a negative predictive value for endometrial cancer of 98%. However, a biopsy is required if the lining is thicker than 5 mm, there is any heterogeneity, the endometrium is not adequately visualized, and/or if the women has any persistent bleeding.

TAKE HOME POINTS

- The primary goal in the evaluation of PMB is to exclude malignancy.
- Both endometrial biopsy and transvaginal ultrasound can be used as an initial test for evaluating the endometrium. However, endometrial thickness of 5 mm or more, heterogeneity, persistent bleeding, or inadequately visualized endometrium requires an endometrial biopsy.
- Endometrial atrophy and endometrial polyps are the most common causes of PMB.
- Endometrial carcinoma is the cause of PMB in about 10% of patients.

SUGGESTED READINGS

Goodman A. The evaluation and management of uterine bleeding in postmenopausal women. In: Rose BD, ed. *UpToDate*, Wellesley, MA: UpToDate; 2008.

Lobo RA. In: Katz VL, ed. *Comprehensive Gynecology*. 5th ed. Philadelphia, PA: Mosby Elsevier; 2007:915–931.

Lu K, Slomovitz CM. In: Katz VL, ed. *Comprehensive Gynecology*. 5th ed. Philadelphia, PA: Mosby Elsevier; 2007:813–837.

120

Osteoporosis: After treatment, you need to monitor

Mark S. Nanes, MD, PhD and Caleb B. Kallen, MD, PhD

Importantly, when assessing results of serial DXA scans for a patient, it is better to assess actual bone density changes (in g/cm^2) rather than to compare present T scores with prior T scores (T scores will vary with patient age, density measurements are age independent). Alternative modalities of BMD testing include quantitative computed tomography, quantitative ultrasound densitometry, and peripheral dual energy x-ray absorptiometry. While these techniques are accurate and reproducible for the purpose of screening, the T scores that they generate cannot be interpreted according to WHO diagnostic classifications obtained using DXA. More importantly, DXA is the only bone density test that is currently useful for assessment of changes in BMD over time and in response to therapy. One unique attribute of quantitative computed tomography is a true 3D measurement that may be more useful for follow-up of anabolic therapies such as teriparatide (discussed in Chapter 122).

A single BMD measurement does not indicate the rate of bone turnover. Serum and urine markers of bone turnover may provide additional information regarding bone turnover. The bone markers currently in clinical use include (1) the bone resorption markers deoxypyridinoline, C-terminal cross-linking telopeptide of type I collagen (or C-telopeptide = CTx), and N-terminal cross-linking telopeptide of type I collagen (or N-telopeptide=NTx) and (2) the bone formation markers bone-specific alkaline phosphate, osteocalcin, and C-terminal propeptide type I collagen (C1CP). Because bone resorption and formation are coupled processes, interpretation of results as "excess resorption" or "reduced formation" is generally not possible. Such specific interpretations require a bone biopsy, which is not recommended in routine cases of osteoporosis. The use of clinical markers of bone turnover remains controversial.

For most patients, avoid BMD testing more often than every 18 to 24 months. In monitoring therapy with DXA results, it is better to compare actual BMD values rather than serial T scores from the same patient, as noted above. The precision of DXA varies by site of measurement. In general, a significant change in BMD is represented by a 2% change from baseline, though the precision can vary by manufacturer of the densitometer and the site of the measurement.

TAKE HOME POINTS

- Clinical markers of bone resorption and formation may be useful in assessing response to therapy and to promote patient compliance with therapy. Results should be interpreted with caution and may not indicate treatment success or failure.
- Interpret follow-up DXA scans by assessing actual bone density changes (in g/cm^2) rather than changes in T scores.
- You rarely need to repeat DXA scans more often than every 18 to 24 months.

SUGGESTED READINGS

Luciano AA. Osteoporosis: an update. *Hospital Physician, Obstetrics and Gynecology Board Review Manual.* 2001;7(4):16–24.

National Osteoporosis Foundation. *Clinician's Guide to Prevention and Treatment of Osteoporosis.* www.nof.org

121

OSTEOPOROSIS: WHO GETS IT AND HOW DO YOU KNOW?

MARK S. NANES, MD, PhD AND CALEB B. KALLEN, MD, PhD

COMMON ERROR: UNDERESTIMATING A PATIENT'S RISK FOR OSTEOPOROSIS

Osteoporosis is generally without symptoms until a clinically significant bone fracture occurs. An important part of diagnosing osteoporosis begins with understanding the risk factors that predispose to fracture (*Table 121.1*, adapted from National Osteoporosis Foundation, NOF). In fact, although changes in bone mineral density (BMD) and in biochemical markers of bone metabolism are reflective of bone turnover, these do not measure bone quality. The central dual x-ray absorptiometry (DXA) is the gold standard tool for assessing bone density. Low BMD measurements account for 40% of the overall fracture risk when applied to individuals, with residual risk attributable to other features of bone quality. Thus, the World Health Organization (WHO) has recommended that all evaluations of fracture risk include assessment of the most important predictors of fracture risk: (1) age, (2) tobacco use, (3) family history of osteoporotic fracture, (4) low body mass index (BMI), (5) chronic estrogen deprivation (or hypogonadism in men), (6) rheumatoid arthritis, and (7) glucocorticoid therapy.

In postmenopausal women, bone resorption cumulatively and chronically exceeds bone formation leading to high rates of osteoporosis. Menopausal women experience, on average, a sustained doubling of bone turnover. This effect is reduced by estrogen replacement.

It is important to recognize that although osteopenia predisposes to osteoporosis and osteoporosis predisposes to bone fractures, most patients with osteoporosis will not experience a fracture. Furthermore, BMD is specific but not sensitive for fracture risk: many patients who experience a fracture will not meet diagnostic criteria for osteoporosis. Thus, over 50% of patients with hip fractures have a T score > -2.5 and over 35% of spine fractures have low or normal BMD (T > -2.5). Nevertheless, there exists a strong correlation between decreasing bone density and increased risk of fracture.

Risk assessment using the WHO risk factors optimizes clinical decision making regarding therapy. To this end, the WHO has recently implemented a web-based tool, FRAX, which can be populated with 12 risk factors, along with the BMD, to produce a 10-year probability of fracture of the hip

---

TABLE 121.1 **RISK FACTORS FOR OSTEOPOROSIS**

Personal history of fracture after age 50

Current low bone mass (T score <−1.5)

History of fracture in a 1! relative

Being female

Being thin and/or having a small frame/Low Body Mass Index (<21 kg/m^2)

Advanced age

A family history of osteoporosis

Estrogen deficiency as a result of menopause, especially early or surgically induced

Absence of menstrual periods (amenorrhea)

Anorexia nervosa

Low lifetime calcium intake

Vitamin D deficiency

Presence of certain chronic medical conditions (Cushing syndrome, anorexia, hypogonadism, IBD, DM, celiac sprue, hyperparathyroidism, hyperthyroidism, and HIV).

An inactive/sedentary lifestyle

Current cigarette smoking

Excessive use of alcohol

Being Caucasian or Asian, although African Americans and Hispanic Americans are at significant risk as well

In males, testosterone deficiency

Potentially modifiable risks are highlighted in bold
Source: Adapted from the NOF.

(www.shef.ac.uk/FRAX). While treatment decisions must be individualized, a general guideline would be to consider pharmacologic therapy for a 10-year fracture probability ≥3% for the hip or ≥20% cumulative risk for fracture combining *all major* osteoporosis-related fracture sites. Prior NOF recommendations included initiation of treatment for postmenopausal women with T scores <−2.0 (with no risk factors) or <−1.5 (with risk factors). By contrast, WHO had recommended a diagnostic threshold for osteoporosis of T score <−2.5. FRAX circumvents this inconsistency in guidelines by relying on population-specific fracture risk calculated from international epidemiologic data.

Which patients should be offered a screening DXA? WHO recommendations include testing BMD for women >age 65, regardless of risk factors, and also for postmenopausal women less than age 65, with one or more risk factors for osteoporosis. BMD testing most commonly employs DXA and the results are expressed as standard deviations from age- and sex-matched standards (Z score) or "young" peak bone mass standards (T score). WHO defines normal bone mass as T score >-1.0, with osteopenia being T scores between -1.0 and -2.5 and osteoporosis being T score ≤-2.5. Because each standard deviation represents a difference of 10% to 15% in BMD, osteoporosis is indicative of $\geq25\%$ loss of peak bone mass. Fracture risk increases approximately 1.7-fold for every standard deviation decrease (-1.0) in T score.

DXA uses x-rays to assess BMD by area (not volume) and the radiation dose is approximately one tenth that of a standard chest x-ray. It is important for patients to get repeat BMD measurements done on the same machine. Error between machines or trying to convert measurements from one manufacturer's standard to another can introduce errors larger than the sensitivity of the actual densitometry measurements. Furthermore, the WHO diagnostic classifications cannot be applied to premenopausal women, men $<$age 50, and children, for whom the International Society for Clinical Densitometry recommends ethnic- or race-adjusted Z scores be used (Z score <-2.0 indicating low bone density).

TAKE HOME POINTS

- Osteoporosis is common. Any "fragility fracture" indicates clinically meaningful osteoporosis, regardless of the T score, and all fractures should be followed by BMD testing to assess level of disease.

- Online risk assessment is easy (www.shef.ac.uk/FRAX), evidence based, and will help the clinician consider the most relevant risk factors for osteoporosis and fracture, including BMD.

- Comprehensive risk assessment simplifies the discussion of when to initiate bone-sparing therapy and can reveal diverse and treatable contributors to osteoporosis.

- For premenopausal women, use Z score not T score, although supportive data are limited with regard to fracture risk assessment and, at younger ages, $Z \approx T$.

- BMD is important, but it is not the only determinant of fracture risk. Use online assessment tools to identify patients who might benefit from bone-sparing therapy.

SUGGESTED READINGS

Khosla S, Burr D, Cauley J, et al. Bisphosphonate-associated osteonecrosis of the jaw: report of a task force of the American Society for Bone and Mineral Research. *J Bone Miner Res.* 2007;22(10):1479–1491.

Looker AC, Orwoll ES, Johnston CC Jr, et al. Prevalence of low femoral bone density in older U.S. adults from NHANES III. *J Bone Miner Res.* 1997;12(11):1761–1768.

Luciano AA. Osteoporosis: an update. Hospital Physician, Obstetrics and Gynecology Board Review Manual. 2001;7(4):16–24.

National Osteoporosis Foundation. *Clinician's Guide to Prevention and Treatment of Osteoporosis.* www.nof.org

Schuit SC, van der Klift M, Weel AE, et al. Fracture incidence and association with bone mineral density in elderly men and women: the Rotterdam Study. *Bone.* 2004;34(1):195–202.

122

THERAPEUTIC APPROACHES: LIFESTYLE, EXERCISE, AND MEDICATIONS

MARK S. NANES, MD, PhD AND CALEB B. KALLEN, MD, PhD

Regular weight-bearing and muscle-strengthening exercise is an important part of bone maintenance. Fall prevention can include measures to improve eyesight, hearing, strength, stability, and home safety (lighting, stairways, shoes, medication adjustments, etc.). Use of tobacco or excessive alcohol consumption should be avoided.

Getting the daily recommended amount of calcium, whether through diet, supplements, or both, is essential to maintaining bone strength and can play a vital role in preventing osteoporosis-related fractures. Often, thrice-daily dosing of over-the-counter preparations is required to adequately replete calcium and vitamin D. According to NOF recommendations, adults under age 50 need 1,000 mg of elemental calcium daily and adults aged 50 and over need 1,200 to 1,500 mg of calcium daily (*Table 122.1*). It can be seen from *Table 122.1* that a 600-mg calcium carbonate pill only provides 240 mg of elemental calcium (600 mg × 40% = 240 mg). Thus, four pills a day in divided doses would be required for nearly 1,000 mg per day elemental calcium. A common error is to assume that only two pills a day meet the 1,000 mg requirement. Similar calculations must be done for other calcium preparations. Dietary calcium should be calculated and subtracted from the pill requirement. The average dairy-free diet contains 250 mg of calcium per day and calcium-rich foods can be considered for motivated patients.

Vitamin D plays a major role in calcium absorption and bone health. Vitamin D_3 (cholecalciferol) is synthesized in the skin following direct exposure to sunlight; however, there are many different factors that affect a person's ability to make adequate amounts of vitamin D. Vitamin D_3 and commercial vitamin D_2 (ergocalciferol) will both support bone health since both are metabolized to 25(OH)D in the liver and finally to the active metabolite $1,25(OH)_2D$ in the kidney. According to NOF recommendations, adults under age 50 need 400 to 800 IU of vitamin D_3 daily and adults aged 50 and older need 800 to 1,000 IU of vitamin D_3 daily for maintenance of normal levels. There is considerable variability of serum vitamin D_3 levels throughout the day due to variable sunlight exposure. Vitamin D_3 is hydroxylated in the liver to 25-hydroxyvitamin D_3 ($25[OH]D_3$) in an unregulated manner and then 1-hydroxylated in the kidney under

TABLE 122.1	ELEMENTAL CALCIUM CONTENT OF ORALLY AVAILABLE CALCIUM SUPPLEMENTS	
CALCIUM PREPARATION		% ELEMENTAL CALCIUM
Calcium carbonate		40
Calcium citrate		21
Calcium lactate		12.8
Calcium gluconate		8.8
Calcium glubionate		6.5

Target daily elemental calcium allowance roughly 1,000 mg/d premenopause and 1,500 mg/d postmenopause.

minute-to-minute regulation by parathyroid hormone. Thus, the stable 25(OH)D$_3$ level best reflects nutritional repletion and is the appropriate test to evaluate the vitamin D status of patients. A common error is to measure the wrong vitamin D metabolite to assess nutritional status. In this regard, the author has observed that up to 30% of resident house staff and primary care physicians obtain a 1,25(OH)$_2$D$_3$ level rather than the 25(OH)D$_3$ level in their prereferral evaluations.

For patients with markedly low 25(OH)D$_3$ values (<30 ng/mL), consider high-dose supplementation using ergocalciferol, 50,000 IU twice per week for 2 to 3 months. Adequate supplementation can be evidenced by suppression of previously elevated serum PTH values or an increase of 24-hour urine calcium from previously low to the midnormal range. Vitamin D can also be obtained from fortified milk, egg yolks, saltwater fish, and liver though nutrition alone is unlikely to replete a markedly deficient patient.

Decreasing fracture risk includes prevention (bone accrual and maintenance) and treatment of osteoporosis (reducing risk of fracture in the setting of established osteoporosis). Current FDA-approved pharmacologic options for osteoporosis prevention and/or treatment are bisphosphonates (alendronate, ibandronate, risedronate, zolendronate), teraparatide (parathyroid hormone1–34), estrogens, the estrogen agonist/antagonist raloxifene, and calcitonin. Treatment decisions must be based upon clinical scenario and intervention thresholds.

Antiresorptive agents: These include bisphosphonates that prevent bone loss and reduce fracture risk of the hip and spine. In recent studies, zolendronate decreased fracture risk and increased overall patient survival. Risks of oral bisphosphonates are mostly GI and esophageal irritation. These medications are theoretically problematic in women of childbearing age (pelvic considerations and fetal considerations). Rarely, the oral agents have been associated with a complication, osteonecrosis of the jaw (ONJ), though this is far more common using IV agents in higher doses and generally in selected patient populations (i.e., oncology patients). Ninety-five percent of reported cases of ONJ are observed with the use of IV zoledronic acid or IV pamidronate for metastatic bone disease (doses used generally 4- to 12-fold higher than what is used for treatment of osteoporosis). Patients should be informed of this low risk and bisphosphonates should be held for several months for dental extraction or orthodontic surgery. Alternative antiresorptive therapies include estrogens (alone or combined with progestins) and raloxifene (a selective estrogen receptor modulator), the former shown to be effective for preventing fractures of the hip and spine and the latter effective for fractures of the spine. Follow-up of the large MORE clinical trial and subsequent RUTH trial showed that raloxifene reduced the incidence of breast cancer, unlike some hormonal preparations that may increase cancer risk. Estrogen and raloxifene increase the risk of deep venous thromboses and stroke.

One clinical error is failure to discontinue hormonal therapy in hospitalized or otherwise immobile patients, since the risk of thromboembolism is increased under such circumstances. Calcitonin is rarely recommended in light of better available agents and the fact that hip fracture protection has never been established for this agent.

Anabolic agents such as teriparatide (PTH 1–34), given by daily subcutaneous injection, potently reduce the risk of fractures of the spine, hip, and other sites. Safety has not been documented beyond 2 years of therapy. Combination therapies (bisphosphonate plus nonbisphosphonate) may confer benefit with regard to BMD; however, the impact on fracture rates is unknown and the approach warrants further investigation including a risk/benefit analysis. Patients should be monitored for hypercalcemia after starting teraparatide. Bisphosphonates may blunt the effect of teraparatide; therefore, a clinical decision on the use of teraparatide should be made early. A common clinical error is to start a bisphosphonate immediately, without first assessing for secondary causes of osteoporosis or considering teraparatide as a therapeutic option. Teraparatide is currently the most expensive approved therapy for osteoporosis in the United States. Fluoride increases fractures when administered in high dose but may reduce fractures at low dose. Fluoride is approved as an osteoporosis therapy in Europe.

TAKE HOME POINTS

■ It is important to identify and treat modifiable risk factors for osteoporosis: tobacco use, low BMI (<21 kg/M^2), physical inactivity, alcoholism, poor nutrition/eating disorder, and estrogen deficiency in the premenopausal patient.

- Calcium citrate is most bioavailable, calcium carbonate should be given with meals (requires acid for absorption), and only the calculated elemental calcium in dosing is relevant.
- When testing for vitamin D deficiency, always check 25-OH–vitamin D, not 1,25 $(OH)_2$-D, the latter of which does not reflect nutritional status. 25-OH–vitamin D < 30 ng/mL indicates nutritional deficiency and <15 ng/mL profound deficiency. These levels require high-dose replacement (50,000 IU weekly for several months) followed by vitamin D maintenance doses (800 IU per day).
- Antiresorptive agents can protect from fractures of the hip and the spine.
- Bisphosphonates may blunt the effect of teriparatide (PTH 1–34), so avoid initiating these prior to establishing that teriparatide would not be better indicated.
- When oral doses of bisphosphonates are used in the noncancer patient population the incidence of ONJ is rare (estimated to be ≤1 case per 100,000 patients). For patients who are unable to swallow or are intolerant of oral bisphosphonates, consider IV zolendronate.

SUGGESTED READINGS

Barrett-Connor E, Mosca L, Collins P, et al. Effects of raloxifene on cardiovascular events and breast cancer in postmenopausal women. *N Engl J Med.* 2006;355(2):125–137.

Khosla S, Burr D, Cauley J, et al. Bisphosphonate-associated osteonecrosis of the jaw: report of a task force of the American Society for Bone and Mineral Research. *J Bone Miner Res.* 2007;22(10):1479–1491.

Martino S, Cauley JA, Barrett-Connor E, et al. Continuing outcomes relevant to Evista: breast cancer incidence in postmenopausal osteoporotic women in a randomized trial of raloxifene. *J Natl Cancer Inst.* 2004;96(23):1751–1761.

National Osteoporosis Foundation. *Clinician's Guide to Prevention and Treatment of Osteoporosis.* www.nof.org

Siris ES, Harris ST, Eastell R, et al. Skeletal effects of raloxifene after 8 years: results from the continuing outcomes relevant to Evista (CORE) study. *J Bone Miner Res.* 2005;20(9):1514–1524.

123

DIAGNOSING SECONDARY CAUSES OF OSTEOPOROSIS

MARK S. NANES, MD, PhD AND CALEB B. KALLEN, MD, PhD

Numerous medications and conditions are known to predispose to osteoporosis and fracture. Failure to assess secondary causes of osteoporosis is a major "error" in care since a large fraction of osteoporotic women have secondary causes that might require additional intervention (such as thiazides to prevent renal calcium leak, vitamin D repletion, or optimal treatment of hyperthyroidism). Secondary causes of osteoporosis should be ruled out as clinically indicated. Common causes include osteomalacia, vitamin D deficiency, and inherited hypercalciuria (~9%–10% of general population) and can be ruled out with serum 25-OH–vitamin D and 24–hour urinary calcium testing. In the setting of osteoporosis, physicians should screen for hyperthyroidism (TSH), hyperparathyroidism (Ca^{2+}/phosphorous), celiac sprue (tissue transglutaminase, endomysial antibody, total IgA, and antigliadin IgA and IgG), cirrhosis (ALT/AST/Alk Phos), kidney failure (serum creatinine), hypercalciuria and hypocalciuria (24–hour urine calcium, creatinine, and sodium), marrow disorders (CBC, possible SPEP for elderly patients), and premature menopause (PRL, FSH, estradiol). A formal medication history for offending medications includes glucocorticoid therapy, excess thyroid hormone replacement, and medications such as phenytoin, phenobarbital, Depo-Lupron, letrozole, cyclosporine, aluminum antacids, Depo Provera, long-term heparinization, excess vitamin A (retinol), lithium, SSRIs, and proton pump inhibitors, all of which are associated with bone loss.

TAKE HOME POINTS

- A few simple questions and tests can identify additional causes of osteoporosis and will guide appropriate therapy.
- Take a history for offending skeletal medications.
- PRIOR to initiating medical therapy for osteoporosis, check 24–hour urinary calcium excretion (the diagnosis of high or low 24–hour urinary calcium excretion is obscured after initiation of some antiresorptive therapies).

- Never check a spot urinary calcium to assess calcium balance since calcium is not uniformly excreted throughout the day.
- In patients receiving hydrochlorothiazide (HCTZ), which can inhibit renal calcium excretion, it is best to measure 24-hour urinary calcium AFTER discontinuing the use of HCTZ for several weeks.
- When screening for hyperparathyroidism, test fasting serum Ca^{2+}/phosphorous first and then PTH if electrolytes are abnormal.
- Consider alternative causes of osteoporosis, especially in younger patients with fracture or in those who fail to respond to therapy.

SUGGESTED READINGS

Luciano AA. Osteoporosis: an update. Hospital Physician, Obstetrics and Gynecology Board Review Manual. 2001;7(4):16–24.

National Osteoporosis Foundation. *Clinician's Guide to Prevention and Treatment of Osteoporosis.* www.nof.org

124

Preoperative evaluation and preparation: Is she ready for surgery?

Long Nguyen, MD and Diana Broomfield, MD, MBA, FACOG, FACS

A 62-year-old G4P4 woman with a history of abdominal pain presented for evaluation. A transvaginal ultrasound and abdominal CT scan reveal a 34-cm adnexal mass with a small amount of free fluid. She was subsequently scheduled for an exploratory laparotomy. Her past medical history is remarkable for chronic atrial fibrillation, for which she has been on Coumadin 5 mg daily for the past year. Her current INR is 2.5. She also has been diagnosed with sleep apnea due to a BMI of 42. The patient is worried and desires immediate surgical removal of the mass.

Preoperative evaluation and preparation for surgery will include a thorough history and physical examination, including preoperative medical clearance and stabilization of her medical comorbidities. A common error to avoid is taking an unprepared or underprepared patient to the operating room; doing so increases morbidity and mortality risks.

Delaying or Postponing Elective Surgery

If the patient cannot be stabilized preoperatively, decision for delay should be based on the risks, benefits, and alternative options. In addition, a determination must be made regarding the urgency for the procedure. Is this an elective procedure? Does the patient's risk worsen with or without postponing the surgery? As the patient's age increases, the incidence of comorbidities increases. Thus, your elderly patients are more at risk for intraoperative and postoperative complications. It is estimated that 13% of patients are 65 years of age or older currently; this number will increase to 20% in 2030. It is imperative that these patients are thoroughly evaluated and get the necessary preoperative medical clearance to avoid or minimize intraoperative and postoperative complications. In a study done by Mangalo in 2002, it was noted that each year approximately 50,000 patients in the United States have perioperative myocardial infarctions (MIs) and about 40% will die.

According to two studies done by Steen and Tarhan, up to 37% of patients with a history of a previous MI will have a significant risk of a reinfarction within 3 months of surgery when undergoing general anesthesia. Patients at highest postoperative risk for MI are those older than 70 years old, those in poor general health, and those with pulmonary or cardiac disorders. Healthy patients undergoing gynecologic (pelvic or abdominal) surgeries are typically considered at an "intermediate" cardiac risk, associated with <5% risk for postoperative MI.

Recommendations for preoperative testing are based on the clinical predictors that can be identified when conducting a thorough history and physical examination. Major clinical predictors for increased perioperative risks include patients with a history of unstable angina, recent MI, significant arrhythmias, severe valvular heart disease, and patients with a history of decompensated congestive heart failure (CHF). Remember that the presence of major predictors may justify a delay or cancellation of an elective surgery until adequate preoperative evaluation and clearance can be done.

Preoperative Evaluation Consists of the following:

Thorough history and complete physical examination (above and below the pelvis)

Basic laboratory testing (βHCG, CBC, chemistry profile)

Other labs to be ordered as indicated

Coagulation profile: PT/PTT/INR as indicated

Thrombophilia studies if indicated: Factor V Leiden, 20210A mutation, lupus anticoagulant, antithrombin, antiphospholipid antibodies

Liver and renal function test, electrolytes, blood sugar test

Electrocardiogram for patients age >50, with a history of known or suspected cardiac pathology

Anesthesiology consultation

Preoperative consultation as indicated

PREOPERATIVE MANAGEMENT

There are three major groups of disorders that increase preoperative risk which is commonly seen in the practice of gynecologic surgery: cardiovascular, pulmonary, and thrombotic disorders. Common errors that are to be avoided usually involve inadequate preoperative risk assessment.

1. Cardiovascular risk:
   Medical disorders that require preoperative testing are unstable or severe angina, myocardial infarction <1 month, class IV NYHA heart failure, significant arrhythmias such as Mobitz II and third-degree AV block, and severe valvular diseases such as severe aortic stenosis and symptomatic mitral stenosis. Other medical disorders

that require preoperative testing include patients on β-blockers for angina, arrhythmias, hypertension, or history of other cardiac disease. Patients with multiple cardiac risk factors may benefit from β-blockers preoperatively. Also note that patients on aspirin or clopidogrel should discontinue these medications 5 days before elective surgery if they meet criteria to stop therapy.

2. Pulmonary risk:

Patients with a history of shortness of breath or wheezing at rest or with modest exertion and patients with history of asthma should undergo preoperative pulmonary testing. These patients may require pulmonary function testing and arterial blood gases. Patients requiring a routine preoperative chest x-ray include patients over age 50 who will be undergoing upper abdominal, thoracic, or abdominal surgery. Thus, gynecologic procedures routinely do not require a chest x-ray preoperatively. Medications for obstructive diseases are recommended to continue through the perioperative period. Compliance is essential to minimize perioperative complications. If the surgical procedure is elective and your patient is noncompliant with the preoperative recommendations, then the surgery should be postponed. Smoking cessation should be completed 6 to 8 weeks before surgery to minimize perioperative risks. Preoperative instructions in the use of the incentive spirometer have proved to be remarkably effective at preventing postoperative atelectasis and pneumonia.

3. Deep venous thrombosis (DVT) risk:

Perioperative prophylaxis is indicated for moderate- to high-risk patients. The time to start can be within 12 hours preoperatively for low molecular weight heparin (LMWH) or 2 hours preoperatively for unfractionated heparin. Another regimen option to consider is to start shortly after incision is closed. Both groups of patients are recommended to continue heparin for at least 3 to 5 days postoperatively. For patients at high DVT risk (patients with gynecologic cancers), transition to warfarin for another 4 weeks is recommended. LMWH should be used with precaution in case of spinal or epidural anesthesia because of the increased risk of spinal hematoma. In these patients, a compression device and early ambulation should be employed. Patients on oral contraceptives/hormone therapy undergoing low risk gynecologic procedures may continue their medications. Those undergoing moderate- to high-risk procedures, should discontinue hormonal therapy 4 to 6 weeks before surgery.

For patients who require surgery and are on warfarin therapy: After warfarin is stopped, it takes approximately 4 days for INR to reach 1.5; at this point, surgery can be performed. It is imperative to reinitiate anticoagulation 4 to 6 hours postoperatively because of the increased risk of recurrence of DVT that is as high as 100-fold increase in patients with history of previous DVT.

In addition to the above disorders, patients at increased preoperative risk also include patients with diabetes, hypertension, and morbid obesity. These patients must undergo preoperative medical clearance. Oral medications (antihypertensive and hypoglycemic agents) can be continued on the morning of surgery with a sip of water. Consult your anesthesiologist prior to surgery. Typically, patients on insulin will be advised to hold their morning of surgery dose and the anesthesiologist will administer it intraoperatively. For elective procedures, diabetes and hypertension should be under control. Patients with both diabetes and hypertension have higher cardiovascular and renal risks. Morbid obesity is a perioperative risk. Tissue perfusion is reduced, healing may be impaired, and ambulation is compromised, all of which also increase risk of DVT.

Patients who are morbidly obese require fasting glucose to detect undiagnosed diabetes.

Those patients with sleep apnea need continuous positive airway pressure (CPAP) treatment while hospitalized.

TAKE HOME POINTS

- Recommendations for preoperative testing are based on the clinical predictors that can be identified when conducting a thorough history and physical examination.
- Failure to complete a thorough history and physical examination can increase your patient's preoperative risks.
- Beta-blockers are recommended for patients with more than one clinical risk factor of cardiovascular disease.
- Aspirin and clopidogrel should be discontinued 5 days before surgery
- Smoking cessation should be 6 to 8 weeks before surgery.
- Give DVT prophylaxis for moderate- and high-risk groups.
- Unfractionated heparin or LWMH can be given before or after incision.
- OCP and hormone therapy should be discontinued preoperatively in patients who are at moderate and high risk for DVT.
- In patients with previous history of DVT with long-term warfarin, it is recommended that warfarin should be stopped 4 days before surgery to reach INR 1.5.
- Remember that the presence of major predictors may justify a delay or cancellation of an elective surgery until adequate preoperative evaluation and clearance can be done.

SUGGESTED READINGS

ACOG Practice Bulletin. Prevention of Deep Vein Thrombosis and Pulmonary Embolism. ACOG Practice Bulletin No. 84, August 2007.

Johnson BE, Porter J. Preoperative Evaluation of the Gynecologic Patient. Considerations for improved outcome. ACOG Practice Bulletin; 111(5), May 2008.

Karnath BM. Perioperative risk assessment. *J Am Fam Phys*. 2002;66(10):1889–1895.

Mangano DT. Perioperative cardiac morbidity. *Anesthesiology*. 1990;72:153–184.

Prolog. *Gynecology and Surgery*. 5th ed. Washington, DC. American College of Obstetrics and Gynecology. 2004.

Rock JA, Jones HW III. *TeLinde's Operative Gynecology*. 10th ed. Philadelphia, PA: Lippincott Williams & Wilkins; 2008.

Steen PA, Tinker JH, Tarhan S. Myocardial rein-farction after anesthesia and surgery. *JAMA*. 1978;239:2566–2570.

Tarhan S, Moffitt EA, Taylor WF, et al. Myocardial infarction after general anesthesia. *JAMA*. 1972;220:1451–1454.

125

PREPARATION BEFORE THE SURGERY

THINH DUONG, MD

The appropriateness and successfulness of a surgical procedure depend on several factors including the ability and sound judgment of the surgeon, the surgeon's knowledge of the disease process, and the likelihood of surgical success depending on the disease process. Thus, the likelihood that a patient will gain benefit from the surgery is guided by a careful and detailed preoperative evaluation with sufficient preparation. Although each surgical candidate may have various nuances, certain common themes are present.

All preoperative evaluation begins with a detailed history and physical examination. A careful evaluation of the patient's presenting symptoms and the various signs of the complaint is important. A careful review of all systems may reveal related symptoms missed if the surgeon is too focused on the specific patient complaint. For example, patients with adnexal torsion may present with fevers, chills, nausea or vomiting, and symptoms that may appear completely unrelated to a torsed ovary. A detailed social and family history may reveal environmental and genetic factors that may change the choice or type of surgery. For the gynecologist, attention must be paid to the obstetrical, gynecological, and sexual history, given that most women may not talk about such things with their primary care providers.

A preoperative physical examination should cover all of the systems. However, special attention needs to be paid to the particular area of complaint and the major systems (e.g., pulmonary and cardiovascular). Although a detailed description of a physical examination is beyond the scope of this discussion, certain features of the various portions of the exam should be noted:

Neck: Note any enlarged masses on the thyroid or deviation of the trachea.

Breast: In general, the breasts should be examined in the upright and supine position. Note the symmetry, size, condition of the nipples, any nipple discharge, any masses, the condition of the skin, and the presence of any enlarged axillary lymph nodes.

Pulmonary: Note any decrease in breath sounds, rales, wheezes, or rhonchis.

Heart: Note any irregularities in the heart rate, rhythm, or additional heart sounds.

Abdomen: Examination includes visualization, palpation, auscultation, and percussion. Note for any abnormal bulges or sites of tenderness. Auscultation may aid in distinguishing between distended bowel, a large tumor, or even pregnancy.

Extremities: Note any asymmetry, weaknesses, or signs of poor perfusion (e.g., decreased pulses, clubbing, cyanosis, or edema).

Evaluation of the pelvis and rectum in detail is paramount to the gynecologist. In general, patients are examined in the dorsal lithotomy position; however, examination in the upright position may be warranted in certain circumstances (e.g., to assess for stress urinary leakage). An empty bladder is essential to an adequate exam. The external genitalia should be inspected for any lesions. The urethra should be inspected for any abnormalities. The patient should be asked to valsalva (i.e., bear down or push) with the labia folds separated to asses for any vaginal or uterine prolapse. All five quadrants of the vagina (anterior, posterior, left, right, and apex) should be gently palpated to evaluate for tenderness or masses. The urethra should be gently milked to assess for any mass or purulent discharge. The cervix should be gently moved to the left, right, anterior, and posterior and the location and intensity of the any pain should be noted. A bimanual examination with one hand palpating the vagina and the second hand palpating the lower abdomen should assess for any tenderness or masses. The ovaries may often be palpated; however, patient discomfort during the exam may limit their palpation. A rectovaginal examination should also be accomplished with the index finger inserted in the vagina and the middle finger placed into the rectum. Ease of rectal placement may be accomplished by advising the patient to bear down like she is having a bowel movement to relax the anal sphincter. Attention should be paid to the ovaries, posterior aspects of the broad ligament, and uterosacral ligaments.

Preoperative laboratory assessment is dependent on the likelihood of identifying a medical problem. However, an excess of laboratories will increase the possibility of a false-positive test, subjecting patients to unnecessary concerns and additional invasive testing. Suggested lab testing includes a urine pregnancy test (unless the patient had a hysterectomy or is postmenopausal), urinalysis, a complete blood count, and evaluation for bleeding disorders (PT, PTT, INR). In the presence of symptoms suggestive of hepatic, renal, or metabolic disease, a chemistry panel with evaluation glucose, liver enzymes, BUN, creatinine, and thyroid functions may be useful. In the presence of an ovarian mass, tumor markers may be appropriate. Furthermore, all patients should have a preoperative Pap smear if none has been done within the past year. Women with abnormal uterine bleeding require a preoperative endometrial biopsy. In addition, a pelvic ultrasound is useful in the presence of abnormal uterine bleeding, an enlarged uterus, or pelvic masses.

The need for a preoperative electrocardiogram (ECG or EKG) remains controversial. For minor procedures, its use may not be necessary.

However, it may be appropriate in women with a history and physical exam suggestive of cardiovascular disease, the presence of hypertension or diabetes, patients taking medications with known cardiac toxicities, patients at risk for electrolyte disturbances, and patients undergoing major surgical procedures. In general, all women over 40 should undergo an ECG prior to a major surgical procedure. Additional imaging studies such as computer tomography, magnetic resonance imaging, or positron emission tomography may be indicated in certain circumstances depending on the disease process.

Although there are no clear guidelines for obtaining preoperative pulmonary assessments, several items should be considered. Baseline preoperative pulmonary function tests may be useful in patients with a history of breathing difficulties or abnormal findings on physical examination. Patients with asthma need to be optimized prior to surgery and inhaler or nebulizer therapy should be considered prior to anesthesia induction.

Patients with cardiac disease need special attention, given the potentially deadly consequences of poor cardiac function. For elective procedures, the American College of Cardiology recommends postponement of the surgery should the patient fall into any of the following categories:

1. Unstable or severe angina
2. Myocardial infarction <1 month ago
3. Decompensated heart failure, defined as worsening or new heart failure or New York Heart Association Class IV heart failure
4. Significant arrhythmias including high-grade atrioventricular block, symptomatic or newly diagnosed ventricular tachycardia, supraventricular tachycardia with conducted heart rates >100 per minute at rest, and symptomatic bradycardia
5. Severe valvular disease including severe aortic stenosis or symptomatic mitral stenosis

Furthermore, cardiac testing should be performed in patients whose operative risks are intermediate to high, whose functional ability is <4 MET, and who have one or more of the following risk factors: (1) history of ischemic heart disease, (2) history of compensated or prior congestive heart failure, (3) history of cerebral vascular disease, (4) diabetes mellitus, or (5) chronic kidney disease.

For patient on anticoagulant therapy, several options exist. Those on warfarin should be converted to low-dose heparin (5,000 U subcutaneously every 12 hours) 4 to 5 days prior to the surgery. This dose should be continued until the patient can tolerate oral feeds, at which time warfarin may be restarted. In addition, the use of preoperative elastic stockings or sequential compression devices in the lower extremities at the beginning of the surgery with continuation until the patient is ambulatory may prevent venous stasis and the formation of deep venous thrombosis (DVT). Although no studies directly support the discontinuation of oral contraceptives prior to surgery for the prevention of DVT, discontinuation of estrogen contraceptives 2 to 4 weeks preoperative is reasonable when there is a high concern for DVT formation. If this is done, patients should be advised to either abstain from intercourse or use another effective method of contraception as to avoid unplanned pregnancy.

Surgical site infections may cause significant morbidity and mortality. Thus, preoperative prevention serves the greatest opportunity to decrease this major morbidity. Several measures may reduce postoperative infections:

- Infections remote from the surgical site should be treated prior to any elective surgery. Should treatment be inadequate or unsuccessful, the surgery should be delayed until the infection is improved.
- Routine removal of hair preoperatively should be avoided, unless it interferes with the surgery. If hair removal is necessary, use electric clippers to remove the hair just before the surgery.
- Diabetic patients should have adequate control of blood glucose levels and hyperglycemia avoided perioperatively.
- Cessation of any tobacco use should be done a minimum of 30 days prior to surgery.
- Advise patients to shower or bathe with an antiseptic agent the night before the surgery.
- Wash and clean the surgical site prior to antiseptic skin preparation to remove gross contamination.
- Apply antiseptic skin preparation in concentric circles moving from the incision site toward the periphery. The extent of the preparation should cover the incision and any potential extension of the incision, new incisions, or site of drain placement.
- Minimize preoperative hospital stays.
- Preoperative antibiotic with a cephalosporin is recommended for both abdominal and vaginal hysterectomies. Antibiotics should be administered 1 to 2 hours before the surgery and repeated for long surgeries (>3 hours) or significant blood loss (>1,500 mL).
- If present, bacterial vaginosis should be treated prior to the surgery.

When bowel entry or injury is of concern, then a preoperative bowel cleansing is recommended. The use of any of the commercially available products will suffice and oral antibiotics are generally unnecessary. The large colon should be emptied with an enema the evening before the surgery and repeated in the morning to ensure complete decompression. In general, all women undergoing laparoscopic surgery, cancer surgery, or have a history of chronic pelvic pain should have complete preoperative bowel preparation of the small and large intestines.

TAKE HOME POINTS

- A thorough history and physical exam are required prior to any surgical procedure.
- Preoperative laboratories and testing should be individualized depending on the surgery and the patient's associated risk.
- A pregnancy test is required in all reproductive-aged women who have not undergone a hysterectomy.
- Elective surgery should be postponed in very high risk patients and appropriate cardiac testing performed depending on the patient's risk history, functional ability, and operative risk.
- The patient on warfarin should be converted to low-dose heparin and continued until she can take oral feeds, at which time warfarin should be restarted.
- Unnecessary hair removal should be avoided and, if necessary, only be done immediately preoperative with electric clippers.
- Preoperative bowel preparation should be done when injury is of concern or when decompressed intestine is surgically useful.

SUGGESTED READINGS

ACOG Educational Bulletin. Antibiotics and gynecologic infections. *ACOG Educational Bulletin*. 1997;237.

Center for Disease Control and Prevention. Hospital Infection Control Practices Advisory Committee. Guidelines for prevention of surgical site infections. *Am J Infect Control*. 1999;27:250–277.

Fischer SP. Cost-effective preoperative evaluation and testing. *Chest*. 1999;115:96S–100S.

Johnson BE, Porter J. Preoperative evaluation of the gynecologic patient. *Obstet Gynecol*. 2008;111:1183–1194.

Kaplan EB, Sheiner LB, Boeckmann AJ, et al. The usefulness of preoperative laboratory screening. *JAMA*. 1985;253:3576–3581.

LeBlond RF, DeGowin RL, Brown DD. *DeGowin's Diagnostic Examination*. 8th ed. New York, NY: McGraw-Hill; 2004.

126

MINOR GYNECOLOGIC SURGERY: INCOMPLETE HISTORY TAKING

KEVIN SCOTT SMITH, MD, FACOG

The commonest error in minor gynecologic surgery is arguably adopting such nomenclature itself. All gynecologic surgeries potentially may result in major complications, and therefore, prudence should be exercised when deeming any gynecologic surgery as minor. With that disclaimer out of the way, what follows are some points of caution for minor gynecologic surgeries.

INCOMPLETE HISTORY TAKING

Prior to performing an endometrial biopsy for evaluation of postmenopausal bleeding, an eager junior resident applies an ample coating of povidone iodine solution to the patient's cervix. As the endometrial biopsy gets underway, the patient reports trouble swallowing. Within minutes, she describes a tightening of her throat. Next, her speech slurs as the resident notes swelling of the patient's lips and tongue. The resident quickly administers Benadryl recognizing the patient's allergic reaction. The patient later recalls a similar incident during an elegant seafood dinner.

Basic medical training emphasizes obtaining a thorough history. This may involve probing for information that the patient does not regard as relevant. Do not make the error of being satisfied with just the limited information that your patients provide. You must elicit history that they may find irrelevant and unnecessary. When reporting their allergy history, many patients (and physicians) only think about allergies to medications. However, allergic reactions to seafood and shellfish are often overlooked. Many patients have seafood allergies, which indeed may be anaphylactic and life threatening. Anaphylaxis, thus, may be triggered by the povidone iodine solution commonly used as a sterile preparation during gynecologic procedures. Alternatives to the betadine solution include chlorhexidine, hydrogen peroxide, or alcohol.

Another integral component to any complete gynecologic history is the patient's recent menstrual history. Despite this well-known fact, a common error is to minimize the need for timing of hysteroscopic procedures. For premenopausal women with regular menstrual cycles, the proliferative phase is best for visualization of the uterine cavity. The thickened secretory endometrium can obscure visualization of smaller submucous fibroids or endometrial polyps. Identification of tubal ostia required for hysteroscopic sterilization or tubal canalization can also be obstructed by a secretory endometrial lining. The endometrium can also be prepared with hormonal manipulation using combination oral contraceptives or progestational agents.

You must also avoid the error of not confirming that your patient is not pregnant prior to any instrumentation of the uterine cavity in all women of reproductive age. This is devastating not only to the patient but also to the physician when the tissue sample is reported as containing chronic villi or products of conception. This can undoubtedly lead to litigious action. Avoid haste and assumptions!

TAKE HOME POINTS

- A thorough history inclusive of drug allergy and menstrual history may minimize complications and optimize procedure yield.
- A pregnancy test is always required prior to instrumentation of the uterine cavity in all women of reproductive age.
- Relating clear and complete expectations to patients is essential for best patient satisfaction.

SUGGESTED READINGS

Abbott JA, Garry R. The surgical management of menorrhagia. *Hum Reprod.* 2002;8:68–78.
ACOG Practice Bulletin No. 81: Endometrial Ablation. *Obstet Gynecol.* 2007;109:1233.
Brill AI. What is the role of hysteroscopy in the management of abnormal uterine bleeding? *Clin Obstet Gynecol.* 1995;38:319.
Copeland LJ. *Textbook of Gynecology.* 2nd ed. Philadelphia, PA: W.B. Saunders; 2000.
Donnadieu AC, Fernandez H. The role of Essure sterilization performed simultaneously with endometrial ablation. *Curr Opin Obstet Gynecol.* 2008;20(4):359–363.
Lo JS, Pickersgill A. Pregnancy after endometrial ablation: English literature review and case report. *J Minim Invasive Gynecol.* 2006;13:88.
Xia E, Li TC, Yu D, et al. The occurrence and outcome of 39 pregnancies after 1621 cases of transcervical resection of endometrium. *Hum Reprod.* 2006;21:3282.

127

MINOR GYNECOLOGIC SURGERY: INCOMPLETE PHYSICAL EXAM

KEVIN SCOTT SMITH, MD, FACOG

The commonest error in minor gynecologic surgery is arguably adopting such nomenclature itself. All gynecologic surgeries potentially may result in major complications, and therefore, prudence should be exercised when deeming any gynecologic surgery as minor. With that disclaimer out of the way, what follows are points of caution for minor gynecologic surgeries.

INCOMPLETE PHYSICAL EXAMINATION

A young newlywed presents to her gynecologist hopeful about the prospect of beginning her childbearing. Despite multiple attempts, it has been very difficult to locate the subdermal contraceptive implant that was placed 2 years prior to presentation by her previous gynecologist. The effort is further complicated by pain and bleeding incurred resulting from aggressive blunt and sharp dissection in a location that was incorrect. After the implant is located on ultrasound, the patient is scheduled for removal under anesthesia.

A common caution with the previously employed Norplant and currently available Implanon subdermal contraceptive devices is to avoid insertion deep to the subdermis. A thorough physical exam is important. This may be difficult when either the patient has gained a lot of weight or the device has been placed inappropriately. Placement too deeply may result in injury to muscle, nerves, or blood vessels. Additionally, removal may be quite difficult. When placed properly, the Implanon rod will be palpable by pressing your fingertips over the skin in the patient's arm where it was placed. Insertion is in the medial aspect of the upper part of the nondominant arm. Correct superficial placement of the rod ensures easy removal in the future. It has been recommended that doctors undergo a recognized training course in the use of the implant.

Awareness of anatomical limits is also paramount when inserting intrauterine contraceptive devices (IUD). Despite the usual practice of uterine sounding prior to IUD insertion, it is quite easy to perform incorrect placement. IUD placement high in the uterus (i.e., at the fundus) minimizes expulsions, accidental pregnancies, and possible bleeding. Adequate placement of the IUD can be confirmed with ultrasound visualization of the uterus in the office setting.

Uterine perforation is a common complication during minor gynecologic procedures. Sounding of the uterus slowly and gently to determine its depth and direction reduces the risk of perforating the uterus, which usually occurs because the sound or IUD is inserted too deeply or at the wrong angle. The bimanual exam determines the size, position, consistency, and mobility of the uterus and identifies any tenderness, which might indicate infection. Hysteroscopic procedures particularly emphasize the need for thorough pelvic exam. Once the uterus has been stabilized utilizing a tenaculum on the anterior cervical lip, excessive force applied to advance the hysteroscope (or IUD) beyond the internal os of the uterus is a common cause of uterine perforation or cervical laceration. This is particularly likely with a severely retroverted uterus.

Knowledge of preprocedure anatomy may require additional testing. For example, all women should have endometrial sampling documenting the absence of premalignant or malignant disease prior to endometrial ablation. The endometrial cavity should also be assessed by either office hysteroscopy or sonohysterography to exclude the presence of submucous myomata or polyps, which can be treated with simple resection. It is also extremely important to avoid excessive dilation of the internal cervical os during hysteroscopic procedures. Doing so will result in leakage of the distending medium around the hysteroscope undermining visualization efforts. Troubleshooting may be achieved by placing a tenaculum on the cervix around the inserted hysteroscope.

TAKE HOME POINTS

- Comprehensive physical examination and applicable testing will enhance safety and effectiveness of gynecologic procedures.
- Knowledge of preprocedure anatomy may require additional testing.

SUGGESTED READINGS

Abbott JA, Garry R. The surgical management of menorrhagia. *Hum Reprod.* 2002;8:68–78.
ACOG Practice Bulletin No. 81: Endometrial Ablation. *Obstet Gynecol.* 2007;109:1233.
Brill AI. What is the role of hysteroscopy in the management of abnormal uterine bleeding? *Clin Obstet Gynecol.* 1995;38:319.

128

MINOR GYNECOLOGIC SURGERY: PATIENT COUNSELING

KEVIN SCOTT SMITH, MD, FACOG

The commonest error in minor gynecologic surgery is arguably adopting such nomenclature itself. All gynecologic surgeries potentially may result in major complications, and therefore, prudence should be exercised when deeming any gynecologic surgery as minor. With that disclaimer out of the way, what follows are some points of caution for minor gynecologic surgeries.

PATIENT COUNSELING

A 46-year-old woman presents to her gynecologist's office 8 months following an endometrial ablation for menorrhagia. She is quite enraged by her continued menstrual cycles although she describes them as much shorter and more regular than preoperatively. She insists that she was promised that she would have no future menses following her procedure. She informs her gynecologist that she is leaving that practice in search of another physician.

This patient was a victim of misinformation. A common mistake when counseling patients regarding expectations following an endometrial ablation is to assure them of amenorrhea. In fact, the reported incidence of postoperative amenorrhea after endometrial ablation has ranged from 23% to 60%, and 6% to 20% of women have required further surgery for control of their symptoms after 1 to 5 years of follow-up. Another common omission when counseling patients regarding postablation outcomes is that pregnancy is possible and can be hazardous (e.g., increased risk of miscarriage, antepartum hemorrhage, preterm delivery, abnormal placental attachment). Infertility after endometrial ablation is probably related to tubal occlusion and impaired endometrial receptivity; however, endometrial ablation should not be regarded as a sterilization procedure.

Attention should be given to the patient's contraceptive management. Concomitant Essure sterilization at the time of global endometrial ablation has also been advocated.

TAKE HOME POINTS

- It is of paramount importance that you communicate with your patients and provide them with accurate information.
- Always be honest with patients.

- Trust is built, developed, and cultivated.
- Relating clear and complete expectations to patients is essential for best patient satisfaction.

SUGGESTED READINGS

Copeland LJ. *Textbook of Gynecology.* 2nd ed. Philadelphia, PA: W.B. Saunders; 2000.

Donnadieu AC, Fernandez H. The role of Essure sterilization performed simultaneously with endometrial ablation. *Curr Opin Obstet Gynecol.* 2008;20(4):359–363.

Lo JS, Pickersgill A. Pregnancy after endometrial ablation: English literature review and case report. *J Minim Invasive Gynecol.* 2006;13:88.

Xia E, Li TC, Yu D, et al. The occurrence and outcome of 39 pregnancies after 1621 cases of transcervical resection of endometrium. *Hum Reprod.* 2006;21:3282.

129

LAPAROSCOPY: THEY GO HOME FASTER IF YOU DO IT RIGHT

ALFRED GENDY, MD

Laparoscopy is an essential diagnostic and therapeutic operative procedure. It is commonly performed in patients with benign diseases as well as gynecologic cancers. Laparoscopic surgical procedures are usually performed in an effort to replicate procedures that have been successful at laparotomy with the potential advantages of the laparoscopy over laparotomy, which include smaller scar, faster recovery, decreased adhesion formation, and decreased cost.

To be better prepared for a laparoscopic procedure, you must know the equipment required for the procedure, which includes mono and bipolar cautery; uterine manipulators (Hulka, HUMI, RUMI); laparoscope (5 and 10 mm sizes) at 0-, 12-, and 30-degree visualization angles; camera head; light cable; CO_2 tubing; Veress needle (standard length 11.5 and 17 cm long); and trocars (5 to 15 mm).

A detailed history of prior abdominal surgeries and radiation therapy which give a hint about possible intra-abdominal adhesions and anatomic distortion is required. When there are concerns about altered anatomy at the umbilicus, an alternative entry method can make laparoscopic entry safer. These techniques include the use of the Hasson open approach, direct intraperitoneal placement of 5-mm trocar, and the use of Palmer's point in the left hypochondrium.

Intraoperatively, the patient should be placed in the modified lithotomy position to allow access to the vagina where the hips will be extended and thighs at the same level of the abdomen, legs should be well positioned and well protected, knees should be deflexed to avoid stretching of the femoral nerve, arms can be adducted, pronated, and tucked to the patient's side with proper protection of the fingers, hands, and elbow with foam pads.

Some positioning injuries can result from improper positions. A brachial plexus injury can be caused by outstretched arms and compression by shoulder braces during steep Trendelenburg positions. This nerve injury can result in sensory loss of the radial two third of the hand and wrist drop if severe. A peroneal nerve injury can be caused by compression of peroneal nerve at the lateral head of the fibula which results in sensory loss of the lateral aspects of the lower leg and foot drop. An exaggerated dorsal lithotomy position will result in femoral nerve and stretch injuries which will lead to sensory loss of the anterior thigh and the inability to raise the leg. An ulnar nerve injury can be caused by over supination of the arm if tucked to the side or over pronation if outstretched on arm board and can result in sensory loss over the medial one and half fingers and claw hands if severe.

It is important to empty the bladder to avoid injury of distended bladder with the trocar or Veress needle insertion and moving the buttocks a few centimeters beyond the edge of the table will avoid undue pressure on the sacrum leading to coccydynia. During the surgery, an orogastric tube can be used by the anesthesia team to decompress the stomach and small bowel to decrease injury and allow for improved visualization of the pelvic cavity. A uterine cannula or manipulator should be used for visualization of structures in the cul-de-sac except when the uterus is absent, anomalies exist that prevent exposure to the cervix, the woman is prepubescent female with small hymenal opening, or an intrauterine pregnancy is suspected.

TAKE HOME POINTS

- Know your patient's prior surgical history and have a plan for abdominal wall entry before the surgery.
- A brachial plexus injury can result in sensory loss of the radial two thirds of the hand and wrist drop.
- Peroneal nerve injury can result in sensory loss of the lateral aspects of the lower leg and foot drop.
- Femoral nerve and stretch injuries can lead to sensory loss of the anterior thigh and the inability to raise the leg.
- Ulnar nerve injury can result in sensory loss over the medial one and half fingers and claw hands.
- Always drain the bladder prior to inserting the Veress needle or trocar.

SUGGESTED READINGS

Hulka JF, Reich H. *Textbook of Laparoscopy*. 3rd ed. Philadelphia, PA: W.B. Saunders Company; 1998.

Pasic R, Levine RL. *A Practical Manual of Laparoscopy: A Clinical Cookbook*. London, UK: Taylor & Francis; 2002.

Rock JA, Jones HW. *Te Linde's Operative Gynecology*. 9th ed. Philadelphia, PA: Lippincott Williams & Wilkin; 2003.

130

"WHAT IS WRONG WITH THE CAMERA, WHY IS MY SUCTION NOT WORKING, AND WHY WILL THE GRASPER NOT FIT THROUGH THIS SCOPE?"

KENAN OMURTAG, MD

Hysteroscopy requires a thorough understanding of the equipment used and how to troubleshoot it. There is a delicate balance between distension, suction, and camera focus required to actually perform the procedure. Preoperative preparation of the equipment is crucial in maximizing operative time and ensuring a successful case.

Prior to scrubbing, the surgeon should assist the circulator in arranging the ancillary equipment. This is the job of the surgeon and also fosters cooperation, leadership, and trust amongst the operative team. The choice of medium should be determined and made available as well as a method of delivery. There are two ways to deliver distension medium: (1) gravity or (2) continuous flow via a fluid pump. Gravity is usually sufficient and consists of the medium hung at an elevated level wrapped with a blood pressure cuff. Continuous flow fluid pumps allow the surgeon to control pressures. Communicate with the circulator and the anesthesia staff about which form of distension delivery you decide to use. If the surgeon decides to use a continuous flow system, both the surgeon and the circulator should be versed in its use and know how to troubleshoot it.

If the particular case is an operative one that requires special equipment such as a resectoscope and/or various energy sources, this is the time to ensure that these devices and their accessories are in the room and ready to be assembled during surgical draping. The distention media for simple diagnostic hysteroscopy may be saline or Ringer lactate. Stay away from hypotonic media such as dextrose 5% in water as its reabsorption can more readily lead to water intoxication. When performing an operative procedure with electrocautery, saline and Ringer lactate can conduct electricity and should be avoided. Glycine is preferred in cases of electrosurgery. Complications from saline and Ringer lactate include fluid overload and pulmonary edema. This is especially likely when the uterine wall is damaged with either endometrial ablation or myomectomy. Glycine overload is associated with congestive failure, pulmonary edema, and ammonia intoxication. Although rarely used today, Hyskon (32% dextran 70 in dextrose) may cause an alarming bleeding diathesis, noncardiogenic pulmonary edema, and an anaphylactoid reaction.

The surgeon should then ensure that the video monitor is in an appropriate field of view for either sitting or standing. While adjusting the monitor, the surgeon should ensure that the video equipment is functioning properly and that images from prior surgeries have been cleared. Doing this simple check will also determine whether the photo printer is working properly. In our experience, reviewing the findings of the surgery with the patient can improve patient satisfaction.

After scrubbing for the case and introducing himself or herself to the scrub technician, the surgeon should inspect the hysteroscopic equipment and assemble it according to the needs of the case. Occasionally, diagnostic hysteroscopic accessories and operative hysteroscopic accessories will be mixed together, and this is why it is **essential** for the surgeon to review the contents of the hysteroscope tray and assemble the hysteroscope prior to using it.

In cases in which operative ports/channels or a resectoscope is used, it is important to ensure that the appropriate accessories are available and preoperative construction of the hysteroscope is simulated to minimize wasted time intraoperatively. When using operative instruments, the surgeon should ensure that the instruments fit through the operative port completely. These simple exercises save intraoperative time and also build communication with the OR staff.

Once the equipment check has been made and the patient has been draped, assembly of the hysteroscope and attachment of the inflow and outflow ports should be performed next so that a functioning hysteroscope is on standby. This preparation also helps the surgeon familiarize himself or herself to the various ports and their respective valves and determine any equipment failures prior to starting the case as these can be remedied by the circulator as the case begins. At this point, it bears mentioning that the surgeon should loudly call for the light to be on "standby" when the scope is not in use. When resting the hysteroscope, ensure that the tip is off the drapes. When on full power, the light source is hot enough to burn a hole in the drape and potentially cause burn injury to the patient in a matter of seconds.

Ultimately, hysteroscopy, with its many applications, is one of the many procedures unique to gynecology. Skill with this procedure usually begins early in a resident's career. Understanding the equipment, its setup, and its pitfalls early on will make these procedures more rewarding and less frustrating.

TAKE HOME POINTS

- Know whether your case is going to be diagnostic or operative.
- Make sure the appropriate distension media is in the operating room.
- Put the hysteroscope together after you have scrubbed.
- Make sure suction is appropriately connected to the hysteroscope prior to starting.
- Loudly call "place scope on standby" when not in use.

SUGGESTED READINGS

Azziz R, Murphy AA. *Practical Manual of Operative Laparoscopy and Hysteroscopy*. 2nd ed. New York, NY: Springer; 1997.

Rock J, Jones H. *TeLindes Operative Gynecology*. Philadelphia, PA: Lippincott Williams & Wilkins; 2003.

131

"I CANNOT SEE A THING!"

KENAN OMURTAG, MD

The best time to perform hysteroscopy, particularly diagnostic, is during the proliferative phase of the menstrual cycle. However, one of the most common indications for hysteroscopy is abnormal uterine bleeding and therefore timing one's cycle to coordinate date of surgery is futile. Visibility, however, is not guaranteed with hysteroscopy and requires an understanding of the mediums used, their interaction with blood, and the various techniques used in hysteroscopy to facilitate maximum visualization.

Visibility is essential in ensuring safe operative hysteroscopy and minimizing perforation. Poor visibility is commonly due to pushing the telescope up to the endometrium, which results in a red blur. There is a tendency to push forward; however, pushing forward may lead to perforation, and in all cases of poor visibility, the operator should pull the scope back when encountering poor visibility.

Oftentimes, blood from dilation or curettage done prior to hysteroscopy results in poor visualization of the cavity. Blood in the cavity can be remedied by balancing aspiration of the cavity with inflow of fresh distension medium to "recycle" the medium. High-viscosity mediums such as Hyskon are immiscible with blood and create a "clear field." Additionally, they are inert and permit electrosurgery to be performed within them. However, there is concern over their toxicities when absorbed resulting in pulmonary edema, anaphylaxis, and/or bleeding diasthesis.

Lower viscosity mediums include normal saline, sorbitol, glycine, and mannitol. Normal saline is commonly used in diagnostic procedures or in operative cases where resection without energy is predictable. Use of energy in normal saline is contraindicated due to the conduction properties of the solution. Unlike Hyskon, though, saline easily flows retrograde from the uterus, therefore requiring high volumes and flow to provide adequate uterine distension.

Sorbitol and glycine are commonly used in male urologic procedures and have been picked up by gynecologic hysteroscopists. These fluids are inert and allow for use of energy; however, absorption of these fluids can lead to acute hyponatremia. Interestingly, a mechanism of cation pumping is unique to neurons in the male brain and provides an electrolyte balance. Therefore, women undergoing operative hysteroscopy are more sensitive to a hypoosmolar and thus cerebral edema and great care should be used when using these mediums. Mannitol is another inert medium commonly used that is more iso-osmolar than the above. Regardless of the medium used, it is imperative that accurate totals of fluid in's and out's are monitored during hysteroscopy by both the surgeon and circulating nurse.

Achieving and maintaining visibility are vital during hysteroscopy, whether by adjusting focus of the camera or manipulating the inflow and outflow of distension media.

TAKE HOME POINTS

- Know how to focus the camera while simultaneously introducing it.
- Never push forward when visibility is poor; instead pull back.
- Know which type of medium the case requires and the advantages/disadvantages of that.
- Energy- and electrolyte-rich mediums such as saline *do not* go together.
- Ensure adequate monitoring of I's and O's.

SUGGESTED READING

Rock J, Jones H. *TeLindes Operative Gynecology*. Philadelphia, PA: Lippincott Williams & Wilkins; 2003.

132

"DID YOU PERFORATE THE UTERUS?"

KENAN OMURTAG, MD

Uterine perforation is the complication most commonly anticipated when placing any rigid instrument into the uterus. Operative hysteroscopy with its use of long operative rigid scopes and various energy sources is a common culprit in perforation injuries. Perforation rates during operative hysteroscopy can affect between 1% and 2% of operative hysteroscopy. Using safe techniques and early identification of perforation as indications for operative hysteroscopy are expanding.

Nearly half of all uterine perforations at the time of hysteroscopy are related to cervical dilation. Dilation is essential not only because it allows adequate dimensions for passage of the scope. Additionally, coupled with exam under anesthesia, it provides the surgeon with the path of the cervical canal.

If the surgeon does not dilate the cervix enough, passage of the rigid hysteroscope becomes difficult. Dilate the cervix too much, and the surgeon runs the risk of losing distention media through the cervix creating poor visibility. Once dilation is complete, the cervical os should be visualized with the naked eye and the distention media should be turned on. The scope should be in focus and then introduced through the cervix under direct visualization supplemented with the surgeon's tactile feedback.

The complexity of the case may dictate whether concomitant laparoscopy may be indicated. Ultimately, this is not mandatory. Uterine perforation during hysteroscopy can usually be identified quickly, for example, while performing a septum resection when loss of uterine distention is encountered in light of heavy volumes of distention medium.

Knowing how the perforation occurred will dictate how the surgeon will manage it. If the perforation is identified and encountered immediately after sharp resection, it may be managed conservatively at the minimum with diagnostic laparoscopy if intra–abdominal/pelvic injury is suspected. Perforation sites are small and heal without need for repair. Most of the time, uterine perforation will result in a stoppage of the case, but if the case must continue, directed laparoscopy should be advised and energy sources should be minimized.

Safe use of energy is essential in minimizing risk of perforation. When perforation is suspected with the use of energy, laparoscopy is necessary to rule out injury to the nearby bowel, ureter, or major vessels due to thermal spread. When using energy with a resectoscope, the surgeon should activate the energy when pulling the resectoscope backward and *not* forward. Activation should only occur when adequate visualization is achieved. Perforation from injury, if not identified intraoperatively, may manifest itself 24 to 48 hours later and both the physician and the patient should be aware of signs of injury (pain, nausea, vomiting, falling blood pressure, abdominal distension, fever, oligo–anuria, etc.). Oftentimes, if injury is suspected, in-house observation for 24 hours may be warranted.

Understanding common points in operative hysteroscopy when uterine perforation may occur is necessary in order to take the appropriate safeguards to minimize its occurrence. In addition to the above, operator awareness of his or her own skill level is also crucial in minimizing complications during complex operative hysteroscopy.

TAKE HOME POINTS

- Half of all uterine perforations occur during dilation.
- Introduce the hysteroscope under direct visualization; do not look at the cervix.
- Sudden difficulty with distention despite heavy volumes may suggest perforation.
- Diagnostic laparoscopy is done to survey abdomen/pelvis in case of perforation.
- Common signs postoperatively of intra–abdominal injury are fever, nausea, abdominal distension/pain.

SUGGESTED READINGS

Azziz R, Murphy AA. *Practical Manual of Operative Laparoscopy and Hysteroscopy*. 2nd ed. New York, NY: Springer; 1997.

Paschopoulos M, Polyzos NP, Lavasidis LG, et al. Safety issues of hysteoscopic surgery. *Ann N Y Acad Sci*. 2006;1092:229–234.

Pasini A, Belloni C. Intraoperative complications of 697 Consecutive Hysteroscopies. *Minerva Ginecol*. 2001;53:13–20.

Rock J, Jones H. *TeLindes Operative Gynecology*. Philadelphia, PA: Lippincott Williams & Wilkins; 2003.

133

MINIMIZE THE RISK OF ASHERMAN SYNDROME BY RESECTING SUBMUCOSAL FIBROIDS IN APPOSITION TO ONE ANOTHER IN MULTIPLE STAGES

JOHN K. PARK, MD, MSc

Approximately 5% of uterine fibroids are submucosal in location. These fibroids often present with menorrhagia, infertility, or recurrent pregnancy loss. Submucosal fibroids should be suspected when there is an intrauterine filling defect on a hysterosalpingogram (HSG) or by visualizing a mass encroaching on the endometrial lining during a routine pelvic ultrasound. In either situation, the differential diagnosis can also include an endometrial polyp or endometrial hyperplasia. The evaluation should proceed with a saline–infusion ultrasound (sonohysterogram) because it is the most cost-effective way to diagnose submucosal fibroids, and this will also allow characterization and mapping of fibroids within the uterine cavity. There are two types of submucosal fibroids that are amenable to hysteroscopic resection. Type 0 fibroids are pedunculated and entirely within the uterine cavity and type 1 fibroids are those with >50% of the volume projecting into the uterine cavity. The information from the sonohysterogram can be used to plan the surgical approach and to appropriately counsel the patient on the expected outcomes of surgical removal.

If more than one submucosal fibroid is present, it is important to perform the sonohysterogram to determine whether any are on direct opposite sides of the endometrial cavity and in apposition to one another. If this is the case, hysteroscopic resection of the two fibroids in question should not be performed during the same procedure because the risk of intrauterine adhesion formation (Asherman syndrome) is as high as 78%. The adhesions result from having two areas of denuded endometrium in contact with one another during the healing process. To maximally decrease the risk of adhesion formation, the hysteroscopy should be performed in two stages. One fibroid should be resected, and after sufficient time for endometrial healing, the second fibroid should be removed. The incidence of adhesions after removal of one fibroid is <5%. By performing two separate procedures to remove apposing fibroids individually, the risk of Asherman's can be drastically reduced.

Once Asherman syndrome has occurred, it is not always possible to restore the cavity to its original condition. Hysteroscopic lysis of adhesions can be performed in an attempt to restore the uterine cavity, and some investigators have tried to use various devices and materials postoperatively to prevent the recurrence of adhesions. A Foley catheter balloon, an intrauterine device, and hyaluronic acid gel have been shown to reduce the incidence of adhesion recurrence, but none of these methods are 100% effective.

Even if all synechiae are removed, it is very likely that some damage has occurred to the endometrium in these areas, which may impair uterine function. This has important implications for those who desire future fertility. Women with Asherman syndrome have reduced fertility and a higher risk of pregnancy complications, such as spontaneous abortion, preterm delivery, intrauterine growth restriction, and placenta accreta or previa. Therefore, the best strategy is to take every measure possible to prevent adhesions before they can form.

TAKE HOME POINTS

- In the workup for submucosal fibroids, the saline–infusion ultrasound is the most cost-effective way to determine their number, size, and location.
- Hysteroscopic resection of submucosal fibroids is possible for type 0 and type 1 fibroids.
- If more than one submucosal fibroid is present, it is important to determine whether two are in apposition to one another because there is a high risk of Asherman syndrome if both fibroids are resected during the same procedure. Resecting the fibroids in two stages can reduce the risk of adhesion formation.

SUGGESTED READINGS

Giatras K, Berkeley AS, Noyes N, et al. Fertility after hysteroscopic resection of submucous myomas. *J Am Assoc Gynecol Laparosc.* 1999;6(2):155–158.

Yang J, Chen M, Wu M, et al. Office hysteroscopic early lysis of intrauterine adhesion after transcervical resection of multiple apposing submucous myomas. *Fertil Steril.* 2008;89:1254–1259.

Yu D, Wong YM, Cheong Y, et al. Asherman syndrome—one century later. *Fertil Steril.* 2008;89(4):759–779.

134

PRIOR TO MYOMECTOMY OR HYSTERECTOMY SECONDARY TO FIBROIDS, CONSIDER PREOPERATIVE TREATMENT WITH A GnRH ANALOG

JOHN K. PARK, MD, MSc

Analogs of GnRH are synthesized with amino acid substitutions to make them resistant to degradation, which increases their half-life. Several GnRH agonists have been studied, which include intramuscular, subcutaneous, and intranasal delivery systems. All forms have been shown to be effective in reducing fibroid volumes, with no evidence to state that one form is superior to another.

The main mechanism of action of a GnRH agonist is the down-regulation of GnRH receptors in pituitary gonadotropes, thereby creating desensitization to further GnRH stimulation. This leads to decreased gonadotropin secretion, and suppressed estrogen and progesterone levels are found 1 to 2 weeks after initial GnRH agonist administration.

Preoperatively, GnRH agonists and the removal of estrogen and progesterone offer several advantages. Because menorrhagia related to fibroids is a common indication for surgery, one benefit of GnRH agonists is the amenorrhea that follows, which often allows for the correction of any anemia that may be present. The ability to correct anemia is improved with the addition of oral iron sulfate. Another advantage to using a GnRH agonist is that the uterine volume may decrease by approximately 50%. However, individual responses vary greatly, from no response to an 80% reduction in uterine size. The vast majority of the reduction in size occurs within the first 3 months. This reduction in uterine volume may allow for a less extensive surgical procedure. For example, hysterectomy or myomectomy may be performed through a smaller laparotomy incision or by a minimally invasive means, such as vaginal hysterectomy, laparoscopy, or hysteroscopy. GnRH agonists have also been found to diminish fibroid vascularity and uterine blood flow. Expression of basic fibroblast growth factor (bFGF), vascular endothelial growth factor (VEGF), and platelet-derived growth factor (PDGF) decreased in GnRH-treated fibroids, together with the total number of blood vessels.

There are some disadvantages to using preoperative GnRH agonists. Leiomyoma degeneration from GnRH agonists may reduce the pseudocapsule interface between the fibroid and the myometrium. A clean dissection between the fibroid and the myometrium may be more difficult. Moreover, studies have shown higher rates of leiomyoma recurrence in women treated with GnRH agonists prior to myomectomy. Fibroids treated with these agents may shrink in volume to the point where they are undetected during surgical removal of the larger tumors. These smaller fibroids can rapidly return once the GnRH agonist has been removed.

GnRH agonists have side effects that result from the drop in estrogen levels, which include vasomotor symptoms, libido changes, and vaginal dryness. More importantly, 6 months of agonist therapy can result in a loss in trabecular bone, not all of which may be regained following discontinuation. As a result, GnRH agonists are not recommended for >6 months without add-back therapy.

For these reasons, GnRH agonists should not be used routinely in all patients undergoing myomectomy. These can be recommended for preoperative use in women with greatly enlarged uteri or preoperative anemia or in cases in which a decrease in uterine volume would allow a less invasive approach to leiomyoma removal.

TAKE HOME POINTS

- The use of GnRH analogs for 3 to 4 months prior to fibroid surgery often reduces both uterine volume and fibroid size.
- A reduction in uterine volume may allow for a less extensive surgical procedure.
- GnRH agonists may help correct preoperative iron deficiency anemia and reduce intraoperative blood loss.

SUGGESTED READINGS

Crosignani P, Vercellini P, Meschìa M, et al. GnRH agonists before surgery for uterine leiomyomas. A review. *J Reprod Med*. 1996;41(6):415–421.

Di Lieto A, De Falco M, Pollio F, et al. Clinical response, vascular change, and angiogenesis in gonadotropin-releasing hormone analogue-treated women with uterine myomas. *J Soc Gynecol Investig*. 2005;12(2):123–128.

Lethaby A, Vollenhoven B, Sowter M. Pre-operative GnRH analogue therapy before hysterectomy or myomectomy for uterine fibroids. *Cochrane Database Syst Rev*. 2001;(2): CD000547.

Vercellini P, Trespidi L, Zaina B, et al. Gonadotropin-releasing hormone agonist treatment before abdominal myomectomy: a controlled trial. *Fertil Steril*. 2003;79:1390.

135

WHEN COUNSELING FOR UTERINE ARTERY EMBOLIZATION, ALWAYS ASK THE PATIENT IF SHE MAY DESIRE FUTURE FERTILITY

JOHN K. PARK, MD, MSc

Uterine artery embolization (UAE) has become an increasingly popular method for the treatment of symptomatic uterine leiomyoma. This procedure is a safe and effective nonsurgical treatment. Given that the procedure was introduced in 1995, there are few studies that have evaluated long-term outcome, but the studies evaluating outcome after 5 years consistently show promising results, with symptom control ranging from 73% to 89.5%.

The procedure is performed by an interventional radiologist, because it involves the insertion of a catheter through a common femoral artery into the uterine arteries and the injection of embolic material to decrease uterine blood flow. The reduction in arterial blood flow causes ischemic injury to the fibroids, initiating necrosis and shrinkage.

The American College of Obstetricians and Gynecologists' Committee on Gynecologic Practice considers the desire for future fertility a relative contraindication for the procedure. There is a paucity of evidence to ensure its safety in women who desire the retention of their fertility. Furthermore, pregnancy-related outcomes are understudied.

Of great concern are the cases of ovarian failure that have been reported following UAE, most of which occur in women older than 45 years. However, several cases of ovarian failure also have been reported in younger women. The purported mechanism involves the embolization of ovarian tissue via the collateral vessels from the uterus. If this is the mechanism of action, UAE may have a detrimental effect on ovarian reserve, which may not be immediately apparent for patients unless damage is severe, as in the cases of ovarian failure. In an attempt to clarify this issue, basal FSH values have been measured prior to UAE and up to 6 months later. Although FSH levels were not significantly different for most patients, those who were 45 to 50 years old had significantly higher FSH values 6 months after UAE. Larger studies with longer follow-up periods are needed to conclusively determine the effect of UAE on ovarian reserve for all ages. It is very possible that younger women also experience an insult to their ovarian reserve, but it may not be detected within a short follow-up period.

There are several case series of pregnancies that have occurred after UAE. These demonstrate that normal term pregnancy can occur after

UAE, but the question of fecundity after UAE still needs to be addressed. The information from published case series suggests that there are higher rates of pregnancy complications, such as spontaneous abortion, preterm delivery, cesarean section, abnormal placentation, and postpartum hemorrhage. This information needs to be interpreted with caution due to the potential for bias in many of these reports, as well as the many confounding factors such as advanced maternal age and other reproductive issues. Patients should be counseled that UAE may increase the risk of such complications on a subsequent pregnancy. A very important clinical question with respect to reproductive outcomes is whether UAE is any different than myomectomy when it comes to fecundability and pregnancy complications.

One randomized trial has been published to address this question, but the number of patients is small. In a cohort of 66 women who attempted conception following UAE or myomectomy, there were more pregnancies and live births with fewer abortions in the myomectomy group after a mean follow-up of 25 months.

The ideal candidates for UAE are women who no longer desire fertility but wish to avoid hysterectomy or myomectomy. However, for women who desire future fertility, UAE may be safer than myomectomy for those in whom surgery is contraindicated or for those with very large fibroids that are difficult to remove.

TAKE HOME POINTS

- When counseling a patient about UAE, always ask if future fertility is desired.
- UAE is relatively contraindicated in women wishing to retain fertility.
- UAE may have an effect on future fecundity as well as a possible increased risk of pregnancy complications, such as spontaneous abortion, preterm delivery, cesarean section, abnormal placentation, and postpartum hemorrhage.

SUGGESTED READINGS

American College of Obstetricians and Gynecologists. Uterine artery embolization. ACOG Committee Opinion No 293. *Obstet Gynecol.* 2004:103;403–404.

Katsumori T, Kasahara T, Akazawa K. Long-term outcomes of uterine artery embolization using gelatin sponge particles alone for symptomatic fibroids. *Am J Roentgenol.* 2006;186:848–854.

Spies JB, Bruno J, Czeyda-Pommersheim F, et al. Long-term outcome of uterine artery embolization of leiomyomata. *Obstet Gynecol.* 2005;106(5 Pt 1):933–939.

Spies JB, Roth AR, Gonsalves SM, et al. Ovarian function after uterine artery embolization for leiomyomata: assessment with use of serum follicle stimulating hormone assay. *J Vasc Interv Radiol.* 2001;12(4):437–442.

Tropeano G, Amoroso S, Scambia G. Non-surgical management of uterine fibroids. *Hum Rep Update.* 2008;14:259–274.

136

POSTOPERATIVE COMPLICATIONS: IS THIS A NORMAL AMOUNT OF DRAINAGE FROM THE INCISION SITE?

LYDIA MAYIDA, MD AND DIANA BROOMFIELD, MD, MBA, FACOG, FACS

A 45-year-old multiparous woman has recently undergone an endometrial biopsy for abnormal uterine bleeding and has been diagnosed with endometrial cancer. She is scheduled to undergo a TAH/BSO/LND. Her past medical history is significant for a diabetes mellitus, sarcoidosis, and asthma. She has been taking oral steroids (prednisolone 5 mg) daily for the past 5 years. Her surgery proceeds uneventfully and she is discharged to home on postoperative day 4. She calls you, her physician, on Saturday night with complaints that something is protruding out of her abdomen and you appropriately ask her to come to the emergency room immediately for evaluation.

DISCUSSION

She has suffered a wound complication. Your differential is wound dehiscence or evisceration, wound separation, wound seroma with serosanguinous fluid drainage. Once she arrives at the emergency department, the staples should be removed and the wound and fascia gently probed with a small Q-tip for complete examination. A common error to avoid is inadequate preoperative evaluation of your patient's risks for intraoperative and postoperative complications.

Risk factors for wound complications are advanced age, obesity, immunosupression, diabetes mellitus, malignancy, prolonged use of corticosteroids, liver failure, uremia, hypoproteinemia, sepsis, chemotherapy, prior radiation, and incision through previous scar tissue.

WOUND INFECTION

The risk of having wound infection in a patient after an abdominal hysterectomy is approximately 5%. Having a wound infection increases not only length of hospital stay but also the cost to the patient, hospital, and insurance company.

Why are some patients at risk for wound separation or breakdown? Bacterial growth is facilitated by decreased tissue oxygen tension in the wound. Incidence of superficial skin infection increases as the duration of the procedure. For every additional hour of surgery, the risk of wound complications, especially infection, doubles. The incidence of postoperative wound infection increases eightfold with obese patients weighing >200 lb. The first symptoms of wound infection may not occur until postoperative day 5 to 10. These patients present with fever, tachycardia, tenderness, swelling, erythema, and edema at the incision. Rare virulent pathogens that can cause toxicity within 48 hours are

1. Acute β-hemolytic *Streptococcus* infection causes an odorless discharge with erythema and edema at the incision.
2. *Clostridium* species may cause a foul-smelling odor, edema, and boggy sensation on palpation and a sweet-smelling discharge.

Management of wound infections involves opening and draining the incision and aerobic and anaerobic cultures should be obtained, followed by periodic copious irrigation and packing.

If a distinct zone of cellulitis is noted, this is likely to be an infection with group B hemolytic *Streptococcus* and antibiotics are recommended. Prevention of wound infection can be achieved with the use of prophylactic antibiotics. Antibiotic doses may be increased with increased duration of the procedure over 2 hours or if there was blood loss >2 L. Delayed primary closure on day 3 or 4 is another technique that may be used to reduce risk of wound infection.

NECROTIZING FASCIITIS
Necrotizing fasciitis is also associated with decreased tissue perfusion. This is a serious complication that presents with local pain, fever, tachycardia, and no obvious skin changes until there is crepitance and bullae formation. Anesthetic areas develop over the wound. Associated mortality is 30% to 50%. A common error is a delay in diagnosis. Because this is a rare occurrence, there is need for a high index of suspicion. Management involves high-dose broad-spectrum antibiotics, debridement of devitalized tissues, and hyperbaric oxygen.

WOUND DEHISCENCE AND EVISCERATION
Wound dehiscence involves separation of the edges of the incision including skin, subcutaneous tissue, and the fascia but not the peritoneum; this occurs especially in the first 14 days of the procedure and is usually noted soon after removal of sutures or staples. The incidence is 1:200. It increases the risk of incisional hernia but does not increase mortality. Dehiscence is decreased with use of synthetic absorbable suture such as vicryl or dexon.

Evisceration involves complete breakdown of the healing process involving the fascia and peritoneum with resultant of the omentum or bowel presenting through the incision. Classically, the wound that eventually eviscerates lacks the healing ridge of tissue that is palpable in normal healing wounds and is also draining serosanguinous fluid by day 5 to 8. Imperative for prevention is appropriately evaluating patients at risk and those patients choosing the proper fascial closure. Particularly in patients at risk, a recommended closure is the Smead-Jones closure. This closure technique is associated with a rate of 1:1,000 wound dehiscences. This is done as a primary mass closure using monofilament permanent suture, nylon, or prolene.

HEMATOMAS

Incidence of hematomas is reduced with increased meticulous hemostasis intraoperatively. Placing patients on low-dose heparin increases the risk but these are usually self-limiting. Retroperitoneal hematomas may carry a large volume of blood and patients may need to be transfused. Clinical features may be tenderness and fever secondary to inflammation around the hematoma. Management is conservative unless the hematoma is larger than 5 cm in which case incision and drainage via the extraperitoneal approach as soon as it liquefies is considered appropriate; otherwise, there is increased risk of infection. Differential diagnosis includes sponge left in situ.

TAKE HOME POINTS

- Incidence of post-op infection increases eightfold in obese patients weighing >200 lb
- Copious intraoperative irrigation is important. Remember that "the solution to pollution is dilution."
- Management of wound infection involves taking aerobic and anaerobic cultures, opening the wound, allowing drainage, periodic irrigation, and packing the wound.
- Prophylactic antibiotics reduce incidence of post-op wound infections, and it is recommended to increase doses with increasing duration of the procedure past 2 hours and also increased blood loss over 2 L.
- Lastly, remember to have a high index of suspicion when any patient presents with postoperative complaints!

SUGGESTED READINGS

American College of Obstetricians and Gynecologists. Compendium of Selected Publications. 2007.

Stenchever MA, Droegemueller W, Herbst AL, et al. (eds) *Comprehensive Gynecology,* 4th ed., 2002, New York, NY, Elsevier.

137

POSTOPERATIVE COMPLICATIONS... IS MY PATIENT INFECTED?

DIANA BROOMFIELD, MD, MBA, FACOG, FACS

Sally is a 45-year-old G5P5 female who is postoperative day 3 status post abdominal hysterectomy, bilateral salipingo-oophorectomy, and Burch procedures. While on call, the nurse asks you to evaluate the patient's temperature of 38.9°C. She still has her Foley catheter, is tachypneic, and complains of progressively worsening abdominal pain. What is your differential diagnosis?

Postoperative complications may include a fever. Fever is defined as the presence of a temperature ≥100.4°F on two occasions at least 4 hours apart (excluding the first 24 hours) or one temperature >101.5°F.

The workup of fevers postoperatively focuses on the five Ws: Wind, Water, Wound, Walking, and Wonder drugs.

Wind, ask if this is atelectasis or pneumonia. *Water*, is this a urinary tract infection (UTI)? UTIs are the most common cause (incidence of 4% to 20%) of post-op fevers. It is usually seen anytime after post-op day 3. *Wound*, take a look at your handy work. Remove the dressings, if needed; is your wound infected? Wound infections may occur anytime after post-op day 5. *Walking*, is this a PE or DVT? DVT and pulmonary emboli usually occurs during post-op days 7 to 10.*Wonder drugs*, this is usually a diagnosis of exclusion and can occur at anytime. Remember to check all the medications that your patient is on. So what should your workup consist of? First, conduct a thorough physical examination and then order a CBC with differential, CXR, two blood cultures, UA, and a urine culture.

Postoperative respiratory infections are uncommon in gynecological patients. If the site of infection is the lungs, pneumonia is usually seen during post-op days 1 to 2. Patients with risk factors for pneumonia include obese patients, patients on a respirator, patients with underlying pulmonary disease (e.g., COPD, asthma) or recent infection, and patients who ate within a few hours of surgery (typically <6 hours). The offending organisms typically are *Pseudomonas* and *Klebsiella*. The drugs of choice are aminoglycosides and penicillin. Aspiration pneumonia may be treated with an NGT for decompression and oxygenation. These patients typically present postoperatively with cough, sputum production, fever, and increased respiration. The finding on the CXR is consistent with an infiltrate. The WBC count is usually elevated.

Is it her urinary tract? UTI usually presents after post-op day 3. Patients who have a Foley catheter are at an increased risk of a post-op UTI. There is a 5% chance for each day the Foley is in. The patient typically presents with dysuria, however, if the Foley catheter is still in the patients do not have dysuria. Risk factors associated with post-op UTI includes patients with diabetes, catheters, intraoperative bladder injury, and urinary retention. The offending microorganisms include *Pseudomonas*, *Serratia*, *Enterococcus*, *E. coli*, *Proteus*, and *Klebsiella*. Laboratory findings are consistent with elevated WBC and the UA is positive for leukocyte esterase and nitrites; the urine culture is positive. Do not forget to check the sensitivity studies. Treatment is dependent on findings. Consider discontinuing the Foley, increase IV fluids, and start antibiotics. Do not be afraid to look at the wound. Discontinue the dressing after post-op day 1.

Look at the incision(s). Are the incisions clean and dry? Probe the incision with a Q-tip, is the incision intact? Wound infections typically occur after post-op day 4 or 5. A wound infection is the second most frequent cause of post-op infection. The typical presentation of patients with wound infections is an incision that is erythematous (usually >2 cm), inflamed with swelling, warmth, and pain around incisional site. The most common offending microorganism in the wound is Staphylococcus aureus. If the etiology of the infection is the gastrointestinal tract, the organisms are typically *E. coli*, *Bacteroides*, or *Enterococcus*. If the origin of the infection is the genitourinary tract, the microorganisms involved are typically *Pseudomonas* and *Proteus*. If the wound is infected, the wound must undergo drainage and debridement. After it has been cleaned, apply wet-to-dry dressings twice daily, culture the wound, and start antibiotics.

Tissue infections such as cellulitis and necrotizing fasciitis may be caused by *S. aureus*, *Streptococcus*, Gram-negative bacteria, and anaerobes. Necrotizing Fasciitis is rare but has a high mortality rate. It is caused by the production of hyaluronidase and lipase in subcutaneous space that destroys the fascia and adipose tissue. If not recognized, it may rapidly progress and cause sepsis, shock, and death.

Check the patient's lines and legs. Is this phlebitis or vasculitis? Is the IV site infected? IVs should be discontinued after 72 hours post-op. These patients usually present with fever, leukocytosis on CBC, bacteremia, or a positive culture from the line tip. The organisms are typically *S. aureus* and *S. epidermidis*. Management includes discontinuing the lines and starting antibiotics. IV antibiotics may be necessary, so place another IV site in a different location from the infected line. Prevention includes changing the lines frequently and the use of intraoperative and postoperative SCD and TEDS. Treatment includes ambulation and anticoagulation and considers antibiotics.

If your patient is or has been on antibiotics and is having diarrhea, you must rule out infection caused by clostridium difficile. The recommended treatment for antibiotic-associated diarrhea with *Clostridium difficile* is oral metronidazole 250 mg q6hrly or vancomycin 125 mg q6hrly orally.

Could the infection be secondary to peritonitis? Remember, the solution to pollution is dilution. Peritonitis may occur if there was perforation of GI tract. Patients typically present with abdominal pain, fever, and sepsis. These patients can deteriorate quickly and have a high mortality rate. Check KUB for free air. These patients may be managed by placing them on an NPO diet with NGT, start antibiotic and IV fluids, and schedule for emergency surgical exploration of the bowel. Consider your gynecologic oncologist or general surgeon to help intraoperatively. Additional complications include abscess formation, which is usually caused by polymicrobial organisms. Abscesses may be drained intraoperatively or via CT guidance.

The differential for intraoperative fever includes transfusion reaction, intraoperative septicemia, and malignant hyperthermia. Etiological factors for malignant hyperthermia include the use of halothane, succinylcholine, MAO inhibitors, and meperidine. This is an emergency. Your patient can die quickly! Surgery and anesthetic agents must be stopped immediately. Patients are managed with muscle relaxants (dantrolene), cooling blanket for rapid cooling, hyperventilation, bicarbonate, and mannitol. Mortality is as high as 60%.

TAKE HOME POINTS

- An easy method to remember the etiology and post-op day of presentation is
  - Wind, Post-op day 1
  - Water, Post-op day 3
  - Wound, Post-op day 5
  - Walking, Post-op day 7
  - Wonder drugs, Any post-op day
- Management of wound infection involves taking aerobic and anaerobic cultures, opening wound, allowing drainage, periodic irrigation, and packing the wound.
- Prophylactic antibiotics reduce incidence of post-op wound infections, and it is recommended to increase doses with increasing duration of the procedure past 2 hours and also increased blood loss over 2 L.
- Recommended treatment for antibiotic-associated diarrhea with *C. difficile* is oral metronidazole 250 mg q6hrly or vancomycin 125 mg q6hrly orally.

- Necrotizing fasciitis is caused by the production of hyaluronidase and lipase may be caused by *S. aureus*, *Streptococcus*, Gram-negative bacteria, and anaerobes.

- Quick infection killers are
  - Necrotizing fasciitis
  - Malignant hyperthermia
  - Peritonitis
  - Sepsis

SUGGESTED READINGS

Lawrence SJ, Kirmani N. Treatment of Infectioius Diseases. Cooper DH, Krainik AJ, Lubner SJ, et al. (eds) *The Washington Manual of Medical Therapeutics*, 32nd ed. Philadelphia, PA: Lippincott Williams & Wilkins; 2007.

Schey D, Salom EM, Papadia A, et al. Extensive fever workup produces low yield in determining infectious eitiology. *Am J Obstet Gynecol*. 2005;192(5):1729–1734.

138

POSTOPERATIVE COMPLICATIONS: WHAT'S THE BIG DEAL ABOUT HAVING ONLY 10 mL PER HOUR OF URINE OUTPUT POSTOPERATIVELY? SHE IS JUST DRY

LYDIA MAYIDA, MD AND DIANA BROOMFIELD, MD, MBA, FACOG, FACS

A 35-year-old otherwise healthy nonpregnant woman is taken to the operating room for an open myomectomy. The duration of her procedure is 2 hours, with an EBL noted at about 1,500 mL. Postoperatively, she complains of dizziness and shortness of breath (SOB) on sitting up, and her blood pressure is noted to be 80/40 with a pulse of 114 bpm.

Postoperative problems: (1) hypotension, (2) dizziness, and (3) SOB.

Following any operative procedure, vital signs are monitored frequently to detect possible complications so that intervention can be implemented in a timely fashion to minimize morbidity or even mortality. Hypotension in a postoperative patient may be a sign of internal hemorrhage and subsequently lead to shock and inadequate tissue perfusion. Although postoperative hypotension may be a result of hypovolemia secondary to hemorrhage, it may also be of cardiogenic, septic, or anaphylactic origin. Commonly, hypotension occurs due to hypovolemia, which may be the result of inadequate fluid resuscitation alone, excessive intraoperative or postoperative blood loss associated with the common error, or not recognizing or addressing the signs of hypovolemia. Expedient management includes adequate fluid replacement and recognizing postoperative or internal hemorrhage necessitating reoperation.

On examination, the observation of a pale, weak patient with hypotension and tachycardia may should trigger concerns of hypovolemia. Orthostatic blood pressure measurements and close urine output monitoring along with lab values for a complete blood count will help with both diagnosis and your plan for management. Significant orthostatic change is noted when there is a significant drop in the systolic blood pressure and diastolic blood pressure of 10 mm Hg from sitting up to standing as compared with lying down suggestive of hypovolemia. An elevation of heart rate by about 15 bpm is also supportive of a hypovolemia diagnosis. A minimum volume for urine output of 30 mL per hour (i.e., 0.5 mL/kg body weight per hour) is acceptable and less than this may indicate possible hypovolemia. Appropriate fluid replacement is in the ratio of 3:1 with crystalloids. Colloids are not indicated unless it is determined the patient needs a blood transfusion and the blood is not immediately available and acceptable ratio is 1:1, which is similar to blood transfusion. Appropriate crystalloids are normal saline and lactated Ringer's because of their electrolyte contents as detailed below:

> Extracellular fluid glucose 1,000 g/L/Na 140/Cl 102/HCO_3 27/ K 4.2/Ca 5/Mg 3 HPO4 0.3
> Normal saline Na 154/Cl 154
> Lactated Ringer's: Na^+ 130/Cl^- 109/HCO_3^- 28/K^+ 4.0/Ca 2.7
> D5W glucose 50g/L

CBC measurement immediately postoperatively may not be accurate due to fluid shifts that occur; however, the decision to transfuse the patient should be determined by the clinical condition of the patient and her hematocrit. Remember that young patients may tolerate a hematocrit of 20% to 22% but a 60-year-old patient may need her hematocrit to be maintained above 28%. Failure of clinical improvement, for example, persistent hypotension and abdominal distention, may indicate continued hemorrhage with need for surgical intervention or consider and reevaluate for a different etiology of hypotension.

TAKE HOME POINTS

- Orthostatic changes are significant if BP drops by >10 mm Hg or the pulse rate increases by 10 to 15 bpm.
- Adequate minimum urine output in a patient is 0.5 mL/kg/hour.
- Fluid resuscitation should be done in the 3:1 ratio for crystalloids versus blood loss and 1:1 if replacing with packed cells; colloids are usually not recommended.
- Be suspicious, and intervene expeditiously when the patient is hemodynamically unstable.

SUGGESTED READINGS

American College of Obstetricians and Gynecologists. Compendium of Selected Publications. 2007.
Rock JA, Jones HW. *TeLinde's Operative Gynecology*. 10th ed. Philadelphia, PA: Lippincott Williams & Wilkins; 2008.
Stenchever MA, Droegemueller W, Herbst AL, et al. (eds) *Comprehensive Gynecology*, 4th ed., 2002, New York, NY, Elsevier.

139

POSTOPERATIVE COMPLICATIONS: PULMONARY EMBOLISM AND VENOUS THROMBOEMBOLISM

LYDIA MAYIDA, MD AND DIANA BROOMFIELD, MD, MBA, FACOG, FACS

Sally is a 55-year-old morbidly obese female with a history of ovarian cancer. She recently underwent major pelvic surgery. Since surgery, she has not been ambulatory, and on postoperative day 7, she complained of shortness of breath, chest pain, and dizziness. She was rushed to the emergency room for evaluation.

According to a nursing research project conducted by Brooks-Brunn, the rate of postoperative pulmonary complications for North Americans is estimated to be as high as 1 million of every 45 million people who undergo nonthoracic surgery. Brooks-Brunn's research also estimated that 8 of every 1,000 patients will experience a postoperative pulmonary embolus.

Patients undergoing pelvic surgery are at risk of developing venous thromboembolism (VTE) and should be given thromboembolic prophylaxis. Specific prophylaxis is determined by the patient's risk factors. Typical risk factors include the duration of surgery, obesity, trauma to the lower extremities, the postoperative period, prolonged immobilization (including air travel), and the use of estrogen-containing medications. Patients with other risk factors include older patients with diabetes mellitus and malignancy and patients with a diagnosis of thrombophilia.

The lowest risk for VTE is when surgery is performed within 30 minutes on a patient of 40 years of age or younger who is otherwise healthy. Patients with known risk factors should receive adequate (both medical and mechanical) prophylaxis with heparin and sequential compression devices. Although precautions are taken, the patient may still present with pulmonary embolism.

The two most common errors are not having a high index of suspicion and not identifying patients who are at increased risk. The symptoms are not specific but may include chest pain, dyspnea with minimal exertion, hemoptysis, palpitations, and low-grade fever. The gold standard for diagnosis is pulmonary angiography (spiral CT), and other tests performed are d-dimer, EKG, and Doppler ultrasound of the lower extremities with a V/Q scan.

Differential diagnoses may include atelectasis, pneumonia, pneumothorax, pulmonary effusion, and cardiac failure, and other tests may be indicated to rule these out.

TAKE HOME POINTS

- Have a high index of suspicion.
- Evaluate the patient in the preoperative, intraoperative, and postoperative periods carefully.
- Identify patients with VTE risk factors.
- Patients at high risk for VTE require both mechanical and medical means for DVT prophylaxis, both heparin and SCDs.
- The gold standard for diagnosis of pulmonary embolism is spiral CT (pulmonary angiography).

SUGGESTED READINGS

American College of Obstetricians and Gynecologists. Compendium of Selected Publications. 2007.

Brooks-Brunn JA. Development of a predictive model for postoperative pulmonary complications after cholecystectomy. *Clin Nurs Res.* 1992;1(May):180–195.

Brooks-Brunn JA. Predictors of postoperative pulmonary complications following abdominal surgery. *Chest.* 1997;111(March):564–571.

Rock JA, Jones HW. *TeLinde's Operative Gynecology.* 10th ed. Philadelphia, PA: Lippincott Williams & Wilkins; 2008.

Stenchever MA, Droegemueller W, Herbst AL, et al. (eds) *Comprehensive Gynecology*, 4th ed., 2002, New York, NY, Elsevier.

140

POSTOPERATIVE COMPLICATIONS: IS THIS AN ILEUS OR AN OBSTRUCTION?

LYDIA MAYIDA, MD AND DIANA BROOMFIELD, MD, MBA, FACOG, FACS

Ms. Salazar is a 35-year-old G3P3 female who is 3 days status postcaesarean section with chief complaints of abdominal pain, bloating, and nausea. You are called to evaluate her and note that she has not ambulated since delivery. You encourage ambulation and change of diet to NPO. Her symptoms resolve promptly and she is subsequently discharged.

An ileus occurs from hypoactivity or hypomotility of the gastrointestinal tract in the absence of mechanical bowel obstruction. This is thought to be a result of transient impairment of bowel activity resulting in failure or compromise in transport of the intestinal contents. This hypoactivity and slow movement of bowel contents lead to an accumulation of gas and fluids within the bowel. Although there are numerous causes of ileus, the typical patient is a postoperative patient. Senagore noted that >50% of postoperative patients develop an ileus.

Postoperatively, the patient may experience bloating, mild to moderate abdominal discomfort, nausea for up to 12 hours, and pass flatus within 24 to 48 hours. These patients may have a bowel movement within 4 to 5 days post-op. The abdomen may be distended and tympanic. On examination, the abdomen may be tender with absent or hypoactive bowel sounds. Risk of developing an ileus is increased with extent of bowel manipulation intraoperatively. Thus, patients undergoing vaginal surgery such as a vaginal hysterectomy compared with abdominal hysterectomy are less likely to experience an ileus. Peritonitis is also a risk factor for development of an ileus.

Usually, an ileus resolves spontaneously with bowel rest and observation. Some patients may need an NG tube. If an ileus is unresolved within 5 days or progressively worsens, then a diagnosis of mechanical bowel obstruction must be considered. Mechanical bowel obstruction commonly occurs due to major abdominal surgery resulting in adhesion formation. Patients with bowel obstruction in contrast have high–pitched bowel sounds on examination with air fluid level on plain film x-rays. Bowel obstruction can be diagnosed with imaging, abdominal x-rays erect and supine (air fluid levels), and CT of the abdomen with contrast (a transition zone may indicate obstruction).

TAKE HOME POINTS

- An ileus occurs from hypoactivity or hypomotility of the gastrointestinal tract in the absence of mechanical bowel obstruction.
- Risk of developing an ileus is increased with extent of bowel manipulation intraoperatively.
- Usually, an ileus resolves spontaneously with bowel rest and observation.
- More than 50% of postoperative patients may develop an ileus.

SUGGESTED READINGS

Rock JA, Jones HW. *TeLinde's Operative Gynecology*. 10th ed. Philadelphia, PA: Lippincott Williams & Wilkins; 2008.

Senagore AJ. Pathogenesis and clinical and economic consequences of postoperative ileus. *Am J Health Syst Pharm*. 2007;64(20 Suppl 13):S3–S7 [Medline].

Stenchever MA, Droegemueller W, Herbst AL, et al. (eds) *Comprehensive Gynecology*, 4th ed., 2002, New York, NY, Elsevier.

141

POSTOPERATIVE COMPLICATIONS: URINARY PROBLEMS

LYDIA MAYIDA, MD AND DIANA BROOMFIELD, MD, MBA, FACOG, FACS

A 33-year-old G4P4 delivers a 10-lb baby girl vaginally. The delivery was complicated by a fourth-degree laceration that was repaired. However, 3 weeks later, she complained of burning on urination and passing gas and feces via her vagina.

INABILITY TO VOID
The inability to void may be due to performance anxiety, mechanical obstruction secondary to swelling or edema, neurological imbalance, and drug-associated detrusor hypotonia. The inability to void may be avoided by providing adequate patient privacy and allowing patients to be in the sitting position and removing the Foley catheter once the patient is ambulating well and has adequate urine output. Intermittent straight catheterization is better than Foley catheter replacement. Ureteral spasm may lead to urinary retention that may be relieved by phenoxybenzamine. Bladder hypotonia may be relieved with bethanechol.

URINARY TRACT INFECTION
Gram-negative bacteremia is the most common hospital-acquired infection. A most frequent cause is Foley catheter–associated urinary tract infection. Silver alloy–coated urinary catheters are more effective in preventing infection than the silver oxide catheters. The recommendation is to treat infection once symptomatic and not to give prophylactic antibiotics in view of risk of developing resistant strains unless the patient is immunosuppressed.

URINARY FISTULA/RECTOVAGINAL FISTULA
Urinary bladder injury versus ureteral injury occurs in the ratio 5:1. Urinary bladder injury occurs once in every 200 abdominal hysterectomies. A urinary fistula causes painless loss of urine from the vagina. The diagnosis of a fistula may involve placing a tampon in the vagina and instilling methylene blue into the bladder; if there is no blue dye seen on the tampon on removal of the tampon, then the test is negative. The diagnosis of an ureterovaginal or vesicovaginal fistula can be done by giving 3 to 5 mL of indigo carmine intravenously while the patient wears a tampon in the vagina.

Blue dye on the tampon may indicate an uretero- or vesicovaginal fistula. IVP or enhanced CT should be obtained for further evaluation.

The primary method for prevention of bladder injury is emptying the bladder preoperatively and sharp dissection in the correct planes. The most important mechanism to avoid the development of fistulas is recognition of injury intraoperatively or soon as symptoms develop postoperatively. Once injury to bladder is suspected, leaving the Foley catheter in for 3 to 5 days usually results in spontaneous healing.

Rectovaginal fistula rarely occurs with gynecological surgery. It results in an abnormal connection between the vagina and the rectum. An estimated 0.1% of vaginal births lead to a rectovaginal fistula (RVF). RVFs may vary greatly in size, but most are <2 cm in diameter. Small-sized fistulas are <0.5 cm in diameter, medium-sized fistulas are 0.5 to 2.5 cm, and large-sized fistulas exceed 2.5 cm. Increased risk is seen with history of cancer and radiation therapy, perirectal abscess, inflammatory bowel disease, Crohn disease, lymphogranuloma venereum, and trauma. Symptoms include passing fecal matter vaginally, foul-smelling vaginal discharge, and subsequent dyspareunia. Diagnosis is usually by a thorough examination. Placing a vaginal tampon, instilling methylene blue into the rectum, and examining the tampon after 15 to 20 minutes can often establish the presence of RVF. If the tampon is unstained, another part of the GI tract may be involved. When the diagnosis is illusive, radiological testing can be done. Barium enema can demonstrate RVF or the more common sigmoid–vaginal cuff fistula observed in diverticulitis. Computed tomography (CT) scanning can also aid in the diagnosis of bowel–reproductive tract pathology.

Treatment for very small fistulas may involve placing the patient on a low-residue diet and giving Lomotil to facilitate spontaneous healing, which occurs in 25% of cases. Larger RVF in patients necessitates surgery.

TAKE HOME POINTS

- The primary method for prevention of bladder injury is by emptying the bladder preoperatively and by sharp dissection.
- Three to five milliliters indigo carmine given IV with a tampon in the vagina helps for diagnosis of vesicovaginal fistula.
- Urinary bladder injury occurs once in every 200 abdominal hysterectomies.
- Silver alloy–coated urinary catheters are more effective in preventing infection than the silver oxide catheters.

SUGGESTED READINGS

American College of Obstetricians and Gynecologists. *Compendium of Selected Publications.* 2007.

Stenchever MA, Droegemueller W, Herbst AL, et al. (eds) *Comprehensive Gynecology,* 4th ed., 2002, New York, NY, Elsevier.

MISCELLANEOUS OFFICE GYNECOLOGY

142

DIAGNOSTIC OFFICE PROCEDURES: LOCATING THE CERVIX

STEPHEN H. WEISS, MD, MPH

The cervix is attached to both the uterus and the vagina. A 36-year-old patient comes in for a Pap smear. She has a massive and irregular fibroid uterus. Multiple attempts to visualize the cervix fail. What will you do?

There are a number of possibilities for having trouble locating the cervix. For example, when there is extreme uterus to cervix flexion/version or the uterus is misshaped, locating the cervix may be difficult. There is a rare congenital condition in which the cervix is not present. That condition can be diagnosed via ultrasound or magnetic resonance imaging (MRI). Occasionally, a patient may have neglected to inform you that she had a hysterectomy. In addition, after multiple cone biopsies, the cervix may be flush with the vagina and difficult to locate. When the walls of the vagina are very relaxed, the view of the cervix may be obstructed. Finally, extreme obesity may make the exam difficult.

There are a few tricks for finding the cervix. First, once the speculum is inserted past the hymenal ring, aim down at a 30-degree angle and pull the handle of the speculum at a right angle to the blades as you advance the speculum until the hinge is even with the labia minus. The lower third of the vagina is the most sensitive, and the closer the hinge is to it, the less it will be spread. Having placed the speculum in this manner, the shorter anterior blade will be under a normally located cervix, and by opening the speculum slightly, the cervix will fall into view.

If the body habitus of the patient will not allow the hinge to reach the labia minus, then the blades may not reach the cervix. While a longer speculum may help, it will stretch the lower vagina and may be painful. A better technique is to place the speculum in upside down since the mons pubis will not protrude as far as the buttocks. Remember to hug the posterior vaginal wall during entry. If the cervix still cannot be located, do a bimanual exam to make sure there is a cervix and where it is located, then try one of the above techniques directed toward it. A "blind" Pap smear can be done by introducing the sampling device with your fingers and directing it to the cervix. If you must see the cervix in addition to locating it:

- Introduce a single-tooth tenaculum with your fingers and direct it to the cervix; then reassemble the speculum around it or use an open-sided speculum.
- If the issue is vaginal wall obstruction, a large latex glove, thumb cut off at the base and tip, may be used like a condom over the speculum to block the open sides. Also, a side wall retractor instrument or a three-bladed speculum can be used.
- Placing the patient in a knee-chest position will allow gravity and air to distend the vagina. With a single-bladed speculum, (Sims' or bottom half of a regular speculum), you can pull the posterior wall upward.

TAKE HOME POINTS

- If the cervix is difficult to find due to the patient's body habitus, place the speculum in upside down since the mons pubis will not protrude as far as the buttocks.
- Do a bimanual exam to make sure there is a cervix and where it is located.
- A blind Pap smear can be done by introducing the sampling device with your fingers and directing it to the cervix.
- If the issue is vaginal wall obstruction, a large latex glove, thumb cut off at the base and tip, may be used like a condom over the speculum to block the open sides. Alternatively, a side wall retractor instrument or a three-bladed speculum can be used.

SUGGESTED READING

Gibbs RS, Karlan BY, Haney AF, et al. *Danforth's Obstetrics and Gynecology*. Philadelphia, PA: Lippincott Williams & Wilkins; 2008.

143

TRANSCERVICAL PROCEDURES

STEPHEN H. WEISS, MD, MPH

A 56-year-old with a history of a cryotherapy of the cervix 20 years ago comes to see you for postmenopausal bleeding. You attempt to perform an endometrial biopsy, but the cervix will not allow the instrument to enter the endometrial cavity. What would you do next?

The cervix can be difficult to traverse for a number of reasons secondary to multiple causes including cervical myomas, extreme flexion between the uterus and the cervix, and, most commonly, cervical stenosis.

Office procedures that require traversing the cervix include endometrial biopsy, hysteroscopy, sonohysterogram or saline infusion sonogram (SIS), and placement of an intrauterine device or IUD.

One concern with transcervical procedures is perforation of the uterus. To decrease the risk, follow these steps. However, these steps are not always necessary for a soft catheter endometrial biopsy or sonohysterogram due to the low risk of perforation. First, perform a bimanual exam to determine the position of the cervix and its relationship to the uterus. Determine the uterine size and shape. Next, place a speculum inside the vagina and cleanse the cervix. Grasp the cervix with a single-tooth tenaculum. Traction will straighten the cervix to the uterus junction. Grasp anterior to the os for anteflexed uteri and posterior for retroflexed uteri. A vertical grasp with one tooth in the os is less likely to tear out with traction than a transverse grasp. Use a uterine sound to determine the depth and direction of the cervical canal and endometrial cavity. Between two fingers, gently hold the uterine sound and any instruments passed through the cervix to allow the instrument to pivot in whatever direction the cervix and uterus take it. Placing your pinky or little finger against the patient's thigh will move the instrument should the patient suddenly change positions.

If the problem seems to be a cervical myoma, an ultrasound (abdominal, vaginal, or endorectal) can allow you to guide instruments following the endocervical and endometrial canals. If the problem is cervical stenosis, use an os finder, which is a flexible and reusable Teflon or disposable plastic rod with a soft but small pointed end. This will help locate, follow, and slightly dilate the cervix. Alternatively, send the patient home and have her return after taking 400 µg of misoprostol orally 12 hours before the procedure. This prostaglandin drug can help soften and dilate the cervix. If the patient cannot tolerate prostaglandins, a laminaria may be inserted 24 hours before the procedure. Finally, often cervical stenosis is at or within a few millimeters of the external os. A 5-mm-by-5-mm LEEP loop used to remove the most distal portion of the cervical canal will open the os for you and avoid a trip to the operating room.

TAKE HOME POINTS

- To decrease the risk of uterine perforation, perform a bimanual exam to determine the position of the cervix and its relationship to the uterus. Determine the uterine size and shape.
- Use an os to locate, follow, and slightly dilate the cervix.
- Prostaglandins can help soften and dilate the cervix.
- A laminaria may be inserted 24 hours before the procedure.
- As a last resort, a 5-mm-by-5-mm LEEP loop used to remove the most distal portion of the cervical canal can open the os.

SUGGESTED READINGS

Christianson, Barker, Lindheim. Overcoming the challenging cervix: techniques to access the uterine cavity. *J Lower Genital Tract Dis.* 12:1;24–31. 11/1/08.

Telinde's Operative Gynecology: Various editions. Chapter on "Normal and Abnormal Bleeding": "Technique of Cervical Dilatation." J.B Lippincott Company.

144

BONUS PEARLS OF WISDOM FOR OFFICE PROCEDURES

STEPHEN H. WEISS, MD, MPH

The following are a few miscellaneous pearls that will help avoid errors in the ambulatory gynecology setting.

During the bimanual exam in a patient who has presented with a "lost tampon," grasp the tampon between two or three fingers and as you retract your hand, peel off the glove so it envelopes the tampon and then tie the glove in a knot and throw away. This will prevent a long-lasting odor from closing down the room. Next, inspect the cervix and vaginal walls for erosions.

When attempting to locate a lost IUD (when no string is visualized), it is important to begin with an ultrasound, a 3D, or a sonohysterogram to confirm cavity placement. If the IUD is not in the uterus, get a flat plate x-ray to see if it is elsewhere in the body. On some occasions, it is possible the IUD fell out and went unnoticed on a pad or tampon. If the IUD is in a normal position, it will work fine without the string exposed and the patient may keep it in until the scheduled date for removal. You may want to invest in an alligator forceps for removing intracavitary lost string IUDs.

When performing a loop electrosurgical excision procedure (LEEP) in the office, it is necessary to provide anesthesia to the cervix. Potocky needles help deliver the local anesthesia to the proper depth and are very small gauge at the end but stiff in the body. These needles provide accurate placement and minimize pain.

TAKE HOME POINTS

- Cover and tie a lost tampon within a glove when extracting it from the vagina to decrease a foul odor in the exam room.
- Always perform an ultrasound to identify a lost IUD within the uterus before hunting for the string.
- Potocky needles will help deliver anesthesia to the cervix before an office procedure.

SUGGESTED READING

Gibbs RS, Karlan BY, Haney AF, et al. *Danforth's Obstetrics and Gynecology*. Philadelphia, PA: Lippincott Williams & Wilkins; 2008.

145

WHEN SHOULD I DO AN ENDOMETRIAL BIOPSY?

FRANCIS KWARTENG, MD AND DIANA BROOMFIELD, MD, MBA, FACOG, FACS

A 65-year-old G2P2 postmenopausal woman presents with a history of spotting for the past 3 months. She has been in excellent health until the onset of this complaint. She has not been sexually active for the past year. She has a history of diabetes mellitus and is on insulin NPH 10 units at bedtime. Her surgical history is significant for a tonsillectomy 20 years ago and cesarean delivery with her last pregnancy. Family history is consistent with an aunt who died at age 51 from ovarian cancer and a paternal uncle who died from colorectal cancer. She tells the physician, "I am scared because my best friend died from endometrial cancer and had similar symptoms." She then asks, "Am I going to die?"

Endometrial biopsy is generally an office procedure for diagnosing abnormalities of the endometrial cavity. In difficult but very few cases, it may be necessary to perform the procedure in the operating room where the patient could be sedated. Indications for endometrial biopsy include

1. All women 35 years or older with any type of abnormal bleeding.
2. Evaluation of the uterine cavity to ascertain the cause of abnormal uterine bleeding regardless of age in patients with unopposed estrogen use.
3. History of abnormal bleeding with risk factors for endometrial hyperplasia regardless of age as in obesity, chronic anovulation associated with PCOS, history of breast or ovarian cancer, and history of selective estrogen receptor such as tamoxifen use.
4. Patients with strong family history of endometrial, ovarian, breast, colorectal cancer (Lynch II), especially if family members were affected at young age.
5. Evaluation of postmenopausal uterine bleeding.
6. Endometrial dating in relation to infertility evaluations and treatments.
7. Patients with findings of atypical glandular cell (on Pap smear report), thus not otherwise specified or cannot rule out high-grade lesions. Such patients require endometrial cavity evaluations especially if they have history of abnormal uterine bleeding or are at age 35 years and above.

CONTRAINDICATIONS
A common error that must be avoided is failing to test for pregnancy. Women health care providers should always obtain at least a urine pregnancy test to

rule out pregnancy in all women who are in the reproductive age group before performing the procedure. Acute purulent cervical-uterine infection should be treated before endometrial biopsies. Performance of the procedure in such conditions may alter the quality of the sample and may affect the results including increasing the risk for disseminated bacteremia. Endometrial biopsies should be avoided in patients with coagulopathies. Hematologic consults including an INR and other hematologic profile may be necessary. These patients should be relatively stable before the procedure. Test should be avoided in cases of documented invasive cervical cancer.

STEPWISE PROCEDURE DESCRIPTIONS

Instrumentation and materials required for endometrial biopsy are

1. Sterile gloves (two pairs)
2. Formalin container, well labeled with patient information (to receive the specimen)
3. Sterile, weighted speculum or self-retaining speculum may be used depending on the physician's preference
4. Twenty percent benzocaine spray at the cervix to minimize patient discomfort (most physicians skip this step)
5. Povidone iodine solutions (if not allergic to iodines and shellfish) to clean the vagina and cervix using small cotton balls
6. Uterine sound
7. Single-tooth cervical tenaculum (A long Allis clamp may be used since it is associated with less bleeding.)
8. Endometrial suction catheter

PROCEDURE

1. An informed consent is obtained.
2. The patient is placed in the dorsal lithotomy position and bimanual examination performed to determine accurately the uterine position. This is an essential step in any procedure involving introduction of instrument across the cervico-uterine junction (isthmus) into the uterine cavity to avoid posterior or anterior uterine perforations (especially in postmenopausal women).
3. Well-lubricated weighted speculum or self-retaining speculum is introduced into the vagina gently.
4. The vagina and cervical fornix are cleaned of any discharges using povidone iodine solution.
5. Single-tooth tenaculum or long Allis clamp is introduced to hold the anterior cervical lip and is gently pulled to straighten the cervico-uterine angle. In patients with a retroverted uterus, the tenaculum or Allis clamp should hold the posterior lip and be pulled to avoid anterior perforations.

6. Some physicians spray 20% benzocaine to the cervix to minimize discomfort. Most physicians do not apply any topical anesthetic agent.

7. Uterine sound is introduced gently and advanced until the fundus of the uterus is reached and gently removed. The depth of the cavity is determined on the centimeter/millimeter calibrations on the uterine sound.

8. The endometrial catheter is inserted through the cervix until the fundus is reached. The piton is removed from the catheter. Some catheters may require a hypodermic syringe to be connected with suction pressure maintained while the catheter is moved forward and backward between the fundus and the internal os of the uterus and turning 360 degrees simultaneously. With moderate to maximal tissue seen in the catheter, the procedure is completed. Sample of the endometrial tissue is pushed into the formalin container for transport to the histopathology laboratory.

9. All instruments are removed from the vagina and homeostasis confirmed.

TAKE HOME POINTS

- Always get a pregnancy test before doing an endometrial biopsy in a reproductive-aged female.
- Do not perform an endometrial biopsy in a patient with documented invasive cancer.
- Always obtain an informed consent.

SUGGESTED READINGS

ACOG Practice Bulletin No. 74. Antibiotic prophylaxis for gynecologic procedures. *Obstet Gynecol.* 2006;108:225.

Bremer CC. Endometrial biopsy. *Female Patient.* 1992;17:15–28.

Dijkhuizen FP, Mol BW, Brolmann HA, et al. The accuracy of endometrial sampling in the diagnosis of patients with endometrial carcinoma and hyperplasia: a meta-analysis. *Cancer.* 2000;89:1765.

Dogan E, Celiloglu M, Sarihan E, et al. Anesthetic effect of intrauterine lidocaine plus naproxen sodium in endometrial biopsy. *Obstet Gynecol.* 2004;103:347.

Einerth Y. Vacuum curettage by the Vabra method. A simple procedure for endometrial diagnosis. *Acta Obstet Gynecol Scand.* 1982;61:373.

Kaunitz AM. Endometrial sampling in menopausal patients. *Menopausal Med.* 1993;1:5–8.

Kaunitz AM, Masciello A, Ostrowski M, et al. Comparison of endometrial biopsy with the endometrial Pipelle and Vabra aspirator. *J Reprod Med.* 1988;33:427.

Livengood CH, Land MR, Addison A. Endometrial biopsy, bacteremia, and endocarditis risk. *Obstet Gynecol.* 1985;65:678–681.

Nesse RE. Managing abnormal vaginal bleeding. *Postgrad Med J.* 1991;89:208;213–214.

Yang GC, Wan LS. Endometrial biopsy using the Tao Brush method. A study of 50 women in a general gynecologic practice. *J Reprod Med.* 2000;45:109.

146

CYTOLOGIC SCREENING

FRANCIS KWARTENG, MD AND DIANA BROOMFIELD, MD, MBA, FACOG, FACS

A 31-year-old female GIPI, whose last menstrual period began a week ago and is still spotting, presented for scheduled annual gynecologic examination. A week prior to this visit, she purchased over-the-counter antifungal cream for vaginal discharge and itching, which she was still using at the time of this visit. The physician sees the patient and performs a pelvic examination first, followed by cervical swab for STD screening and cervical cytology in this order, and asks the patient to follow-up in 2 weeks for results.

The Papanicolaou smear (Pap smear) was introduced into clinical medicine between 1939 and 1943 by Dr. George Papanicolaou. Its impact on reducing incidence of cervical cancer is huge. Prior to its introduction, cervical cancer was the leading cause of mortality among gynecologic malignancies. Two decades after its introduction, cervical cancer dropped from first to third place of gynecologic cancer death. The incidence of cervical cancer was 44/100,000 prior to the introduction of this screening test. Currently, it is 7/100,000. This current incidence is as a result of irregular follow-up for screening on the part of patients and false-negative screening test reporting from testing centers. The purpose of this document is to outline the basic steps required for the procedure and common mistakes that could be avoided to reduce false-negative reporting.

Currently, a Pap smear is recommended for every sexually active female, including lesbians, within 3 years after becoming sexually active or by age 21 years.

Human papillomavirus (HPV) affects superficial squamous epithelial cells with the DNA encoding into host DNA. Eventually, the basal layers of the superficial cells are affected as well. Superficial, proliferating cells infected by HPV show no significant inflammatory-mediated response, and the host immune system is stimulated in <20% of its immunocompetency. Infected cells remain in the basal layer of the superficial cells of the cervix, vaginal walls, or vulvovaginal epithelium.

It is, therefore, important to obtain superficial cells (which are likely to show most abnormalities) regardless of the technique used. This enhances true-positive results and lowers false-negative reporting. In order to obtain an adequate amount of superficial cells in the Pap test, you should avoid excessive use of gels on the examining speculum. Warm running water may be used to rinse the speculum. Thick excessive vaginal or cervical discharge should be gently removed with cotton swabs prior to obtaining specimen. The physician should avoid taking smears during menstruation or periods of abnormal uterine bleeding. Generally, pelvic resting is ideal 48 to 72 hours prior to cytologic testing (no sexual intercourse, douching, and tampon use).

For cervical smears, excessive pelvic activity changes the integrity of the most superficial squamous epithelial cells resulting in smears being obtained from normal underlying cells. This has the potential of rendering the cytology results as false negative. Furthermore, if the Pap smear is being obtained during annual gynecologic examinations that will also screen for sexually transmitted infections, the clinician should always obtain cervical cytology before the smears for STI.

TAKE HOME POINTS

- Any activity that would alter the integrity of superficial cells of the lower genital tract should be avoided. This includes but is not limited to sexual intercourse prior to testing, douching, menstruation, or abnormal bleeding.
- Excessive amount of discharge may be rinsed with warm saline.
- Pap smear first before STI testing.
- Lesbians should be tested the same way as heterosexual individuals.
- Testing should be initiated by 3 years after the first sexual encounter, including rape.
- Patients with history of total abdominal hysterectomies for benign reasons, such as fibroids, do not require further screening if they did not have any cervical abnormalities prior to their hysterectomy.
- Patients with h/o TAH and prior cervical epithelial abnormality should continue screening until three consecutive negative cytological results are obtained.
- Cervical cytologic screening should discontinue at age 70 by ACS or 65 years as recommended by ACOG if such patients are immunocompetent and no history of abnormal cytologic for three consecutive times within the last 10-year period.

SUGGESTED READINGS

ACOG Practice Bulletin: clinical management guidelines for obstetrician-gynecologists. Number 45, August 2003. Cervical cytology screening (replaces committee opinion 152, March 1995). *Obstet Gynecol.* 2003;102:417.

Amies AM, Miller L, Lee SK, et al. The effect of vaginal speculum lubrication on the rate of unsatisfactory cervical cytology diagnosis. *Obstet Gynecol.* 2002;100:889.

Bernstein SJ, Sanchez-Ramos L, Ndubisi B. Liquid-based cervical cytologic smear study and conventional Papanicolaou smears: a metaanalysis of prospective studies comparing cytologic diagnosis and sample adequacy. *Am J Obstet Gynecol.* 2001;185:308.

Cibas ES, Alonzo TA, Austin RM, et al. Then MonoPrep test for the detection of cervical cancer and its precursors. Part I: results of a multicenter clinical trial. *Am J Clin Pathol.* 2008;129:193.

Fremont-Smith M, Marino J, Griffin B, et al. Comparison of the Surepathtrade mark liquid-based Papanicolaou smear with the conventional Papanicolaou smear in a multisite direct-to-vial study. *Cancer.* 2004;102:269.

Harrison DD, Hernandez E, Dunton CJ. Endocervical brush versus cotton swab for obtaining cervical smears at a clinic: a cost comparison. *J Reprod Med.* 1993;38:285.

Makino H, Sato S, Yajima A, et al. Evaluation of the effectiveness of cervical cancer screening: a case-control study in Miyagi, Japan. *Tohoku J Exp Med.* 1995;175:171.

Marshall Austin, R. The detection of precancerous cervical lesions can be significantly increased. *Arch Pathol Lab Med.* 2003;127:143.

Martin-Hirsch P, Lilford R, Jarvis G, et al. Efficacy of cervical-smear collection devices: a systematic review and meta-analysis. *Lancet.* 1999;354:1763.

National Cancer Institute Workshop. The 1988 Bethesda System for reporting cervical/vaginal cytological diagnoses. *JAMA.* 1989;262:931.

Papanicolaou GN, Traut HF. The diagnostic value of vaginal smears in carcinoma of the uterus. *Am J Obstet Gynecol.* 1941;42:193.

Ronco G, Cuzick J, Pierotti P, et al. Accuracy of liquid based versus conventional cytology: overall results of new technologies for cervical cancer screening: randomized controlled trial. *Br Med J.* 2007;335:28.

Sung HY, Kearney KA, Miller M, et al. Papanicolaou smear history and diagnosis of invasive cervical carcinoma among members of a large prepaid health plan. *Cancer.* 2000;88:2283.

147

Colposcopy: How does it really look?

Francis Kwarteng, MD and Diana Broomfield, MD, MBA, FACOG, FACS

A 48-year-old G2P2002, last menstrual period 2 weeks ago, presented for a scheduled colposcopy after a Pap smear showed low-grade squamous intraepithelial lesion. She is divorced but has two sexual partners. She denies drug and alcohol use but smokes a pack of cigarettes daily. She was scheduled for colposcopy and directed biopsy.

In 1925, Hinselmann developed the idea of using a binocular dissecting microscope and an intense light source to evaluate the cervix and vagina, and this has evolved into modern day colposcopy. This procedure has allowed clinicians to detect and manage benign preinvasive malignant conditions of the cervix, vagina, and vulva with an ultimate reduction in mortality. The sole purpose of colposcopy is to aid in identifying potential pathological sites for biopsy in the cervix, vagina, and vulva.

Colposcopy with biopsy is required in the diagnosis and management of benign, premalignant, and malignant conditions of the lower genital tract. Indications include the following Pap smear findings: recurrent or persistent atypical squamous cells of undetermined significance (ASCUS), atypical squamous cells (ASC) suggestive of high-grade lesions, low-grade squamous intraepethelial lesions (LGSIL), atypical glandular cells of undetermined significance (AGUS), malignant cells present in cytology and ASCUS with positive HPV (reflex typing) for high-risk HPV especially in patients older than 30 years, atypical cytological changes in the upper and lower vagina, and lesions of the vulva with high suspicion of malignancy.

The major components of the colposcope include a binocular dissecting microscope, an intense light source, and a focal length. The binocular view of the dissecting microscope allows the colposcoper to appreciate a 3D view of the object being focused. The light source could be xenon or halogen powered. Xenon light source has a more natural color spectrum compared to halogen. It emits spectral temperatures of 6,000 K. However, most colposcope use halogen light source with its yellowish beam compensated for by the instrument to white. Halogen light source operates with spectral temperatures of 3,200 K. The focal length is the distance between the object and the lens and is normally 25 to 40 cm (250 to 400 mm) with an average of 30 cm (300 mm). Always ensure that the intraocular distance is well adjusted before the procedure. The eyepiece is an essential as it magnifies from 10 to 30 depending on the type of colposcope. With the patient positioned, the scope can be adjusted away and toward the patient until an appropriate focus is obtained.

As in all procedures, a detailed but pertinent history and physical examination are essential before performing colposcopy. A family and personal history of benign or preinvasive malignant conditions in the lower genital tract or prior therapy for any of these conditions increases the index of suspension for a recurrent or persistent disease. A history of smoking, low socioeconomic status, multiple sexual partners, DES, and immunocompromised status are associated with the development of a preinvasive disease. A pregnancy test is required before the colposcopy as an endocervical curettage (ECC), probing of the endocervical canal, and biopsies of the endocervical canal (extension from the transition zone) should be avoided if the patient is pregnant. Always obtain an informed consent to allow the patient time to ask questions about the procedure.

To perform the procedure, the patient is placed in the dorsolithotomy position on the examination table and the bed should be adjusted to a comfortable height for the colposcopist. The colposcope is brought into position, light is turned on, and then move forward and backward while the attached dial is adjusted to achieve appropriate intraocular distance and focus. At the beginning of the evaluation, the external genitalia, including the perianal area, are thoroughly examined for any abnormality or suspicious lesions. Next, place a self-retaining sterile speculum into the vagina and open as wide as possible so the cervix stays midsection between the blades of the speculum. Then, visualize the cervix without acetic acid and inspect the ectocervix, transformation zone, and surrounding vaginal fornices. This examination is done at a sixfold magnification. Next, generously apply 3% to 5% acetic acid to the cervix. It is important for clinicians to note that no single colposcopic abnormality is directly associated with malignancy. The diagnosis of malignancy or premalignant condition is invariably the product of a biopsy. In the absence of any suspected abnormality, Lugol iodine (Schiller's) solution is applied to the cervix. Normal squamous epithelium will take up the stain (glycogen-containing cells), whereas atypical squamous epithelium and normal columnar epithelium will not stain.

Finally, clinicians should exercise lots of circumspection in interpreting colposcopy findings in postmenopausal women. Deprived estrogen states may produce false-positive cytological findings in these women and it behooves women's health care providers to incorporate the history, physical examination finding, cytology, and colposcopy in arriving at an informed diagnosis.

TAKE HOME POINTS

- ECC, probing of the endocervical canal, and biopsies of the endocervical canal (extension from the transition zone) should be avoided if the patient is pregnant.
- Normal squamous epithelium will take up the stain (glycogen-containing cells), whereas atypical squamous epithelium and normal columnar epithelium will not stain.
- Hypoestrogenic states may produce false-positive cytological findings.

SUGGESTED READINGS

ACOG Practice Bulletin number 66, September 2005. Management of abnormal cervical cytology and histology. *Obstet Gynecol.* 2005;106:645.

Alvarez RD, Wright TC Jr. Increased detection of high-grade cervical intraepithelial neoplasia utilizing an optical detection system as an adjunct to colposcopy. *Gynecol Oncol.* 2007;106:23. www.ASCCP.org. (Accessed March 2009).

Baggish MS. High power density carbon dioxide laser therapy for early cervical neoplasia. *Am J Obstet Gynecol.* 1980;136:117–125.

Baggish SM. *Colposcopy of Cervix, Vagina and Vulva: A Comprehensive Textbook.* Philadelphia, PA: Mosby; 2003.

Cantor SB, Cardenas-Turanzas M, Cox DD, et al. Accuracy of colposcopy in the diagnostic setting compared with the screening setting. *Obstet Gynecol.* 2008;111:7.

Cronje HS, Parham GP, Cooreman BF, et al. A comparison of four screening methods for cervical neoplasia in a developing country. *Am J Obstet Gynecol.* 2003;188:395.

Gupta J, Pilottisshak KV, et al. Human papillomavirus-associated early vulva neoplasia investigated by in situ hybridization. *Am J Surg Pathol.* 1982;11:430–436.

Hopman EH, Voorhorst FJ, Kenemans P, et al. Observer agreement on interpreting colposcopic images on CIN. *Gynecol Oncol.* 1995;58:206.

Maclean AB. Acetowhite epithelium. *Gynecol Oncol.* 2004;95:691.

Mitchell MF, Schottenfeld D, Tortolero-Luna G, et al. Colposcopy for the diagnosis of squamous intraepithelial lesions: a meta-analysis. *Obstet Gynecol.* 1999;91:626.

Papanicolau GN, Traut HF. Diagnosis of uterine cancer by vagual smear. New York Commonwealth Fund, 1943.

148

PUT THE BOOKS AND THE SCALPEL DOWN... HAVE YOU THOUGHT ABOUT WHAT YOU ARE DOING? ETHICAL DECISION MAKING

VICTORIA GREEN, MD, MHSA, MBA, JD

As exponential advancements in technology in the specialty of obstetrics and gynecology surpass/shatter the boundary/bounds of human knowledge and science, the complexity of medical care and thus the intricacy of the physician–patient relationship intensify. Although, the importance of moral development and biomedical ethics is espoused by the developers of the educational component and core competencies of our specialty including the Association of Professors of Obstetrics and Gynecology (APGO), the Council on Resident Education in Obstetrics and Gynecology (CREOG), the Accreditation Council of Graduate Medical Education (ACGME), and the American Board of Obstetrics and Gynecology (ABOG). The goal is not necessarily to improve moral character (which is likely developed by the time of entering medical school) but to provide those of sound moral character the intellectual tools and interactional skills to give their ethical character its best behavioral expression. The quality of the physician–patient relationship was listed as a concern in the oath, but as the field of medicine has expanded, we see a "dehumanizing of medical education, a diversity of cultures and medical malpractice that prompt the need for ethical decision making."

This ideology was actually manifested at least 2,500 years ago in the Hippocratic tradition and oath. The recitation of this oath that typifies the graduation, investiture, inauguration, and elevation of students into the brotherhood of medicine emphasized the virtues expected to characterize and guide the behavior of burgeoning student doctors. Specifically, "...I will remember that there is art to medicine as well as science. And that warmth, sympathy, and understanding may outweigh the surgeon's knife or the chemist's drug..."; "...I will not be ashamed to say 'I know not' nor will I fail to call in my colleagues when the skills of another are needed for a patient's recovery...." The Florence Nightingale Pledge of Nursing promotes, endorses, and sanctions these principles as well citing "I solemnly pledge myself before God,... to pass my life in purity and to practice my profession faithfully...."; "...I will abstain from whatever is deleterious and mischievous..."; "I will do all in my power to maintain and elevate the standard of my profession, and will hold in confidence all personal matters committed to my keeping...." These ethical underpinnings continue and are a necessary requirement of membership in the American College of Obstetricians and Gynecologists whose code of Professional Ethics recites "Obstetrician-gynecologists, as members of the medical profession, have ethical responsibilities not only to patients, but also to society, to other health professionals, and to themselves."

Pioneering and innovative technology in the field of women's health have thrust multifaceted ethical dilemmas into the forefront of routine medical care. Assisted reproductive technologies, surrogate motherhood, stem cell research, prenatal diagnosis and selective abortion, medical care at the beginning and end of life, and the use of genetic information lay the groundwork for a minefield of bioethical issues for women's health practitioners. Additionally, the law and legal system often interact with the fluid practice of obstetrics and gynecology with questions about reproductive health and maternal-fetal-neonatal outcomes encompassing 50% of the court decisions involving medical care. The law is often said to be the minimum expression of obligation between human beings. Conversely, ethics is the maximum expression of those same individual obligations. Clearly, women's health is an area that reveals deeply felt obligations, beliefs, and values both personal and societal that shape daily medical decisions and frame personal perspective. Thus, we see that ethical issues can actually be framed in the context of conflicting obligations in women's health.

The specialty of women's health portends a multitude of conflicts particularly due to the duality of pregnancy concerning both the mother and the fetus and innovative technologies of procreation including abortion, selective termination, amniocentesis, fetoscopy, CVS, PUBS, in vitro fertilization, sex selection, research on fetal tissue, and cloning. The laws have ranged from Roe v. Wade to parental consent for abortions for a minor. They have dated from antiquity in the bible with "Give me children or I will die" to IVF for postmenopausal women.

When practitioners find themselves in unclear situations, uncertainties, or conflicts, they must appeal to ethical analysis for guidance or justification. Providers should first identify all the decision makers, collect available data and establish the facts upon which the ethical situation revolves, identify all of the appropriate options considering the medical status of the patient, and then evaluate these according to the most appropriate ethical approach available. The ethical conflicts that are elicited through this process are then prioritized with selection of the best-justified option. Once acted upon, the decision is revisited at a later date to ensure issues have not changed and a new option is more appropriate.

The major principles of autonomy, beneficence, nonmaleficence, and justice are commonly invoked to guide professional action in resolving conflicting obligations in women's health and this is termed principle-based ethics. These may serve as an initial point of reference in examining ethical issues. Other principles such as fidelity, honesty, privacy, and confidentiality are often thought to be derived from these four broad principles.

In practice, the autonomy principle implies a respect for patients' ability to govern their care based on their own personal values and beliefs. This includes freedom from controlling influences as well as the ability to make meaningful choices without limitations such as lack of understanding due to health literacy, language barriers, etc. The principle of beneficence dictates that health care personnel should act in the best interest and for the benefit of the patient. Nonmaleficence means providers have an obligation not to cause harm or injury. Justice is the most complex of the principles as it speaks not only to the physician's obligations to render equally what is due to each patient but also to recognize our important role in allocation of limited medical resources in the broader community. This principle is often applied to issues at the societal level such as insurance and access to care, allocation of kidney dialysis and transplantation resources, etc. Each principle may not be absolute as resultant conflict with other principles may dictate acquiescence.

Many mistakes occur in navigation of the relationship of health care professionals to the larger societal goals. These errors are seen in our greater fiduciary role to use our education and knowledge to promote the common good through education of the lay public, consultants to public officials, health advocates, and as expert witnesses. Thus, our relationship with the industry often comes under fire due to monumental compensation, accepting gifts, sample drug usage, and research support. In general, physicians must recognize and understand the potential influence of gifts (even those of nominal value) from industry and ensure that gifts entail benefit for the patient and are related to one's duties as a health care provider. If sample drugs are to be dispensed, they should be on the basis of a true need and for a full course of therapy. Support of any particular product should be evidence based. Other conflicts include incentives to limit diagnostic testing through the managed care company when deemed necessary by the physician and financial interests such as referral for profit. Disclosure of financial interests and support including research support is mandatory although reasonable compensation for speaking, consulting, and lecturing is permissible. Under these circumstances, the virtues of truthfulness, fidelity, trustworthiness, and integrity should steer one along the proper channel.

Expert witness testimony is another area of potential concern in which physicians should testify truthfully and solely in accordance with their own judgment (without unnecessary and inappropriate influence of legal counsel or reimbursement potential); providers should not disparage care that falls within accepted evidence-based standards since maloccurrence does not equal malpractice, should not support obviously deficient practices, and should ensure the standards they proffer do not narrowly reflect their own personal views but that of the specialty as a whole. Additionally, their compensation should be consistent to those customary for this service without the use of a fee based on the outcome of the trial (contingency fee).

Informed consent (IC) doctrines have significant legal and ethical underpinnings that can make attempts at full disclosure often challenging and unduly burdensome. IC must be viewed as more than signing the consent form or telling the patient the relevant facts but telling those facts conscientiously and helpfully based on the perceived expectations of the patient. It, thus, becomes more than just a process of providing information but a shared dialogue in which the patient's questions are answered, consent is obtained, and appropriate documentation of the process takes place. The discourse covers the reason why a particular course of treatment has been suggested, the risks and benefits of the proposed treatment as well as nontreatment, and alternatives to treatment. As the primary provider, one must ensure the patient comprehends the proposed treatment plan taking into allowance the patient's level of health literacy and cultural background. To ensure comprehension (and thus prevent mistakes), it is crucial to have the patient articulate her understanding of essential elements. The most important goals of IC include the patient having an adequate understanding and active participation in the decision-making process voluntarily and free from coercion. Although providers may believe the patient bears some responsibility in gaining an understanding of her medical treatment, the law places the burden on the shoulders of the providers and has determined the patient has no affirmative obligation to try to obtain information about her treatment. Thus, it may be helpful to include family members and significant others in the discussion, use lay language and printed materials, allow enough time for questions, and base the interchange on current date or guidelines. The discussion of the likelihood of success should include the reasonable alternatives, including their cost and whether the patient's insurance plan will cover the cost. Importantly, the prognosis if the treatment is rejected and any risks to the procedure should be reviewed. Additionally, it is mandatory that providers understand the options available when the patient is unable to consent including two doctor consent, third-party consent, and durable power of attorney and health care power of attorney. Particularly in the field of women's health, court-authorized consent has been utilized in rare circumstances, particularly with maternal refusal of treatment.

As online communication between patients and physicians has become a more traditional form of communication, providers should consider obtaining a specific-information consent and consider developing policies regarding avoidance for emergency communication, use with highly sensitive medical topics, and expectations for response times. Appropriate patient selection criteria should be developed to identify those patients most suitable for email correspondence as well as a discussion of disclaimers, service terms, and consultation fees if any.

Inadvertent and intentional disclosure of patient information prompts many ethical errors and has been codified in the Health Insurance Portability and Accountability Act (HIPAA) of 1996. This federal act prevents nonconsensual use or disclosure of patient information except as necessary for patient care and with a few limited exceptions such as for the treatment, payment for health and operation of the clinic/hospital, emergencies, and public health and law enforcement activities. Authorizations must be obtained for disclosure outside of the limitations and signed by the patient. Providers should submit their HIPAA policy for review to all employees and new hires to ensure individually identifiable information is not released and moreover to incorporate these principles into their routine practice to prevent inadvertent disclosure.

Ultimately, we see that ethical and legal issues abound in the field of medicine. It is critical that practitioners become familiar with ethical and legal principles and incorporate them into routine clinical care.

TAKE HOME POINTS

- Remember that there is art to medicine as well as science.
- Assisted reproductive technologies, surrogate motherhood, stem cell research, prenatal diagnosis and selective abortion, medical care at the beginning and end of life, and the use of genetic information lay the groundwork for a minefield of bioethical issues for women's health practitioners.
- Questions about reproductive health and maternal–fetal–neonatal outcomes encompass 50% of the court decisions involving medical care.
- The major principles of autonomy, beneficence, nonmaleficence, and justice are commonly invoked to guide professional action in resolving conflicting obligations in women's health, and this is termed principle-based ethics.

SUGGESTED READINGS

American College of Obstetricians and Gynecologists. *Code of Professional Ethics of the American College of Obstetricians and Gynecologists*. Washington, DC: Author; 2008.

American College of Obstetricians and Gynecologists. Relationships with industry. ACOG Committee Opinion #401, Washington, DC. *Obstet Gynecol.* 2008;111:799–804.

American College of Obstetricians and Gynecologists. Ethical Decision making in obstetrics and gynecology. ACOG Committee Opinion #390, Washington, DC, December 2007. *Obstet Gynecol.* 2007;110:1479–87.

American College of Obstetricians and Gynecologists. Ethics in Obstetrics and Gynecology. 2nd ed. Washington, DC: Author; 2004.

Association of Professors of Obstetrics and Gynecology and the APGO Medical Education Foundation. Exploring medical-legal issues in obstetrics and gynecology. Washington, DC: Author; 1994.

Culver CM, Clouser KD, et al. Basic curricular goals in medical ethics. *N Eng J Med.* 1985;312(4):253–256.

Florence Nightingale Pledge. www.nursingworld.org/FunctionalMenuCategories/AboutANA/WhereWeComeFrom_1/FlorenceNightingalePledge.aspx. Accessed November 3, 2008.

Hippocratic Oath. www.indiana.edu/~ancmed/oath.htm. Accessed November 2, 2008.

The Bible: King James Version. Genesis 30:1

Wazana A. Physicians and the pharmaceutical industry: is a gift ever just a gift? *JAMA.* 2000;283:373–380.

149

PRIORITIZING THE P-VALUE

SUSANNAH D. COPLAND, MD, MSCR

The p-value is the probability of obtaining the study's data given the null hypothesis (that there is no difference between study groups) is true. A higher p-value will result when study groups are similar (supporting the null hypothesis of no difference). A lower p-value will result when the study groups are more different (providing evidence against the null hypothesis of no difference). The p-value does not indicate "truth" or reflect magnitude or direction of association.

A study's power is the probability of correctly rejecting the null hypothesis or correctly reporting a difference between study groups. Power increases with sample size. If the sample size is small, a study may not have the power to detect a difference between groups; the groups may be different, but without a larger number of observations, the p-values will not be statistically significant. If the sample size is very large, a study may be able to detect very small differences between groups with very small, statistically significant p-values. In some cases, the differences detected in large data sets are so small that while they are statistically significant, they are not clinically significant.

The association of preterm birth with subsequent reproduction did not become evident until a large registry study provided the number of observations needed to detect the difference that prior small case-control studies had lacked. Hack and colleagues reported lower pregnancy rates for women but not for men in 242 very low birth weight survivors compared to 233 normal birth weight controls. Saigal and colleagues did not detect a difference in parenthood between 149 extremely low birth weight and 145 normal birth weight young adults. Using Norwegian registry data from over five hundred thousand births, Swamy and colleagues reported that 25% of women born between 22 and 27 weeks reproduced compared to 68% of women born at term (relative risk [RR] 0.33, 95% confidence interval [CI], 0.26 to 0.42), and 13.9% of men born between

22 and 27 weeks reproduced compared to 50.4% born at term (RR 0.24, 95% CI, 0.17 to 0.32). Larger data sets allow the detection of smaller differences between groups. Therefore, the absence of a statistically significant difference in a small study should not deter further investigation.

Confidence intervals provide more information than p-values because they provide information on magnitude and direction of association. The Maternal-Fetal Medicine Units Network study of long-term outcomes after repeated doses of antenatal corticosteroids did not detect a statistically significant difference in cerebral palsy between children exposed to repeated doses of corticosteroids in utero and children exposed to an initial course followed by placebo. The p-value was 0.12. The RR of 5.7, 95% CI 0.7 to 46.7 raises concern, however, since the direction of effect is toward harm (six children who received repeat corticosteroids had cerebral palsy as compared to one child who received placebo after an initial course of corticosteroids). Though this is a "negative study," without statistical significance, the direction of effect in the CIs being toward harm rather than benefit supports the need for additional studies.

TAKE HOME POINTS

- A lower p-value will result when the study groups are more different.
- A study's power is the probability of correctly reporting a difference between study groups.
- Power increases with sample size.

SELECTED READINGS

Hack M, Flannery DJ, Schluchter M, et al. Outcomes in young adulthood for very-low-birth-weight infants. *N Engl J Med*. 2002;346(3):149–157.

Peipert JF, Hogan JW. Research design and fundamental biostatistics. In: Seifer DB, Samuels P, Kniss DA, eds. *The Physiologic Basis of Gynecology and Obstetrics*. Philadelphia, PA: Lippincott Williams & Wilkins; 2001:137–157.

Saigal S, Stoskopf B, Streiner D, et al. Transition of extremely low-birth-weight infants from adolescence to young adulthood: comparison with normal birth-weight controls. *JAMA*. 2006;295(6):667–675.

Swamy GK, Ostbye T, Skjaerven R. Association of preterm birth with long-term survival, reproduction, and next-generation preterm birth. *JAMA*. 2008;299(12):1429–1436.

Wapner RJ, Sorokin Y, Mele L, et al. Long-term outcomes after repeat doses of antenatal corticosteroids. *N Engl J Med*. 2007;357(12):1190–1198.

150

COMMUNICATING STATISTICAL CHANCES TO PATIENTS: DOES ANYONE UNDERSTAND WHAT YOU JUST SAID?

SUSANNAH D. COPLAND, MD, MSCR

Marcoux et al. reported that laparoscopic resection or ablation of endometriosis improved the chance of pregnancy for infertile women with minimal or mild endometriosis.(Marcoux et al., 1997) Women were randomized to resection or ablation of endometriosis or to diagnostic laparoscopy only and then followed for 36 weeks for pregnancy outcomes. The improvement in pregnancy chance with ablation/resection can be quantified in many ways. The cumulative probability of pregnancy after 36 weeks was 30.7% in the treatment group and 17.7% in the diagnostic group. Therefore, the cumulative probability of a pregnancy increased by 73% ([30.7%–17.7%]/17.7%) over the 36 week period. This sounds like a dramatic increase in pregnancy chance. When expressed as cycle fecundity, however, treatment increased pregnancy chance from 2.4% per month to 4.7% per month. Summarizing the same data using cycle fecundity makes the improvement attributed to laparoscopy resection/ablation of endometriosis sound more modest.

Communicating fertility chances in terms of cycle fecundity allows patients to compare treatments. Average cycle fecundity is 20%. The cycle fecundity associated with in vitro fertilization (IVF) in a 31-year-old (the average age of the study population in the Marcoux paper) is 44.7% (www.sart.org, Society for Assisted Reproductive Technology 2006 report). Consistently speaking in terms of cycle fecundity shows that laparoscopic treatment of endometriosis results in a modest improvement in pregnancy chance, still lower than normal fecundity, while IVF results in the highest cycle fecundity.

Another common pitfall is made when calculating and communicating posttest probability. When interpreting screening tests, medical professionals should communicate the posttest probability of disease given a positive screening result. Unfortunately, studies of physicians show that frequently sensitivity (proportion of positive tests among people with disease) is confused with positive predictive value (proportion of people with disease among people with positive tests), and physicians are, thus, not able to adequately counsel patients with positive screening tests. One approach that improves accuracy is to convert probabilities to natural frequencies. Out of

1,000 women in their early forties, 8 will have breast cancer. The sensitivity of mammography is at best 90% so 7 of the 8 with breast cancer will have a true positive test result and one of the 8 will have a false negative test. The specificity of mammography is at best 95%; so 942 of the 992 without breast cancer will test true negative and 50 will test false positive. Therefore, the positive predictive value of the test is 7/57 or 12%; a woman with a positive mammogram has a 12% chance of breast cancer. When given natural frequencies, more medical and legal professionals correctly discern positive predictive value. (Hoffrage, et al., 2000; Gigerenzer, 2002).

TAKE HOME POINTS

- Consistently speaking in terms of cycle fecundity allows comparison. In this example, laparoscopic treatment of endometriosis results in a modest improvement in pregnancy chance, still lower than normal fecundity, while IVF results in the highest cycle fecundity.
- When given natural frequencies, more medical and legal professionals correctly discern positive predictive value.

SUGGESTED READING

Gigerenzer G. *Calculated Risks: How to Know When Numbers Deceive You*. New York, NY: Simon & Schuster; 2002.

Hoffrage U, Lindsey S, et al. Medicine. Communicating statistical information. *Science*. 2000;290(5500):2261–2262.

Marcoux S, Maheux R, Berube S. Laparoscopic surgery in infertile women with minimal or mild endometriosis. Canadian Collaborative Group on Endometriosis. *N Engl J Med*. 1997;337(4):217–222.

NEGLECTING TO TAKE THE STUDY POPULATION INTO ACCOUNT WHEN EXTRAPOLATING TO YOUR PRACTICE

SUSANNAH D. COPLAND, MD, MSCR

Acknowledging the study population is essential to interpreting randomized controlled trials. The Women's Health Initiative Estrogen Plus Progestin Trial (WHI E+P) findings regarding postmenopausal hormone therapy resulted in a dramatic decrease in hormone therapy prescriptions. The findings of increased risk of breast cancer, coronary heart disease, and stroke with estrogen/progestin hormone therapy compared to placebo can be applied with statistical rigor only to the group studied, postmenopausal women average age 63 who did not have vasomotor symptoms. As younger perimenopausal women with severe vasomotor symptoms were excluded from the trial, we cannot adequately counsel these women on their individual risk using the WHI E+P results. The North American Menopause Society (NAMS) currently recommends lowest dose, shortest duration of hormone therapy until we have more data for symptomatic women.

TAKE HOME POINT

- Data can only be applied to patients who are identical to the population studied.

SELECTED READINGS

Gass M. Highlights from the latest WHI publications and the latest North American Menopause Society position statement on use of menopausal hormone therapy. *Cleve Clin J Med*. 2008;75(Suppl 4):S13–S16.

Majumdar SR, Almasi EA, Stafford RS. Promotion and prescribing of hormone therapy after report of harm by the Women's Health Initiative. *JAMA*. 2004;292(16):1983–1988.

Peipert JF, Hogan JW. Research design and fundamental biostatistics. In: Seifer DB, Samuels P, et al., eds. *The Physiologic Basis of Gynecology and Obstetrics*. Philadelphia, PA: Lippincott Williams & Wilkins; 2001:137–157.

Rossouw JE, Anderson GL, Prentice RL, et al. Risks and benefits of estrogen plus progestin in healthy postmenopausal women: principal results from the Women's Health Initiative randomized controlled trial. *JAMA*. 2002;288(3):321–233.

The Women's Health Initiative Study Group. Design of the Women's Health Initiative clinical trial and observational study. *Control Clin Trials*. 1998;19(1):61–109.

DIFFERENT DENOMINATORS: COMPARING TO APPLES TO APPLES, NOT ORANGES

SUSANNAH D. COPLAND, MD, MSCR

When interpreting and comparing summary statistics, we should be mindful of the outcomes being compared. Ideally, the primary outcome in research studies should be the outcome of most interest to patients and physicians. Using intermediate outcomes can be misleading. The early comparisons of metformin to clomiphene citrate focused on ovulation, an intermediate outcome. The supposition was that if a medicine was successful in achieving ovulation, pregnancy would follow. When the Reproductive Medicine Network reported a randomized controlled trial showing clomiphene citrate to be superior to metformin in achieving live birth, it became clear that differences in ovulation did not always result in differences in live birth. Combination therapy with both clomiphene citrate and metformin was superior to clomiphene citrate alone or metformin alone in achieving ovulation but only resulted in differences in live birth when compared to metformin, not to clomiphene citrate. This difference highlights the need to design studies with the primary outcomes of most interest, even though doing so necessitates higher numbers of subjects.

The denominator in comparisons is likewise essential to interpreting statistics. A patient may be counseled that her chance for live birth from a single in vitro fertilization (IVF) cycle is 39% or 42% or 45%. All these numbers are accurate representations of the data, but they differ in denominator. She has a 39% chance of live birth if she starts an IVF cycle, a 42% chance of live birth if she makes it to egg retrieval, and a 45% chance of live birth if she makes it to embryo transfer (www.sart.org; 2006 national data). Another accurate representation is that she has a >50% chance of live birth if she uses all of the embryos from her fresh cycle in future frozen transfer cycles.

Since different centers transfer different numbers of embryos, the pregnancy rate per embryo becomes helpful. As research begins to focus on egg freezing, the pregnancy rate per oocyte becomes most relevant. Patrizio and Sakkas applied the "per oocyte" and "per embryo" metric to 572 oocyte retrievals for IVF and reported that the live birth rate ranges from 1% (women 41 to 42) to 6.8% (egg donors) per oocyte and from 2.7% (women 41 to 42) to 22% (egg donors) per embryo. Using "per oocyte" and "per embryo" denominators allows us to make better comparisons of the efficiency of IVF. When we counsel patients, it is best to use the denominator that applies to the stage of the process that they are in (per cycle before they start a treatment cycle, per transfer if they have made it to the day of embryo transfer).

Statistical methods allow researchers to summarize data in a way that physicians and patients can use to understand probabilities related to different treatments. Taking care to understand the study population and how the data were collected and presented can facilitate better communications between scientists, physicians, and patients.

TAKE HOME POINTS

- Use the denominator that best fits your patient when applying the data to her situation.
- Understand how the data were collected and the primary and intermediate outcomes of the study.

SUGGESTED READINGS

Legro RS, Barnhart HX, Schlaff WD, et al. Clomiphene, metformin, or both for infertility in the polycystic ovary syndrome. *N Engl J Med.* 2007;356(6):551–366.

Patrizio P, Sakkas D. From oocyte to baby: a clinical evaluation of the biological efficiency of in vitro fertilization. *Fertil Steril.* 2009;91(4):1061–1066.

Tiitinen A, Hyden-Granskog C, Gissler M. What is the most relevant standard of success in assisted reproduction? The value of cryopreservation on cumulative pregnancy rates per single oocyte retrieval should not be forgotten. *Hum Reprod.* 2004;19(11):2439–2441.

Note: Page numbers in *italics* denote figures; those followed by a t denote tables.